Cosmetics

Peter Elsner • Shari R. Lipner • Howard Maibach
Editors

Cosmetics

Controlled Efficacy Studies and Regulation

Second Edition

Springer

Editors
Peter Elsner
Jena University Hospital
Jena, Thüringen, Germany

Howard Maibach
Department of Dermatology
University of California, San Francisco
San Francisco, CA, USA

Shari R. Lipner
Department of Dermatology
Weill Cornell Medicine
New York, NY, USA

ISBN 978-3-032-14643-4 ISBN 978-3-032-14644-1 (eBook)
https://doi.org/10.1007/978-3-032-14644-1

This Springer imprint is published by the registered company Springer Nature Switzerland AG
The registered company address is: Gewerbestrasse 11, 6330 Cham, Switzerland

Contents

About the Editors

Shari R. Lipner is a Professor of Clinical Dermatology, Attending Physician, and Director of the Nail Division at the New York-Presbyterian Hospital/Weill Cornell Medical Center. She completed her undergraduate studies at Dartmouth College where she obtained a Bachelor of Arts in Chemistry and graduated Phi Beta Kappa and Summa Cum Laude. She completed her medical training at Albert Einstein College of Medicine, where she received both MD and PhD degrees and graduated Alpha Omega Alpha. She completed her residency training in Dermatology at the New York-Presbyterian Hospital/Weill Cornell Medical Center.

Dr. Lipner is a member of the American Academy of Dermatology, Women's Dermatologic Society, Council for Nail Disorders, American Dermatologic Association, and is chair of multiple committees. She is also past President of the Dermatologic Society of Greater New York, President of the New York State Society of Dermatology and Dermatologic Surgery, and Founding Editor in Chief of *JAAD Reviews*.

Dr. Lipner is board certified in dermatology and is one of the few experts in nail disorders in the world. She is also the Primary Investigator on clinical trials utilizing novel treatments for nail disorders. She is also an expert in telemedicine and has published widely on this topic.

Dr. Lipner is one of the leading researchers in dermatology. She has authored over 670 peer-reviewed publications, numerous books and book chapters, lectures nationally and internationally, and is frequently featured by the media, including CNN, NPR, *Self*, *Allure*, *The Washington Post*, and *The New York Times*, for her expertise.

Peter Elsner is Professor Emeritus of Dermatology, Friedrich Schiller University, Jena University Hospital, Jena, Germany. His research interests include occupational dermatoses, contact dermatitis, dermatotoxicology, dermatopharmacology, and noninvasive methods in dermatology. He participates in research nationally and internationally in dermatoepidemiology, as well as in clinical studies in contact and hand dermatitis.

Professor Elsner received his medical degree from Wuerzburg University, Germany. After completing his residency in dermatology and allergology at the Wuerzburg University Hospital, Germany, he received his lectureship ("Habilitation") and worked as a research dermatologist at the Department of Dermatology, University of California San Francisco, under the leadership of Professor Howard Maibach, one of the founders of the ICDRG. Thereafter, he was appointed as senior physician at the Department of Dermatology, University Hospital Zurich, Switzerland, under the leadership of Professor Günter Burg, before he was appointed Professor of Dermatology and Chairman of the Department of Dermatology at the University Hospital Jena, Germany.

Professor Elsner has been a long-standing Board Member of the German Society of Dermatology (DDG) and of the European Dermato-Epidemiology Network (EDEN) and has been President of the International Society for Dermatology in the Tropics (ISDT).

Howard Maibach is a dermatologist with expertise in treating contact dermatitis (a rash caused by touching an irritating substance) and occupational dermatitis (a rash resulting from workplace exposure to an irritating substance). His specialties include allergic skin disorders and skin conditions caused by exposure to toxic substances. He also has an interest in dermatopharmacology, the study of medications for skin disorders.

Maibach earned his medical degree from Tulane University School of Medicine. He completed a residency as well as a fellowship in dermatology at the Hospital of the University of Pennsylvania. He has served on the editorial boards of more than 30 scientific journals. He is a member of 19 professional societies, including the American Academy of Dermatology, San Francisco Dermatological Society, and International Commission on Occupational Health.

Chapter 1
The Food and Drug Administration and Modernization of U.S. Cosmetic Regulations

Renee Stover, Prashiela Manga, Elizabeth H. Anderson, and Linda M. Katz

Abbreviations

CFR	Code of Federal Regulations
CPSC	U.S. Consumer Product Safety Commission
DOJ	Department of Justice
FD&C Act or the Act	Federal Food, Drug, and Cosmetic Act
FDA	United States Food and Drug Administration
FPLA	Fair Packaging and Labeling Act
FR	Federal Register
GMP	Good Manufacturing Practice
MoCRA	Modernization of Cosmetics Regulation Act of 2022
PFAS	Perfluoroalkyl and Polyfluoroalkyl Substances
PPPA	Poisons Prevention Packaging Act
SAHCODH	Serious Adverse Health Consequences or Death to Humans
U.S.C.	United States Code
USDA	United States Department of Agriculture

Overview

The Food and Drug Administration (FDA) is an agency within the U.S. Department of Health and Human Services (HHS) whose mission is to enhance the health and well-being of all Americans. In 1906, the Food and Drugs Act (also known as the

R. Stover · P. Manga (✉) · E. H. Anderson · L. M. Katz
U.S. Food and Drug Administration, Silver Spring, MD, USA
e-mail: Renee.Stover@fda.hhs.gov; Prashiela.Manga@fda.hhs.gov; Elizabeth.Anderson@fda.hhs.gov; dr.lindamkatz@gmail.com

P. Elsner et al. (eds.), *Cosmetics*, https://doi.org/10.1007/978-3-032-14644-1_1

Table 1.1 Selected FD&C Act sections added by MoCRA and their citations in the United States Code[a]

Key MoCRA amendments	The FD&C Act	United States Code
Definitions	section 604	21 U.S.C. 364
Adverse Events	section 605	21 U.S.C. 364a
Good Manufacturing Practice	section 606	21 U.S.C. 364b
Registration and Product Listing	section 607	21 U.S.C. 364c
Safety Substantiation	section 608	21 U.S.C. 364d
Labeling	section 609	21 U.S.C. 364e
Records	section 610	21 U.S.C. 364f
Mandatory Recall Authority	section 611	21 U.S.C. 364g
Small Businesses	section 612	21 U.S.C. 364h

[a]This table excludes some MoCRA amendments to the FD&C Act such as section 613, section 614, and conforming amendments to existing sections of the FD&C Act

Pure Food and Drug Act and the Wiley Act) was passed to address serious safety concerns found in tainted foods and drugs. The Federal Food, Drug, and Cosmetic Act (FD&C Act, the Act) was enacted by Congress in 1938 and included cosmetics after certain unregulated products caused serious health consequences and at least one death [1–9]. The Act has had over 30 significant amendments [10], and it remains the founding legislation of FDA's authority to regulate food, drugs, medical devices, cosmetics, and other classes of products in the United States.

The 1938 Act provided for limited post-market authority over cosmetic products that, today, include shampoos, body washes, lotions, shaving creams, nail polishes, baby powders, baby wipes, deodorants, perfumes, and makeup. Other laws with notable impact on cosmetic regulations are the 1966 Fair Packaging and Labeling Act (FPLA), that granted FDA authority over cosmetic labeling requirements, and the 1960 Color Additive Amendments which modified the FD&C Act and established regulations for the use of color additives in cosmetics.

The cosmetic industry has undergone increasing growth and innovations over the past several decades. In 2025, the U.S. cosmetics industry is expected to account for approximately 18% of the global cosmetics market, which is projected to reach around $115 billion [11]. This growth prompted Congress to enact the Modernization of Cosmetics Regulation Act of 2022 (MoCRA). MoCRA is the most significant law impacting cosmetics regulation since the 1938 FD&C Act [12]. This new law amended the FD&C Act and expanded FDA's authority, as shown in Table 1.1.

Historical Perspective: Leading up to the FD&C Act

Prior to 1938, there was no federal regulation of cosmetics and limited federal regulation of food and drugs despite passage of the 1906 Food and Drugs Act. The Bureau of Chemistry, an agricultural research laboratory within the U.S. Department of Agriculture (USDA), had been investigating food and drug safety since 1879. As consumer goods usage grew, accounts like Upton Sinclair's shocking but accurate, portrayal of the U.S. meatpacking industry in *The Jungle*, along with press coverage of Harvey Wiley's alarming "Poison Squad" study on chemical preservatives in food, heightened public awareness of the need for regulation. The USDA had initial authority to enforce the 1906 Food and Drugs Act. In 1927, the Bureau's agricultural research and regulatory components were separated, with the regulatory component becoming the Food, Drug, and Insecticide Administration, which was renamed the Food and Drug Administration 4 years later [13].

Cosmetics were included in the earliest drafts of the 1906 Food and Drug Act under the definition for drugs, but were removed in subsequent revisions [14] since it comprised only a small fraction of interstate commerce and had limited impact on public health in comparison to foods and drugs. Makeup, if used at all, was predominantly homemade and used subtly and secretively. Obvious makeup in nineteenth century America was unfashionable and associated with the stigmatized female occupations of prostitution and acting [15]. Even though cosmetics were being purchased, albeit at a low rate, removing them from the bill was one of the trade-offs to secure industry's support [14, 16]. These factors quickly changed in the early twentieth century. At the start of the century, U.S. cosmetic sales were around $7 million [17]. When the U.S. entered World War I in 1917, women's presence in the workforce increased. As a result, women began to care more about their appearance and had discretionary income. Mass-produced cosmetics were a more convenient and cheaper option for young women. Furthermore, the film industry stars of the 1920s glamorized makeup use, offsetting old stigmas. Women were no longer ashamed to purchase and wear cosmetics openly. In turn, these products were widely discussed and advertised in magazines [18]. Consequently, during this time frame, cosmetic sales rose to $200 million [19], and companies including Helena Rubinstein, Elizabeth Arden, Max Factor, Maybelline, and Madam C.J. Walker were founded [20–23].

The importance of the cosmetics industry to its customers is reflected in how the industry weathered the Great Depression. From 1929 to 1931, the cosmetics industry reportedly declined only 17% in production, whereas industry on average declined by 41% [24]. This economic resilience may have been because many women were using cosmetics to help them gain employment and increase their likelihood of financial success. In fact, in 1937, it was estimated that around 200,000 women were employed as beauticians [25].

As consumption of cosmetics increased, so did their impact on public health. There were no restrictions on what ingredients could be used in cosmetics or legal repercussions for companies knowingly including harmful components. For example, Koremlu (Fig. 1.1), a depilatory cream, which contained thallium acetate—an ingredient commonly found in rat poison [8], and Lash Lure (Fig. 1.2), an eyelash/eyebrow dye, which contained the aniline dye paraphenylenediamine that caused severe dermatitis, conjunctival edema, corneal ulceration, and blindness [26], were legally marketed in the 1930s. However, serious injuries and one death caused by Lash Lure [1], brought widespread public attention to the need for cosmetics regulation [27].

The 1938 FD&C Act made it illegal to sell adulterated or misbranded cosmetics in interstate commerce and gave FDA the authority to seize and remove unsafe products from the market. FDA exerted this new authority quickly after the Act's

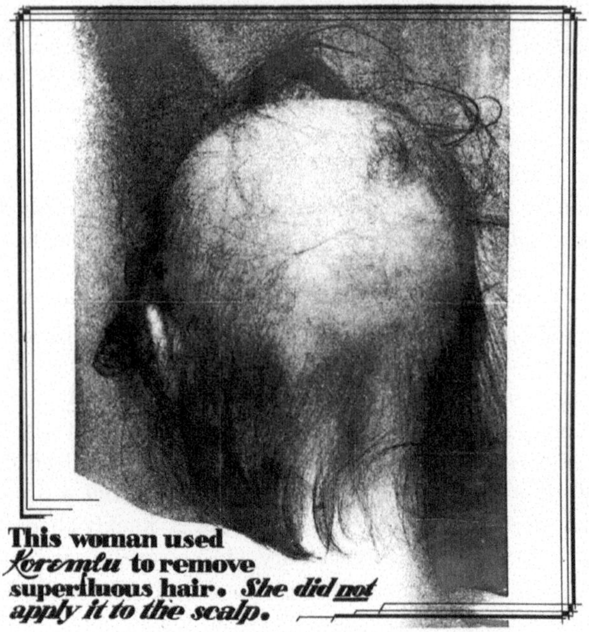

Fig. 1.1 Image from FDA's display at the 1933 Chicago World's Fair. Depicts a woman's hair loss to demonstrate the systemic injuries she suffered because of using Koremlu. (Image obtained from FDA's Flickr account (Flickr/FDA))

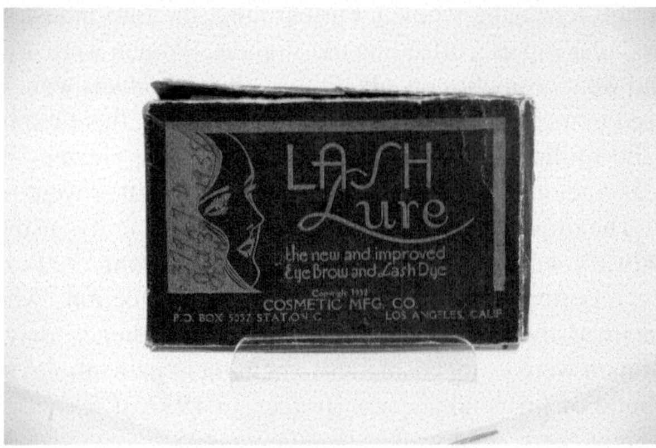

Fig. 1.2 An image of the packaging in which Lash Lure was sold. (Image obtained from FDA's Flickr account (Flickr/FDA))

passage by seizing and removing Lash Lure from shelves—the first cosmetic seizure under the FD&C Act [28]. By 1940, FDA had seized and removed several eyelash/eyebrow dye products containing paraphenylenediamine and lipsticks containing cadmium and selenium [29].

From Legislation to Regulation

The FD&C Act and its amendments, including MoCRA, provide the primary legal authority for the FDA's oversight of cosmetics. FD&C Act sections of interest and their corresponding citations in the United States Code (21 U.S.C. §§ 301-399) can be found in Tables 1.1 and 1.2 [30]. The Fair Packaging and Labeling Act (FPLA) also provides the FDA with authority to require specific labeling information on certain FDA-regulated products.

As a federal agency, FDA implements, interprets, or prescribes what Congress grants by law. It makes operational the provisions in the legislation through rulemaking by developing and implementing regulations (also called rules), adjudication, and publication of guidance. Final rules are published in the Code of Federal Regulations (CFR). FDA's rulemaking authority extends to labeling requirements, manufacturing practices, marketing and advertising restrictions, and safety evaluations for several product categories under the Act.

FDA has published regulations and guidances for the cosmetic industry, including regulations prohibiting or restricting harmful ingredients and the Cosmetic Labeling Guide [31, 32]. MoCRA, in amending the FD&C Act, mandated FDA to establish regulations for (1) standardized testing methods for detecting and identifying asbestos in talc-containing cosmetic products, (2) fragrance allergen labeling requirements, and (3) good manufacturing practice (GMP) requirements for facilities that manufacture cosmetic products. Following the passage of MoCRA, FDA has published a proposed rule for talc-containing cosmetics [33], and made available multiple guidances pertaining to the new provisions under the FD&C Act [34].

Table 1.2 Selected FD&C Act sections that preexisted MoCRA and their citations in the United States Code

Referenced sections	The FD&C Act	United States Code
Prohibited Acts	section 301	21 U.S.C. 331
Adulterated Cosmetics	section 601	21 U.S.C. 361
Misbranded Cosmetics	section 602	21 U.S.C. 362
Factory Inspection	section 704	21 U.S.C. 374
Listing and Certification of Color Additives for Foods, Drugs, and Cosmetics	section 721	21 U.S.C. 379e

FDA's Authority Over Cosmetics

Post-market Interstate Commerce

The FD&C Act specifies that FDA's authority lies over commodities in interstate commerce. FDA cosmetic regulations published in the CFR would not apply, for example, to a homemade lotion sold in a local farmer's market and made from local (meaning within the same state) ingredients and materials, including the packaging. The FD&C Act prohibits the distribution of cosmetics that are adulterated or misbranded only if they have moved, are moving, or will be moving in interstate commerce, which includes products intended for import and export. In today's economy, most cosmetics move in interstate commerce.

FDA's authority over cosmetics is post-market, meaning the agency's role is to regulate cosmetics after they are introduced to the market, rather than pre-approving them before they are sold [35]. Color additives (e.g. dyes and pigments) are the only cosmetic ingredients that must be pre-approved ("listed") by FDA, while coal-tar hair dyes are subject to special regulatory requirements. Other cosmetic ingredients are not pre-approved, meaning a cosmetic manufacturer may use almost any raw material, with the exception of those prohibited or restricted by law, as an ingredient and market the product, provided the manufacturer has substantiated its safety [36]. Prohibited and restricted cosmetic ingredients are listed in 21 CFR § 700 [31]. Each listing is a separate regulation promulgated under notice and comment rule-making procedures. In contrast, drugs and their ingredients must be approved by FDA or comply with the Over-the-Counter Drug Monograph system before being marketed.

As noted above, FDA does not approve cosmetics post-market either. A cosmetic formulation cannot be "*FDA Approved*" since this is not a service FDA provides for the cosmetic industry. Additionally, a cosmetic product or a cosmetic manufacturing facility cannot be "*FDA Certified*" because FDA does not issue any certificates confirming compliance with FDA cosmetic regulations.

Color Additive Amendments

The Color Additive Amendments of 1960 to the FD&C Act defined "color additive" as "(A) a dye, pigment, or other substance made by a process of synthesis or similar artifice, or extracted, isolated, or otherwise derived, with or without intermediate or final change of identity, from a vegetable, animal, mineral, or other source, and (B) when added or applied to a food, drug, or cosmetic, or to the human body or any part thereof, is capable (alone or through reaction with other substance) of imparting color thereto... The term "color" includes black, white, and intermediate grays" [37, 38].

The color additives used in 1960 were provisionally listed and a petition process was established for permanently listing the color additives as "suitable and safe" for the intended use (e.g. use in a cosmetic) in FDA-regulated products [39]. In addition, the 1976 Medical Device Amendments to the FD&C Act added FDA oversight of color additives in direct contact with the body for a significant period of time (such as sutures and contact lenses). Today, color additives are used to impart color to foods, drugs, cosmetics, and certain medical devices; unapproved color additive use would render FDA-regulated products adulterated under the FD&C Act. Each approved color additive is listed in Title 21 of the CFR, in part 73, part 74, and part 82 [40–42].

The dye in Lash Lure, paraphenylenediamine, belongs to a class of dyes called coal-tar colors—so called because they were first produced as byproducts of the coal industry. Today, most of these synthetic organic dyes are made from petroleum. The 1938 FD&C Act mandated the listing of coal-tar colors that were found to have met the standard of "harmless and suitable", as determined by FDA, for use in foods, drugs, and cosmetics. As a result of the 1960 Color Additive Amendments, the term coal-tar colors and its safety standard in the 1938 FD&C Act were replaced by the broader term color additives and the enhanced safety standard of "suitable and safe". Section 601(a) of the FD&C Act states that a cosmetic is adulterated if it contains any deleterious substance that could harm the user when the product is used according to the labeling or customary use. However, this prohibition does not apply to coal-tar colors used in hair dyes if their labels bear the prescribed caution statement: "Caution - This product contains ingredients which may cause skin irritation on certain individuals and a preliminary test according to accompanying directions should first be made. This product must not be used for dyeing the eyelashes or eyebrows; to do so may cause blindness" [43]. If the label lacks the caution statement and patch test directions, FDA can take regulatory action.

The FD&C Act and 21 CFR § 70.5(a) have specific requirements for color additives allowed for use in products applied to the eye area. Color additives must be specifically authorized for this use. In 2021, FDA approved, based on scientifically sound safety data, the first color additive, silver nitrate, to color eyebrows and eyelashes for professional use only [44].

Definitions and Product Claims

Product definitions are crucial to FDA's function. For example, they are used to determine jurisdiction, both within the agency and across other agencies. For FDA to have authority over a product and determine which regulations apply to it, the product must meet one of the product definitions provided in the FD&C Act.

Section 201(i) of the FD&C Act defines cosmetics as "articles intended to be rubbed, poured, sprinkled, or sprayed on, introduced into, or otherwise applied to the human body ... for cleansing, beautifying, promoting attractiveness, or altering the appearance." In comparison, drugs are, among other things, "articles intended for use in the diagnosis, cure, mitigation, treatment, or prevention of disease" and "articles (other than food) intended to affect the structure or any function of the body of man or other animals" [45]. These definitions have not changed since 1938.

If a product has more than one intended use, it may meet multiple product definitions, for example, being both a cosmetic and a drug [46]. A face wash containing salicylic acid may be intended for cleansing the skin, meeting the definition of a cosmetic, but it may also be intended to treat acne, meeting the definition of a drug. A lotion intended only for skin moisturization is a cosmetic. However, a lotion with an SPF component intended to provide moisturization and sun protection is a cosmetic and a drug. In general, products meeting both definitions are subject to the regulatory requirements applicable to both product categories.

Despite the term "cleansing" in the cosmetic definition, traditional soap is not considered a cosmetic (or a drug) [47] and is regulated by the U.S. Consumer Product Safety Commission (CPSC), not FDA. Soaps in the traditional category consist mainly of an alkali salt of fatty acids made by reaction of fats with a lye (i.e. sodium hydroxide or potassium hydroxide); and are sold only as soap [48]. Claims such as moisturizing or antibacterial, for example, would provide evidence that the product is intended for use as a cosmetic or a drug respectively.

FDA may review claims from product labeling or advertising, including from the internet, to establish evidence of intended use and therefore product type. If a product is marketed as a cosmetic but claims it will cure, treat, or prevent disease, or affect the structure or function of the body, these claims will provide evidence of the intended use of the product as a drug. For example, a cream claiming to reduce cellulite or treat wrinkles may be a drug. If it also makes a cosmetic claim, such as moisturizing, then it may be a cosmetic and a drug. Evidence of intended use can also be established by ingredient(s) in the product having a well-known therapeutic use. Additionally, common consumer perception of a product can provide evidence of intended use. In other words, if people expect the product to behave like a drug/cosmetic, then FDA may regulate the product as a drug/cosmetic.

New Definitions in the Modernization of Cosmetics Regulation Act (MoCRA)

By adding definitions of cosmetic related terms to the FD&C Act, MoCRA provided additional clarity for the implementation of its provisions. The following definitions are found in section 604 of the FD&C Act (21 U.S.C. § 364(1)-(5)):

Adverse Event: "any health-related event associated with the use of a cosmetic product that is adverse."

Cosmetic Product: "means a preparation of cosmetic ingredients with a qualitatively and quantitatively set composition for use in a finished product."

Facility: "any establishment (including an establishment of an importer) that manufactures or processes cosmetic products distributed in the United States."

Responsible Person: "the manufacturer, packer, or distributor of a cosmetic product whose name appears on the label of such cosmetic product in accordance with section 609(a) of the FD&C Act or section 4(a) of the Fair Packaging and Labeling Act."

Serious Adverse Event: "an adverse event that:

A. results in:
   - death;
   - a life-threatening experience;
   - inpatient hospitalization;
   - a persistent or significant disability or incapacity;
   - a congenital anomaly or birth defect;
   - an infection; or
   - significant disfigurement (including serious and persistent rashes, second- or third-degree burns, significant hair loss, or persistent or significant alteration of appearance), other than as intended under conditions of use that are customary or usual; or

B. requires, based on reasonable medical judgment, a medical or surgical intervention to prevent an outcome described in (A) above."

Prohibited Acts: Old and New

Chapter III-*Prohibited Acts and Penalties* of the FD&C Act [49] lists all the activities this law makes illegal, and the procedures FDA can use for enforcement of this law. Specifically, section 301 (*Prohibited Acts*) in Chapter III prohibits the manufacture, distribution, selling, or importation of adulterated or misbranded cosmetics—as well as food, drugs, medical devices, and tobacco products. It also prohibits the refusal of FDA inspections [50], and the use of FDA inspection reports on product labels or to promote sales [51]. When section 301 prohibits the act of refusing an FDA inspection, it refers to the section in the FD&C Act in which FDA's inspection authority is provided—in this case, section 704 (*Factory Inspection*) in Chapter VII -*General Authority* (see Table 1.2).

In 2022, MoCRA added new prohibited acts related to cosmetics under the FD&C Act, including the following:

1. Failing to provide FDA access to records, including safety substantiation records, under specific authorities [52].
2. Failing to report or maintain records of a serious adverse event [52].
3. Failing to register a facility or list a cosmetic product [53].
4. Failing to comply with a recall order issued by FDA [54].

These prohibited acts are tied to authorities and requirements MoCRA established in new sections 604–614 of Chapter VI-*Cosmetics* to the Act (see Table 1.1).

MoCRA also added conditions that would render a product adulterated or misbranded, thereby prohibiting such products from interstate commerce.

FDA can take action against a product only if it is adulterated or misbranded. Examples of FDA actions to remove non-compliant products from the market include mandatory recalls, seizures, and injunctions. The conditions that cause a cosmetic to be adulterated or misbranded are outlined in Chapter VI-*Cosmetics* of the FD&C Act.

Adulteration

Under the FD&C Act, a cosmetic is adulterated if it fails to meet certain safety and purity standards. These standards are outlined in section 601 (*Adulterated Cosmetics*) of the FD&C Act and include:

(a) "If it bears or contains any poisonous or deleterious substance which may render it injurious to users under the conditions of use prescribed in the labeling thereof, or under such conditions of use as are customary or usual, except that this provision shall not apply to coal-tar hair dye, …"
(b) "If it consists in whole or in part of any filthy, putrid, or decomposed substance."
(c) "If it has been prepared, packed, or held under insanitary conditions whereby it may have become contaminated with filth, or whereby it may have been rendered injurious to health."
(d) "If its container is composed, in whole or in part, of any poisonous or deleterious substance which may render the contents injurious to health."

While the 1938 FD&C Act provision (e) mandated the batch certification of "coal-tar colors", this paragraph was amended in 1960 under the Color Additive Amendments to use the term "color additive" and to refer to section 721(a) for safety stipulations:

(e) "If it is not a hair dye and it is, or it bears or contains, a color additive which is unsafe within the meaning of section 721(a) [(a) of *Listing and Certification of Color Additives for Foods, Drugs, and Cosmetics*]."

Following the enactment of MoCRA in 2022, non-compliance with good manufacturing practices (GMP) and safety substantiation requirements now constitutes adulteration under the FD&C Act:

(f) "If it has been manufactured or processed under conditions that do not meet the good manufacturing practice requirements of section 606 [*Good Manufacturing Practice*]."
(g) "If it is a cosmetic product, and the cosmetic product, including each ingredient in the cosmetic product, does not have adequate substantiation for safety, as defined in section 608(c) [*(c)* of *Safety Substantiation*]."

Examples of adulteration include the presence of prohibited ingredients, uncertified or non-permitted color additives, microbial contamination levels equal to or over 100 CFU/g (mL) for eye-area products and equal to or over 1000 CFU/g (mL) for all other products, and pathogens such as *pseudomonas aeruginosa* and *staphylococcus aureus* [55, 56]. Prohibited ingredients are ingredients that FDA finds generally unsafe in cosmetics and therefore promulgated a regulation under the authority of section 601(a) to prohibit their use. When such a regulation is in place, then enforcement action against products that contain the prohibited ingredient can occur without having to reprove the underlying evidence that supported the regulation. There may also be cases where FDA has concerns about the safety of an ingredient or potential contaminant and engages in extended research, product testing, and evaluations for better determination of the posed health risk. For examples, see FDA's webpages on lead in lipstick and tattoo ink safety [57–59].

Good Manufacturing Practice (GMP) and Safety Substantiation

MoCRA added section 606 (*Good Manufacturing Practice*) to the FD&C Act, requiring the establishment of GMP regulations for facilities to protect the public health and ensure cosmetic products are not adulterated. Currently, FDA is engaged in the rulemaking process. The GMP regulations are to be consistent, as far as is possible, with national and international standards [60]. In establishing the regulations, FDA must take into account the size and scope of businesses manufacturing cosmetics and the risks posed to the public by such cosmetics [61]. Section 606 also states that the GMP regulations may allow for records access to demonstrate compliance with GMPs during inspections.

The addition of section 608 (*Safety Substantiation*) to the FD&C Act by MoCRA established the requirement for industry to have records substantiating the safety of a product and each ingredient in the product, which may be accessed during inspection under certain conditions. If a cosmetic product does not have adequate substantiation records, it could be deemed adulterated within the meaning of section 601(g) of the Act.

The responsibility of ensuring adequate substantiation of safety and maintaining such records lies with the responsible person for a product. MoCRA defined "adequate substantiation of safety" and "safe" as follows:

Adequate substantiation of safety: "means tests or studies, research, analyses, or other evidence or information that is considered, among experts qualified by scientific training and experience to evaluate the safety of cosmetic products and their ingredients, sufficient to support a reasonable certainty that a cosmetic product is safe" [62].

Safe: "means that the cosmetic product, including any ingredient thereof, is not injurious to users under the conditions of use prescribed in the labeling thereof, or under such conditions of use as are customary or usual." Additionally, a cosmetic product or cosmetic ingredient will not be considered injurious to users solely because it can cause minor and transient reactions in some users [63].

Talc and Perfluoroalkyl and Polyfluoroalkyl Substances (PFAS)

MoCRA introduced stricter oversight of talc-containing cosmetics. Asbestos is found in the same rock types that host talc deposits and may be inseparable from talc in the mining process. MoCRA requires FDA to establish and require standardized testing methods for detecting and identifying asbestos in talc-containing cosmetic products. The proposed rule for talc-containing cosmetics, published in the Federal Register (89 FR 105490) on December 27, 2024, if finalized, would require manufacturers of talc-containing cosmetic products to test their products for asbestos using specified standardized testing methods. FDA has proposed that failure to operate in compliance with the testing or recordkeeping provisions of the rule would render the talc-containing cosmetic product adulterated within the meaning of section 601(a) of the FD&C Act.

MoCRA also mandates that FDA assess the safety of the use of PFAS in cosmetics, including any risks associated with such use, and publish a report of the findings [64].

Misbranding

Through its misbranding provisions, the FD&C Act aims to protect consumers by ensuring labels and packaging present consumers with clear and accurate information that is not misleading about the content and quantity of a product. These labeling and packaging standards are outlined in section 602 (*Misbranded Cosmetics*) of the FD&C Act. A cosmetic is misbranded:

(a) "If its labeling is false or misleading in any particular."

Examples of misbranding under section 602(a) could be a product declaring an ingredient that it does not actually contain or a product being labeled as sterile when it contains microorganisms.

MoCRA established new labeling requirements for industry and amended paragraph (b) by adding part (3) before "*Provided*":

(b) "If in package form unless it bears a label containing (1) the name and place of business of the manufacturer, packer, or distributor; (2) an accurate statement of the quantity of the contents in terms of weight, measure, or numerical count; and (3) the information required under section 609 [*Labeling*]: *Provided*, That under clause (2) of this paragraph reasonable variations shall be permitted, and exemptions as to small packages shall be established, by regulations prescribed by the Secretary."

(c) "If any word, statement, or other information required by or under authority of this chapter to appear on the label or labeling is not prominently placed thereon with such conspicuousness (as compared with other words, statements, designs, or devices, in the labeling) and in such terms as to render it likely to be read and understood by the ordinary individual under customary conditions of purchase and use."

(d) "If its container is so made, formed, or filled as to be misleading."

In 1960, the Color Additive Amendments added paragraph (e):

(e) "If it is a color additive, unless its packaging and labeling are in conformity with such packaging and labeling requirements, applicable to such color additive, as may be contained in regulations issued under section 721 [*Colors*] of this title. This paragraph shall not apply to packages of color additives which, with respect to their use for cosmetics, are marketed and intended for use only in or on hair dyes (as defined in the last sentence of section 601(a) [(a) of *Adulterated Cosmetics*])."

Paragraph (f) was added in 1970 to align the FD&C Act with the Poisons Prevention Packaging Act of 1970 (PPPA), which was enacted to reduce the risk of children ingesting hazardous household substances by requiring child-resistant packaging for certain products. The PPPA is codified into Title 15 of the USC:

(f) "If its packaging or labeling is in violation of an applicable regulation issued pursuant to section 3 or 4 of the Poison Prevention Packaging Act of 1970."

Section 602 of the FD&C Act lists provisions that make a cosmetic product misbranded under the FD&C Act; however, the FPLA includes additional provisions, which may be enforced by the FDA, that make a cosmetic product misbranded within the meaning of the FD&C Act.

Fair Packaging and Labeling Act (FPLA)

FPLA was intended to assist consumers in making informed purchases. As such, the FPLA only requires label information to appear on the outer container of a cosmetic product. Under the FPLA, any consumer commodity which is a food, drug, device, or cosmetic and which is introduced or delivered into commerce in violation of FPLA provisions is misbranded [65]. Section 10(a) of the FPLA defines "consumer commodity." The cosmetic labeling and packaging requirements of the FPLA largely overlap with those of the FD&C Act, but the FPLA adds the following requirements: the product label must specify the identity of the commodity, must have a principal display panel, and must display specific information on that panel [66].

The FPLA also authorizes FDA to implement regulations that are necessary to prevent the deception of consumers to facilitate value comparisons as to any consumer commodity which is a food, drug, device, or cosmetic, such as regulations that require label information and ingredient declaration, and prevent deceptive packaging [67]. Under this authority, FDA promulgated an important ingredient labeling regulation for cosmetics, which generally requires the label on each package declare each ingredient in descending order of predominance, except for fragrance or flavor [68].

New Labeling Requirements After MoCRA

MoCRA introduced new labeling requirements under section 609 of the FD&C Act to boost consumer safety and transparency. Cosmetic product labels must now include contact information—a domestic address, phone number, or electronic contact—that allows consumers to report adverse events [69]. Products intended solely for professional use, like those in salons, must clearly state that they are for use only by licensed professionals [70]. In addition, fragrance allergens must be identified on product labels, although the specific allergens and any required thresholds for disclosure will be defined in future rulemaking [71]. These updates ensure that labels provide modern, accessible safety information for consumers.

Beyond Adulteration and Misbranding: Change After MoCRA

Adverse Events and Record Access

An adverse event is an undesirable reaction that occurs after using a cosmetic, whether the symptoms are minor or significant. Rash, redness, burns, and hair loss are examples of adverse events. If these outcomes escalate to require or cause inpatient hospitalization, significant disfigurement, congenital abnormalities, death, etc., then they become serious adverse events. In 2024, about 49% of FDA-evaluated cosmetic adverse event reports were serious adverse events.

MoCRA requires a responsible person to maintain records of reports of adverse events and to submit any report received of a serious adverse event to FDA, as outlined in section 605 (*Adverse Events*) of the FD&C Act. Responsible persons (manufacturers, packers, or distributors) receive reports of adverse events through the contact information required on each cosmetic label—address, telephone, or electronic contact information [72]. For serious adverse events, submission of a report to FDA within 15 business days is mandatory and must include a scan of the label on or within the retail packaging of the associated cosmetic product [73]. Any additional material medical information that is related to a serious adverse event report and is received within the first year of the serious adverse event report must be reported to the FDA within 15 business days as well [74]. FDA is developing an electronic process specifically for the mandatory submission of cosmetic serious adverse event reports. However, the current process for submitting adverse event reports (non-serious) and serious adverse event reports to FDA is the same and can be done via email or mail. Forms and information on how to submit an adverse event or serious adverse event can be found online at Modernization of Cosmetics RegulationRegulation Act of 2022 (MoCRA) | FDA [12].

MoCRA includes new recordkeeping requirements and provides for the FDA's access to these records during inspections. Responsible persons must maintain records of all adverse event reports—both serious and non-serious—associated with their cosmetic products for 6 years. Businesses that qualify for the small business exemption under section 612 of the FD&C Act are required to retain such records for only 3 years [75]. During an inspection pursuant to section 704 of the FD&C Act, FDA is authorized to access adverse event records required to be maintained under section 605 of the FD&C Act.

Regulations promulgated under section 606 of the FD&C Act for good manufacturing practices may allow FDA, during an inspection, to access records to demonstrate compliance with such regulations.

Section 610 (*Records*) also provides FDA with authority to access records if certain criteria are met. If FDA has reasonable belief that

1. a cosmetic product,
2. or its ingredients,
3. or another cosmetic product likely to be affected in a similar manner,

are likely adulterated and the use or exposure to such product(s) presents a threat of serious adverse health consequences or death to humans (SAHCODH), and all other authorizing circumstances are met, then all records FDA needs to determine safety of the affected product(s) must be made available to FDA upon request [76]. For example, FDA could access safety substantiation records required under section 608 of the FD&C Act. Such records would not include, for example, cosmetic formulas, financial data, or research data other than safety substantiation data.

If FDA becomes aware of or receives product recalls, adverse event reports, consumer complaints, or sampling results which indicate a product is likely adulterated and could cause SAHCODH, FDA could exercise its authority under section 610.

Registration and Listing

Before MoCRA, FDA administered a voluntary cosmetic registration program [77], which was sunset on March 27, 2023. After MoCRA, owners or operators of facilities (both domestic and foreign) that manufacture or process cosmetic products for distribution in the U.S. must register their facilities and responsible persons must list their cosmetic products. As discussed elsewhere in this chapter, there are certain limited exceptions to these cosmetic product listing and facility registration requirements. FDA has made available various submission methods including paper forms and electronic submission portals (e.g. Cosmetics Direct, Electronic Submission Gateway, and X-Forms) to facilitate the submission and receipt of both the registration and listing information required under section 607 (*Registration and Product Listing*) of the FD&C Act.

In December 2023, FDA published a registration and listing guidance for industry followed by an update in December 2024 [78]. This guidance explains, among other things, who is responsible for making the registration and listing submissions, what information to include, what an FDA Establishment Identifier (FEI) is and how to obtain one, how to make submissions, and certain exemptions to the registration and listing requirements [79].

Facility registrations must be renewed every 2 years [80] and any updates to cosmetic product listings must be submitted annually [81]. FDA has the authority to suspend a facility's registration if it determines that a cosmetic product manufactured or processed by the facility has a reasonable probability of causing SAHCODH, and if FDA has a reasonable belief that other cosmetic products manufactured or processed by the facility may be similarly affected because of a failure that cannot be isolated to a product or products, or is sufficiently pervasive to raise concerns about other products manufactured in the facility [82]. If the facility's registration is suspended, distributing or selling cosmetic products from the facility in the U.S. is prohibited [83].

Small Business Exemption

MoCRA included provisions that exempt some small businesses from GMP, registration, and product listing requirements. To qualify for the exemption under section 612 (*Small Businesses*) of the FD&C Act, a business must meet the following criteria:

- The business must have gross annual U.S. sales of cosmetic products averaging less than $1,000,000 over the previous 3 years, adjusted for inflation [84], and
- The business must not manufacture or process the following products:
  - Cosmetic products that regularly come into contact with the mucus membrane of the eye under customary or usual conditions of use.
  - Cosmetic products intended for internal use.
  - Cosmetic products injected into the body.
  - Cosmetic products that alter appearance for more than 24 hours under customary or usual conditions of use and for which removal by the consumer is not part of such conditions of use [85].

While businesses meeting the criteria for the small business exemption are exempt from GMP requirements and registration and product listing requirements, they must still ensure compliance with all other applicable laws and regulations.

Mandatory Recall Authority

MoCRA established mandatory recall authority for cosmetics under section 611 of the FD&C Act, significantly enhancing FDA's ability to protect public health. This provision empowers the agency to require the removal of hazardous cosmetics from the market, thereby reducing potential consumer harm and strengthening overall safety oversight.

Under this authority, FDA can order a mandatory recall if it determines that there is a reasonable probability that a cosmetic is adulterated or misbranded and the use or exposure to such cosmetic will cause SAHCODH, and the responsible person fails to voluntarily cease distribution and recall the product when provided the opportunity [86]. The opportunity to voluntarily cease distribution and recall the cosmetic must be provided before FDA may order a recall. If the responsible person does not act, FDA may issue an order requiring immediate cessation of distribution.

If the order is given, the responsible party must be offered an informal hearing to assess whether sufficient evidence supports the action within 10 days of the order. The hearing will provide the responsible person the opportunity to address whether adequate evidence exists to justify the order [87]. After the hearing, FDA may vacate the order, maintain it for a set time, or amend it to require a recall with specific conditions and timelines [88]. Persons subject to a recall order must immediately cease distribution of a cosmetic, ensure and facilitate the removal of the unsafe product from the market, and provide notice of such recall order as ordered [89]. Additionally, during a recall, FDA will ensure the public is notified by press release and, as appropriate, other disseminated media [90].

As mentioned in *Prohibited Acts: Old and New* of this chapter, failure to comply with a mandatory recall order is a prohibited act [91]. Therefore, a responsible person who refuses or fails to follow such order could be subject to a criminal prosecution or injunction.

Enforcement

Domestically manufactured and imported cosmetics must meet the same requirements. FDA engages in post-market international surveillance through record inspection, consumer complaints, adverse event reports, label reviews, product sampling and testing, and import examination to monitor the safety of the cosmetics in the U.S. market. FDA has the authority to inspect facilities internationally and cite them for violations of the Act [92].

Domestic enforcement actions include seizures, injunctions, civil money penalties, and criminal prosecution. As noted previously, MoCRA provides FDA with mandatory recall authority for cosmetics as well. FDA does not have independent litigating authority, and pursues actions like seizures, injunctions, and criminal prosecution, through the Department of Justice (DOJ) [93]. Without the DOJ, FDA can issue safety alerts, warning letters, import alerts, recalls, civil money penalties, and other administrative tools.

Warning letters, typically FDA's first and preferred course of official action, advise individuals or firms that FDA has identified regulatory violations and give recipients the opportunity to voluntarily come into compliance with the law [93]. A few warning letters providing examples of cosmetics cited for adulteration due to microbial contamination can be found online [94].

Evidence that justifies a mandatory recall, where the firm retains the product, may support a seizure, where the government confiscates the product; however, a seizure is considered a harsher legal action against a firm [93]. FDA does not have to provide prior notice or allow for voluntary compliance before initiating a seizure. There have been cases where public protection required seizures of cosmetics starting with the seizure of Lash Lure in 1938. Other examples would include seizures in 1989 of oral "Tanning Pills" containing canthaxanthin [95] and in 1995 of Rio "natural" hair, which caused adverse events for multiple users [96].

Cosmetics offered for import must be compliant at the time of entry to the U.S. FDA, working closely with U.S. Customs and Border Protection, may refuse entry to products that appear violative [97]. Import Alerts provide notice to a company or country that FDA has evidence the intended import appears to violate U.S. law and may detain the product without inspection. Supporting evidence for detentions without physical examination may include a history of violations or inspectional findings [93]. Imported products that appear violative and are detained without physical examination must be brought into compliance, destroyed, or re-exported.

FDA has multiple official enforcement tools but prefers to bring industry into voluntary compliance through negotiations, guidance, and education. Moreover, FDA may exercise enforcement discretion for certain violations of the FD&C Act [93].

Conclusion

On average, men use 6 cosmetic products and women use 12 cosmetic products per day [98]. MoCRA marks a transformative step in FDA's oversight of cosmetics, helping to enhance the safety of products consumers use daily and aligning regulations with the evolving cosmetics industry. By introducing new requirements for facility registration, product listing, safety substantiation, labeling, and mandatory recall authority, MoCRA addresses longstanding gaps in the FD&C Act.

FDA has published or intends to publish regulations and guidances for the new MoCRA provisions [34]. As the implementation of MoCRA progresses, the continued collaboration between regulators, industry stakeholders, and consumers will be essential to ensure its success. This modernization reflects a critical recognition of the importance of cosmetic safety in the daily lives of millions and sets the foundation for a more regulated and responsible cosmetics market in the United States.

Additional Reading

The U.S.C. and the electronic Code of Federal Regulations (eCFR) can be found online:

- Office of the Law Revision Counsel of the United States House of Representatives. United States Code [Internet]. 2025. https://uscode.house.gov/.
- National Archives and Records Administration's Office of the Federal Register, Government Publishing Office. Electronic Code of Federal Regulations [Internet]. 2025. https://www.ecfr.gov/

Another overview of MoCRA:

- Wells N. FDA Regulation of Cosmetics and Personal Care Products Under the Modernization of Cosmetics Regulation Act of 2022 (MoCRA). Report No.: R47826. Washington, DC: Congressional Research Service; 2023. Available from: https://crsreports.congress.gov/product/details?prodcode=R47826.

References

1. Forbes SB, Blake WC. Fatality resulting from the use of Lashlure on the eyebrow and eyelashes. JAMA J Am Med Assoc. 1934;103(19):1441–2.
2. McCally AW, Farmer AG, Loomis EC. Corneal ulceration following use of Lash-Lure. JAMA J Am Med Assoc. 1933;101(20):1560–1.
3. Harner CE. Dermato-ophthalmitis due to the eyelash dye Lash-Lure. JAMA J Am Med Assoc. 1933;101(20):1558–9.
4. Jamieson RC. Eyelash dye (Lash-Lure) dermatitis with conjunctivitis. JAMA J Am Med Assoc. 1933;101(20):1560.
5. Greenbaum SS. Reports of thallium acetate poisoning following the use of Koremlu. JAMA J Am Med Assoc. 1931;96(22):1868.
6. Hollander L. Dermatitis produced by cosmetics (La Gerardine). JAMA J Am Med Assoc. 1933;101(4):259–61.
7. Lane JE, Strauss MJ. Toilet water dermatitis: with especial reference to Berlock dermatitis. JAMA J Am Med Assoc. 1930;95(10):717–9.
8. JAMA Bureau of Investigation. Koremlu: a dangerous depilatory containing thallium acetate. JAMA. 1931;96:629–31. https://jamanetwork.com/journals/jama/fullarticle/249787. Accessed 19 Feb 2025
9. Waring TP. Another case of thallium poisoning following use of Koremlu cream. JAMA J Am Med Assoc. 1931;97(10):703.

10. U.S. Food and Drug Administration. Selected Amendments to the FD&C Act; 2018. https://www.fda.gov/regulatory-information/laws-enforced-fda/selected-amendments-fdc-act. Accessed 19 Feb 2025.
11. Cosmetics - Worldwide. Statista; 2024. https://www.statista.com/outlook/cmo/beauty-personal-care/cosmetics/worldwide. Accessed 13 Jun 2025.
12. U.S. Food and Drug Administration. Modernization of Cosmetics Regulation Act of 2022 (MoCRA); 2025. https://www.fda.gov/cosmetics/cosmetics-laws-regulations/modernization-cosmetics-regulation-act-2022-mocra. Accessed 13 Mar 2025.
13. Janssen WF. The story of the laws behind the lables. FDA Consumer; 1981. Available from: https://www.fda.gov/about-fda/office-commissioner/office-chief-counsel.
14. Jackson CO. Food and drug legislation in the new deal. Princeton, NJ: Princeton University Press; 1970. p. 4.
15. Kay G. Dying to be beautiful: the fight for safe cosmetics. The Ohio State University; 2005. p. 10–6.
16. Oscar E, Anderson J. Pioneer statute: the pure food and drugs act of 1906. J Pub Law. 1964;13(1):189–96.
17. Department of Commerce. Druggists' preparations, patent medicines and compounds, and perfumery and cosmetics. In: Biennial census of manufacturers: 1921. Washington, DC: U.S. Government Printing Office; 1924. p. 745–64. Table 623, "Summary For the Industry and Its Branches, For the Unites States: 1849 to 1921"; p. 746.
18. Kay G. Dying to be beautiful: the fight for safe cosmetics. The Ohio State University; 2005. p. 30–53.
19. Department of Commerce. Druggists' preparations, patent or proprietary medicines and compounds, perfumes, cosmetics, and other toilet preparations. In: Fifteenth census of the United States, manufactures: 1929, vol. 2. Washington, D.C.: Government Printing Office; 1933. p. 667–77. Table 3, "Products, By Class, Kind, And Value, For the United States: 1923 to 1929"; p. 673.
20. Terrell E. Research guides: business of beauty: a resource guide: history of the beauty business. Library of Congress; 2010. https://guides.loc.gov/business-of-beauty/history. Accessed 19 Feb 2025.
21. Clayman A. Maybelline Company, est. 1915. Made In Chicago Museum; 2018. https://www.madeinchicagomuseum.com/single-post/maybelline-co/. Accessed 19 Feb 2025.
22. Basten FE. Max factor's Hollywood: glamour, movies, make-up; 1995. p. 26–37.
23. Our Heritage. Max factor; 2025. https://www.maxfactor.com/en-gb/our-brand/our-heritage. Accessed 19 Feb 2025.
24. Concannon CC. Drugs and cosmetics in the depression. Drug Cosmet Ind. 1933;32(3).
25. McDonough EG. The truth about cosmetics. New York: The Drug and Cosmetic Industry; 1937. p. 300.
26. Gasch AT. Lash Lure and Paraphenylenediamine: toxic beauty past and present. American Academy of Opthalmology; 2017. https://www.aao.org/lifetime-engaged-ophthalmologist/perspective/article/lash-lure-paraphenylenediamine-toxic-beauty. Accessed 7 Mar 2025.
27. Kay G. Dying to be beautiful: the fight for safe cosmetics. The Ohio State University Press; 2005. p. 71–3.
28. Junod SW. The class of '39: implementing the 1938 Food, drug, and cosmetic act. J Assoc Food Drug Off U S. 1988;52(4):10–25.
29. Kay G. Dying to be beautiful: the fight for safe cosmetics. The Ohio State University; 2005. p. 107–18.
30. Office of the Law Revision Counsel of the United States House of Representatives. United States Code [Interenet]; 2025. https://uscode.house.gov/. Accessed 30 May 2025.
31. U.S. Food and Drug Administration. Prohibited & restricted ingredients in cosmetics; 2022. https://www.fda.gov/cosmetics/cosmetics-laws-regulations/prohibited-restricted-ingredients-cosmetics. Accessed 19 Mar 2025.

32. U.S. Food and Drug Administration. Cosmetics labeling guide; 2022. https://www.fda.gov/cosmetics/cosmetics-labeling-regulations/cosmetics-labeling-guide. Accessed 19 Mar 2025.
33. U.S. Food and Drug Administration. FDA proposes rule to require standardized testing methods for detecting and identifying asbestos in talc-containing cosmetic products; 2024. https://www.fda.gov/news-events/press-announcements/fda-proposes-rule-require-standardized-testing-methods-detecting-and-identifying-asbestos-talc. Accessed 1 Apr 2025.
34. U.S. Food and Drug Administration. Cosmetics guidance documents; 2024. https://www.fda.gov/cosmetics/cosmetics-guidance-regulation/cosmetics-guidance-documents. Accessed 26 Feb 2025.
35. U.S. Food and Drug Administration. FDA authority over cosmetics: how cosmetics are not FDA-approved, but are FDA-regulated; 2022. https://www.fda.gov/cosmetics/cosmetics-laws-regulations/fda-authority-over-cosmetics-how-cosmetics-are-not-fda-approved-are-fda-regulated. Accessed 19 Mar 2025.
36. Katz LM, Lewis KM, Spence S, Sadrieh N. Regulation of cosmetics in the United States. Dermatol Clin. 2022;40(3):307–18.
37. Food and Drug Administration. Color additives; 2024. https://www.fda.gov/industry/color-additives. Accessed 18 Mar 2025.
38. Federal Food, Drug, and Cosmetic Act, 21 U.S.C. § 321(t)(1) (2025).
39. Federal Food, Drug, and Cosmetic Act, 21 U.S.C § 379e(b) (2025).
40. Barrows JN, Lipman AL, Bailey CJ. Color additives history. Food Safety Magazine; 2003. Available from: https://www.fda.gov/industry/color-additives/color-additives-history#authors. Accessed 9 Mar 2025.
41. Zajac AJ, Barrows JN. FDA's regulation of color additives. Food Safety Magazine; 2017. Available from: https://www.food-safety.com/articles/5508-fdae28099s-regulation-of-color-additives#:~:text=The%201960%20Color%20Additive%20Amendments%20established%20four%20factors%20that%20FDA,the%20availability%20of%20analytical%20methods. Accessed 18 Mar 2025.
42. Barrows JN, Lipman AL, Belai N. History of U.S. regulation of color additives and colorants. In: Komolprasert V, Turowski P, editors. Food additives and packaging. Washington, DC: American Chemical Society; 2014.
43. Federal Food, Drug, and Cosmetic Act, 21 U.S.C. § 361(a) (2025).
44. Listing of Color Additives Exempt From Certification; Silver Nitrate, 86 FR 55494 (Oct. 6, 2021) (codified at 21 CFR Part 73). https://www.federalregister.gov/documents/2021/10/06/2021-21755/listing-of-color-additives-exempt-from-certification-silver-nitrate
45. Federal Food, Drug, and Cosmetic Act, 21 U.S.C. § 321(g)(1) (2025).
46. U.S. Food and Drug Administration. Is it a cosmetic, a drug, or both? (Or is it soap?); 2024. https://www.fda.gov/cosmetics/cosmetics-laws-regulations/it-cosmetic-drug-or-both-or-it-soap. Accessed 19 Mar 2025.
47. Federal Food, Drug, and Cosmetic Act, 21 U.S.C. § 321(i)(2) (2025).
48. 21 CFR § 701.20 (2025).
49. Federal Food, Drug, and Cosmetic Act, 21 U.S.C. § 331-337a (2025).
50. Federal Food, Drug, and Cosmetic Act, 21 U.S.C. § 331(f) (2025).
51. Federal Food, Drug, and Cosmetic Act, 21 U.S.C. § 331(n) (2025).
52. Federal Food, Drug, and Cosmetic Act, 21 U.S.C. § 331(e) (2025).
53. Federal Food, Drug, and Cosmetic Act, 21 U.S.C. § 331(hhh) (2025).
54. Federal Food, Drug, and Cosmetic Act, 21 U.S.C. § 331(iii) (2025).
55. U.S. Food and Drug Administration. Microbiological safety and cosmetics; 2024. https://www.fda.gov/cosmetics/potential-contaminants-cosmetics/microbiological-safety-and-cosmetics#Resources. Accessed 7 Mar 2025.
56. Huang J, Hitchins AD, Tran TT, McCarron JE. BAM chapter 23: methods for cosmetics; 2024. Available from: https://www.fda.gov/food/laboratory-methods-food/bam-chapter-23-methods-cosmetics. Accessed 7 Mar 2025.

57. U.S. Food and Drug Administration. Limiting lead in lipstick and other cosmetics; 2022. https://www.fda.gov/cosmetics/cosmetic-products/limiting-lead-lipstick-and-other-cosmetics#expanded_survey. Accessed 7 Mar 2025.
58. U.S. Food and Drug Administration. Think before you ink: tattoo safety; 2024. https://www.fda.gov/consumers/consumer-updates/think-you-ink-tattoo-safety. Accessed 7 Mar 2025.
59. U.S. Food and Drug Administration. Product testing of cosmetics; 2022. https://www.fda.gov/cosmetics/cosmetics-science-research/product-testing-cosmetics#Using. Accessed 9 Mar 2025.
60. Federal Food, Drug, and Cosmetic Act, 21 U.S.C. § 364b(a) (2025).
61. Federal Food, Drug, and Cosmetic Act, 21 U.S.C. § 364b(b) (2025).
62. Federal Food, Drug, and Cosmetic Act, 21 U.S.C. § 364d(c)(1) (2025).
63. Federal Food, Drug, and Cosmetic Act, 21 U.S.C. § 364d(c)(2) (2025).
64. Consolidated Appropriations Act, Pub. L. No. 117-328, 136 Stat. 4459, 5859-60 (March 14, 2022).
65. Federal Food, Drug, and Cosmetic Act, 15 U.S.C. § 1456 (2025).
66. Federal Food, Drug, and Cosmetic Act, 15 U.S.C. § 1453 (2025).
67. Federal Food, Drug, and Cosmetic Act, 15 U.S.C. § 1454 (2025).
68. 21 CFR § 701.3 (2025).
69. Federal Food, Drug, and Cosmetic Act, 21 U.S.C. § 364e(a) (2025).
70. Federal Food, Drug, and Cosmetic Act, 21 U.S.C. § 364e(c)(2) (2025).
71. Federal Food, Drug, and Cosmetic Act, 21 U.S.C. § 364e(b) (2025).
72. Federal Food, Drug, and Cosmetic Act, 21 U.S.C. § 364a(d) (2025).
73. Federal Food, Drug, and Cosmetic Act, 21 U.S.C. § 364a(b)(1) (2025).
74. Federal Food, Drug, and Cosmetic Act, 21 U.S.C. § 364a(b)(2) (2025).
75. Federal Food, Drug, and Cosmetic Act, 21 U.S.C. § 364a(e)(1) (2025).
76. Federal Food, Drug, and Cosmetic Act, 21 U.S.C. § 364f(a) (2025).
77. 21 CFR (2025).
78. U.S. Food and Drug Administration. Guidance for industry: registration and listing of cosmetic product facilities and products; 2024. https://www.fda.gov/regulatory-information/search-fda-guidance-documents/guidance-industry-registration-and-listing-cosmetic-product-facilities-and-products. Accessed 26 Feb 2025.
79. U.S. Food and Drug Administration. Cosmetics direct; 2024. https://www.fda.gov/cosmetics/registration-listing-cosmetic-product-facilities-and-products/cosmetics-direct. Accessed 19 Mar 2025.
80. Federal Food, Drug, and Cosmetic Act, 21 U.S.C. § 364c(a)(2) (2025).
81. Federal Food, Drug, and Cosmetic Act, 21 U.S.C. § 364c(c)(5) (2025).
82. Federal Food, Drug, and Cosmetic Act, 21 U.S.C. § 364c(f)(1) (2025).
83. Federal Food, Drug, and Cosmetic Act, 21 U.S.C. § 364c(f)(6) (2025).
84. Federal Food, Drug, and Cosmetic Act, 21 U.S.C. § 364h(a) (2025).
85. Federal Food, Drug, and Cosmetic Act, 21 U.S.C. § 364h(b) (2025).
86. Federal Food, Drug, and Cosmetic Act, 21 U.S.C. § 364g(a (2025).
87. Federal Food, Drug, and Cosmetic Act, 21 U.S.C. § 364g(b) (2025).
88. Federal Food, Drug, and Cosmetic Act, 21 U.S.C. § 364g(c) (2025).
89. Federal Food, Drug, and Cosmetic Act, 21 U.S.C. § 364g(d) (2025).
90. Federal Food, Drug, and Cosmetic Act, 21 U.S.C. § 364g(f) (2025).
91. Federal Food, Drug, and Cosmetics Act, 21 U.S.C. § 331(iii) (2025).
92. U.S. Food and Drug Administration. Inspection basics; 2024. https://www.fda.gov/inspections-compliance-enforcement-and-criminal-investigations/inspection-basics. Accessed 26 Feb 2025.
93. Staman JA. Enforcement of the food, drug, and cosmetic act: select legal issues. Report No.: R43609. Washington, DC: Congressional Research Service; 2018. Available from: https://crsreports.congress.gov/product/details?prodcode=R43609

94. U.S. Food and Drug Administration. Warning letters cited for cosmetics adulterated due to microbial contamination; 2022. https://www.fda.gov/cosmetics/warning-letters-related-cosmetics/warning-letters-cite-cosmetics-adulterated-due-microbial-contamination. Accessed 25 Feb 2025.
95. U.S. Food and Drug Administration. Tanning pills; 2022. https://www.fda.gov/cosmetics/cosmetic-products/tanning-pills. Accessed 25 Feb 2025.
96. Swee W, Klontz KC, Lambert LA. A nationwide outbreak of alopecia associated with the use of a hair-relaxing formulation. Arch Dermatol. 2000;136(9):1104–8.
97. U.S. Food and Drug Administration. Cosmetics importers; 2022. https://www.fda.gov/cosmetics/cosmetics-international-activities/cosmetics-importers#Imports1. Accessed 25 Feb 2025.
98. Survey finds use of personal care products up since 2004—what that means for your health. Environmental Working Group; 2023. https://www.ewg.org/research/survey-finds-use-personal-care-products-2004-what-means-your-health. Accessed 19 Feb 2025.

Chapter 2
The Contribution of the European Cosmetics Directive Towards International Harmonization: Impact on the Evaluation of Safety and Efficacy of Cosmetics

Peter Elsner

Introduction

The cosmetics industry is a dynamic economic sector with a global market value exceeding €200 billion. Ensuring the safety and efficacy of cosmetic products is paramount, necessitating robust regulatory frameworks. The European Cosmetics Directive (76/768/EEC), and its successor, Regulation (EC) No 1223/2009, have been instrumental in shaping these frameworks, not only within the European Union (EU) but also influencing international standards.

Historical Development of the European Cosmetics Directive

Adopted in 1976, Directive 76/768/EEC aimed to harmonize cosmetic regulations across EU member states to ensure a high level of consumer protection and facilitate the free movement of goods. Over three decades, the Directive was amended multiple times to reflect advancements in toxicology, public health policy, and consumer demand. According to European Union law, directives have to be put into national law by membership parliaments which proved to be a cumbersome and time-consuming process. In addition, a uniform application of regulations is difficult to ensure.

The culmination of the mentioned amendments led to the adoption of Regulation (EC) No 1223/2009, which came into force on July 11, 2013. Unlike directives,

P. Elsner (✉)
Dermatology, Allergology, Dermatopathology, Gera, Germany

Legal Associates Prof. Dr. Peter Elsner Rolf-Peter Dröge, Hamburg, Germany
e-mail: elsner@rechtsanwaltskanzlei-elsner-droege.de

P. Elsner et al. (eds.), *Cosmetics*, https://doi.org/10.1007/978-3-032-14644-1_2

regulations are directly applicable in all member states, ensuring uniformity. This transition marked a significant milestone in the legal governance of cosmetic products in Europe.

Regulatory Structure and Objectives

Article 1 of Regulation (EC) No 1223/2009 states the objective of the regulation which is to "ensure the functioning of the internal market and a high level of protection of human health." The latter is specified in Article 3 "Safety": "A cosmetic product made available on the market shall be safe for human health when used under normal or reasonably foreseeable conditions of use."

To achieve this objective, the Regulation contains several key elements:

- The Responsible Person (RP): Each product must have an RP within the EU responsible for compliance with the Regulation.
- Product Information File (PIF): A detailed dossier containing safety assessments, manufacturing methods, proof of claimed effects, and adverse event records.
- Cosmetic Product Safety Report (CPSR): A mandatory document evaluating a product's safety through toxicological data and risk assessment.
- Notification and Surveillance: Products must be notified through the Cosmetic Products Notification Portal (CPNP) prior to marketing.
- Market Surveillance: National authorities may conduct random inspections and risk-based audits.

Cosmetic Safety Evaluation according to Regulation (EC) No 1223/2009

Only cosmetic products for which a legal or natural person is designated within the EU as 'responsible person' shall be placed on the market. Only professionals with specific qualifications in toxicology, pharmacy, medicine, or related sciences are permitted to serve as a safety assessor of cosmetics which ensures scientific credibility and accountability.

The 'responsible person' has to ensure that the cosmetic product has undergone a safety assessment on the basis of the relevant information and that a cosmetic product safety report is set up.

According to Annex 1 of the Regulation, the cosmetic product safety report has to contain the following information:

Part A: Cosmetic Product Safety Information

1. Quantitative and qualitative composition of the cosmetic product
2. Physical/chemical characteristics and stability of the cosmetic product
3. Microbiological quality
4. Impurities, traces, information about the packaging material
5. Normal and reasonably foreseeable use
6. Exposure to the cosmetic product
7. Exposure to the substances contained in the cosmetic product
8. Toxicological profile of the substances
9. Undesirable effects and serious undesirable effects
10. Information on the cosmetic product, e.g. existing studies from human volunteers

Part B: Cosmetic Product Safety Assessment

This part must contain a statement on the safety of the cosmetic product and on the need to label any particular warnings and instructions of use, signed by the responsible safety assessor. A specific assessment for cosmetic products intended for use on children under the age of three and for cosmetic products intended exclusively for use in external intimate hygiene has to be provided.

Alternatives to Animal Testing in Cosmetic Safety Evaluation

The EU has been a global leader in promoting non-animal testing. The Cosmetics Directive banned animal testing for finished products in 2004 and for cosmetic ingredients in 2009.

In 1991, under Council Directive 86/609/EEC, the "European Centre for the Validation of Alternative Methods" (ECVAM) was established to further the development of alternative methods to animal testing. The new entity followed the "3Rs principle" of replacement, reduction, and refinement of animal methods. In 2010, ECVAM became the EU Reference Laboratory for the validation of alternative methods to animal testing, acquiring the new formal designation EURL ECVAM.

In the 2000s, ECVAM validated and promoted key in vitro methods for skin irritation, phototoxicity, and cytotoxicity. Yearly progress reports have been published with the last dating of 2024 [1].

The following alternative methods were validated by ECVAM and are currently in use for cosmetic safety testing in Europe [2] (Table 2.1):

Table 2.1 Alternative methods for cosmetic safety testing validated by ECVAM and currently in use in Europe

Toxicity endpoint	Validated method(s)
Skin irritation/ corrosion	RhE models (EpiSkin™, EpiDerm™, SkinEthic™)
Eye irritation	BCOP, ICE, RhCE (EpiOcular™, SkinEthic™ HCE)
Skin sensitization	DPRA, KeratinoSens™, h-CLAT
Phototoxicity	3 T3 NRU Phototoxicity Test
Genotoxicity	Ames, In vitro MN test, Chromosomal aberration assay
Acute systemic toxicity	Not fully replaced – reduction and non-animal strategies

Role of the Scientific Committee on Cosmetic Safety

In 1978, the SCC (Scientific Committee on Cosmetology) was established to provide expert advice for the EU Commission on cosmetic ingredients. In 1997, the committee received a broader mandate covering also other consumer products such as toys, and was renamed SCCNFP (Scientific Committee on Cosmetic Products and Non-Food Products Intended for Consumers). In 2008, the SCCS (Scientific Committee on Consumer Safety) was set up which is focused on cosmetic product safety and related areas (tattoos, personal care). The SCCS produces its reports usually in response to a specific request by the Commission, but it may also, at its own initiative, publish statements on specific topics. The final opinions of the SCCS on specific cosmetic ingredients are an important basis for the safety assessment of cosmetic products. All the reports and the meeting minutes of the SCCS are published on its website thus ensuring transparency.

The SCCS has regularly published "Notes of Guidance for the Testing of Cosmetic Ingredients and their Safety Evaluation" with the latest edition dating to 2023 [3]. These notes highlight the usefulness of human testing by stating that tests with human volunteers (e.g. skin compatibility tests) confirm that there are no harmful effects when applying a cosmetic product for the first time to human skin or mucous membranes. "If considered scientifically and ethically necessary, human tests can only be envisaged when the toxicological profiles of the components are available and no concern is raised. A high degree of safety needs to be ensured." They refer to irritancy tests that are less problematic, but also to predictive testing of potentially skin sensitising cosmetic (mixtures of) substances which may induce a long-lasting or permanent immunological sensitisation in the individual thus causing serious ethical questions [3].

Monitoring of Cosmetic Safety

Monitoring of cosmetic safety remains in the competence of the Member States.

If a manufacturer or distributor becomes aware of a serious undesirable effect, they must report it immediately to the competent authority of the Member State in which the serious undesirable effect occurred.

In many cases, however, manufacturers do not learn of adverse reactions to their products. Neither patients who experience such adverse reactions nor dermatologists who treat these patients are obliged to report them in Germany - unlike in France, for example [4]. Unlike for medicinal products, there is also no reporting system for cosmetic side effects by the medical profession in Germany.

The European Commission has established a rapid alert system in which it publishes a weekly overview of reported alerts, information on the dangerous products found, the risks identified and the measures taken in the country of notification ("Rapid Alert System for Dangerous Non-food Products" ("RAPEX notifications")). However, these notifications probably only account for a fraction of the incidents [5]. According to an evaluation of the years 2005–2017, only 157 cosmetic products from Germany were reported to the RAPEX database [5]. Thus, while cosmetic safety is the main objective of the European legislation and while being centrally regulated in Europe, with its everyday management remaining in the competence of the Member States, there may remain differences in application of the Community law between Member States.

Cosmetic Efficacy Evaluation According to Regulation (EC) No 1223/2009

The Cosmetics Regulation states that the consumer should be protected from misleading claims concerning efficacy and other characteristics of cosmetic products. The claims that may be made for cosmetics are defined in more detail in Regulation (EC) No 655/2013. The responsible person shall ensure that the claim is consistent with the documentation proving the effect claimed for the cosmetic product in the product information file.

The criteria for making claims are general in nature and are given in the Annex to the mentioned Regulation (EC) No 655/2013. Thus, cosmetic product claims in the EU must be truthful, clear, and based on verifiable evidence. They must not mislead consumers, exaggerate benefits, or unfairly criticize competitors. All claims should help the average consumer make an informed and honest purchasing decision.

The Regulation mentions that where studies are being used as evidence, they shall be relevant to the product and to the benefit claimed, shall follow well-designed, well-conducted methodologies (valid, reliable and reproducible) and shall respect ethical considerations. However, no specific methods (e.g. bioengineering) are prescribed.

The following study methodologies a.o. may be considered for efficacy evaluation:

- Instrumental Studies, e.g., corneometry for moisturization, profilometry for wrinkle reduction
- Clinical Trials (on human volunteers)
- Consumer Use Tests
- Real-life settings with subjective feedback from users.
- Bibliographic Review
- Scientific literature (e.g., published studies on active ingredients).
- Expert Assessments
- In vitro/Ex vivo Testing

When interpreting the scientific requirements for cosmetic efficacy studies, the courts are more generous than, e.g., for drug studies or health claims. In a well publicised German case regarding the claim for a caffeine-containing shampoo stating that "caffeine may prevent alopecia", the Federal Court of Germany asserted that sufficient scientific substantiation in this context does not require that the effect attributed to the advertised product has become the subject of a general scientific discussion. Rather, sufficient scientific substantiation can already result from an individual study, provided that it is based on convincing methods and findings. That was confirmed in 2016 in a decision considering the claim of a "moisturizing gel reservoir" for a wet razor ([CSL STYLE ERROR: reference with no printed form.]).

In conclusion, the legal requirements for cosmetic claim substantiation are not clearly defined, e.g. by recommended study methodologies for specific claims. On the one hand, this leaves room for interpretation and application of innovative methods, on the other hand, a risk remains for manufacturers being challenged by competitors for unsubstantiated claims.

Contribution of the EU Cosmetics Regulation to International Harmonization

The EU framework has influenced countries like South Korea, Brazil, and members of ASEAN, many of which have adopted similar regulatory models. China is gradually reforming its laws to reduce animal testing, aligning with EU practices.

The EU works with international bodies like the OECD and International Cooperation on Cosmetics Regulation (ICCR) to align safety testing guidelines and terminology, fostering consistency.

While harmonization is progressing, discrepancies still exist. For example, the US FDA does not require pre-market approval or mandatory safety testing for cosmetics, unlike the EU.

References

1. Zuang V, Baccaro M, Barroso J, et al. Non-animal methods in science and regulation. EURL ECVAM status report 2024; 2025. https://publications.jrc.ec.europa.eu/repository/handle/JRC141304. Accessed 31 May 2025.
2. Filaire E, Nachat-Kappes R, Laporte C, et al. Alternative in vitro models used in the main safety tests of cosmetic products and new challenges. Int J Cosmet Sci. 2022;44:604–13.
3. Scientific Committee on Consumer Safety. The SCCS notes of guidance for the testing of cosmetic ingredients and their safety evaluation 12th revision; 2023.
4. Vigan M, Castelain F. Cosmetovigilance: definition, regulation and use "in practice". Eur J Dermatol. 2014;24:643–9.
5. Elsner P, Schliemann S. Dangerous cosmetic products in Germany: analysis of the RAPEX database of the European Commission. Hautarzt. 2017;68:885–9.

Chapter 3
Claim Support: Ethical Aspects for Conducting Human Studies: Why Are Human Volunteers Used in Cosmetic Testing?

Gabrielle Minta, Shivani Sinha, Albert E. Zhou, and Jane M. Grant-Kels

History of Cosmetics Regulations and Why Human Volunteers Are Used in Cosmetic Testing

The United States (US) Federal Food, Drug, and Cosmetic Act (FD&C Act) deems a cosmetic product to be safe if: "the cosmetic product, including any ingredient thereof, is not injurious to users under the conditions of use prescribed in the labeling thereof, or under such conditions of use as are customary or usual. The Secretary shall not consider a cosmetic ingredient or cosmetic product injurious to users solely because it can cause minor and transient reactions or minor and transient skin irritations in some users" [1]. Currently, there are 11 chemicals that are banned or restricted from cosmetic use. The FD&C Act does not specify required testing of cosmetic products or ingredients, except for color additives, prior to the distribution to consumers, only that they are not "adulterated" or "mislabeled". The US Food and Drug Administration (FDA) advises cosmetic manufacturers to conduct whatever testing they deem appropriate and effective to ensure the safety of their product [2]. Neither the FDA nor the FD&C Act require the use of animal (including human)

G. Minta
Frank H. Netter MD School of Medicine at Quinnipiac University, North Haven, CT, USA
e-mail: gminta@uchc.edu

S. Sinha · A. E. Zhou
Dermatology Department, University of Connecticut, Farmington, CT, USA
e-mail: shivsinha@uchc.edu; azhou@uchc.edu

J. M. Grant-Kels (✉)
Dermatology Department, University of Connecticut, Farmington, CT, USA

Department of Dermatology, University of Florida, Gainesville, FL, USA
e-mail: grant@uchc.edu

P. Elsner et al. (eds.), *Cosmetics*, https://doi.org/10.1007/978-3-032-14644-1_3

testing and they support the use of alternative methods that do not employ animal experimentation.

The Modernization of Cosmetic Regulation Act of 2022 (MoCRA) expanded the regulations of cosmetics, creating new authorities for the FDA and new obligations for manufacturers and suppliers [3]. Under MoCRA, the FDA can have products recalled and distribution ceased if there is reasonable probability that the product is adulterated. The FDA can also suspend a facilities registration if there is reasonable probability of the cosmetics manufactured or processed at the facility causing serious adverse health consequences. Under MoCRA, manufacturers and suppliers must register their facilities with the FDA, report any adverse events within 15 days, and maintain records of adequate substantiation of safety using scientifically supported evidence. With this expansion there is still no requirement for the substantiation of safety to involve animal testing, only that it is derived from scientifically robust methods.

As mentioned above, the FDA has issued a general framework to assess the safety of cosmetic products in lieu of issuing specific guidelines. The FDA advises that "the safety of a product can be adequately substantiated through (a) reliance on already available toxicological test data on individual ingredients and on product formulations that are similar in composition to the particular cosmetic, and (b) performance of any additional toxicological and other tests that are appropriate in light of such existing data and information. Although satisfactory toxicological data may exist for each ingredient of a cosmetic product, it will still be necessary to conduct some toxicological testing with the complete formulation to assure adequately the safety of the finished cosmetic" [4].

Similarly, the European Union Cosmetics Regulation (EUCR) requires that: "A cosmetic product made available on the market shall be safe for human health when used under normal or reasonably foreseeable conditions of use, taking account, in particular, of the following: presentation, labeling, instructions for use and disposal" [5]. To ensure the safety of a cosmetic product, an assessment is required which ensures that: "the intended use of the cosmetic product and the anticipated systemic exposure to individual ingredients in a final formulation are taken into account in the safety assessment; an appropriate weight-of-evidence approach is used in the safety assessment for reviewing data from all existing sources; the cosmetic product safety report is kept up to date in view of additional relevant information generated subsequent to placing the product on the market" [5]. Currently, there are over 1700 chemicals that are prohibited or restricted from cosmetic use. The EUCR prohibits the distribution of cosmetic products that have been subject to animal testing or contain ingredients subject to animal testing.

To mitigate the regulatory variations between nations, the International Cooperation on Cosmetics Regulations (ICCR) was established in 2007. The mission of this voluntary group of regulatory authorities is "to maintain the highest level of global consumer protection, while minimizing regulatory barriers to international trade…[and] engage in information sharing, regulatory cooperation, training, and other activities aimed at advancing science and knowledge internationally in this area" [6]. The organization is structured into four sectors, each with different core responsibilities, that include representatives from industry, regulatory governances, and other stakeholders. Both the FDA and the European Commission are part of this regulatory authority. The "Working Group" focuses on cosmetic interests including allergens, safety assessments, and alternatives to animal testing.

Documented cosmetic testing on animals dates back to the early 1940s. Of note, the early foundational work conducted then included The Draize test, which involved applying chemicals to the eyes or skin of rabbits to measure the resulting, if any, irritation. The Draize test was criticized at that time due to variation in test results, difference between humans and rabbits, and the extensive animal suffering caused during the testing [7]. Alternatives to animal testing can be traced back to the 1980s, followed soon after by the development of the European Centre for the Validation of Alternative Methods (ECVAM) which sought to "support the development, validation and acceptance of methods which could reduce, refine or replace the use of laboratory animals" [8]. The US followed suit with the Interagency Coordinating Committee on the Validation of Alternative Methods (ICCVAM) Authorization Act of 2000. Similar to the ECVAM, the ICCVAM sought to develop and validate alternative testing methods to reduce or replace animal testing methods [9]. The ICCVAM is supported by the National Toxicology Program Interagency Center for Evaluation of Alternative Toxicological Methods (NICEATM) which helps evaluate the alternatives to animal use for chemical safety testing. The NICEATM groups novel alternative methods falls into three general categories of technology: in silico, *in chemico,* and in vitro [10]. In silico techniques involve the use of mathematical modeling or machine learning, *in chemico* uses biological molecules outside of cells to study the interactions, and in vitro uses cells or organoids outside of the body. These three techniques serve as an alternative to the use of live animal testing and testing with human volunteers.

Nonetheless, human volunteers have been used in the evaluation of skin irritation for many years. A human 4-h patch test has been developed for acute dermal irritation testing of chemicals. The test was specifically designed to address the issue of the classification and labelling (irritant/non-irritant) of pure chemicals and preparations [11, 12]. Prior to human testing, chemicals and preparations must be demonstrated to be non-corrosive and free from other toxicologically unacceptable hazards using commercially available rat skin transcutaneous electrical resistance (TER) or Episkin™ assays. Assuming these tests are performed satisfactorily, it is possible to conduct a subsequent human test similar to the Draize rabbit skin irritation tests, that is designed to limit the intensity of any skin reactions [13].

Once the ingredients of a formulation have been tested, cosmetic manufacturers generally prefer to have in vivo human data available to confirm the compatibility and tolerance of their finished products in the intended consumer population. Manufacturers are able to release a finished cosmetic product to carefully monitored groups of human subjects first, before exposing larger populations. Smaller groups allow monitoring and the ability to register adverse effects, which becomes difficult or unfeasible during wide commercial launches [14]. Additionally, user trials which reenact the real use conditions of products can identify problems with misuse due to badly designed or defective packaging, and are of significant value for a detailed description of the finished product's safety.

Neither animal tests nor alternative non-animal test methods can confirm product efficacy accurately. For product efficacy testing, the only valuable and appropriate model is the human in vivo model. However, an in vitro approach based on physicochemical or biological endpoints such as ceramide metabolism in human skin pieces, may be used at different stages of product development in order to formulate efficient products [15]. Despite these advances, there is an increasing use of human volunteers in cosmetics testing to provide assurance of tolerance to topical exposure of the finished product and to confirm product efficacy.

Ethical Framework and History

In addition to regulatory bodies, there is an ethical framework related to human testing that is relevant to cosmetics research. The Nuremberg Code, developed in 1947 after the case of US vs. Karl Brandt et al., sets forward a ten-point statement about medical experimentation on human subjects [16]. Under this code, the idea of voluntary consent and the ability of subjects to withdrawal from the study was proposed, while balancing the benefits to science of the experiment with the risk and suffering caused to the experimental subjects.

In 1964 the Declaration of Helsinki was developed, building upon the ideas set forth in the Nuremberg Code, to help "guide [physicians] in biomedical research involving human subjects" [17]. The Declaration of Helsinki was last updated in 2008 and is now the accepted basics for clinical trial ethics; it is advocated that all engaged in research on human beings should follow these recommendations [18]. The Declaration of Helsinki states that non-therapeutic biomedical research involving human subjects is ethically acceptable only under certain conditions. Most importantly, biomedical research involving human subjects cannot legitimately be carried out, unless the inherent risk to the subject is in proportion to the expected benefit for the volunteer, or for society at large.

Ethical concerns persisted due not only to the unethical and cruel Nazi medical research experiments but also the Tuskegee Syphilis Study (1932–1972). The US Department of Health and Human Services was founded in April 1953 under President Dwight D. Eisenhower. The main goal of this organization was to protect the health of Americans and provide essential human services, especially for those who were less capable. The US developed additional protections for human research subjects under the US Department of Health and Human Services (HHS) regulation 45 CFR part 46, which includes the Federal Policy for the Protection of Human Subjects, or the "Common Rule".

Institutional Review Boards (IRBs) were established in the US in 1974. IRBs were mandated to be implemented at institutions conducting human subject research. Ultimately, these ethical principles for human research were outlined and systematized in the "Common Rule" and Belmont Report. The "Common Rule" regulations were published in 1991, last updated in 2018, and were heavily influenced by the Belmont Report of 1979. The Belmont Report outlined three basic principles relevant to research involving human subjects: the principles of respect for persons, beneficence, and justice [19]. The "Common Rule", which is subpart A of HHS regulation 45 CFR part 46, outlines the elements of obtaining and documenting informed consent, and requirements of the Institutional Review Board (IRB) membership, functions and operations, and review of research [20]. Subparts B through D detail additional protections for special research subjects including: pregnant women, human fetuses, neonates, children, and prisoners. All the principles outlined in this regulation are expected to be upheld by the 20 agencies who have official signatories. The FDA is not included in these agencies as their regulations differ from the "Common Rule", but they have set out their own regulations for informed consent and IRB [21] (See Fig. 3.1 Review of historical time line).

The European Commission also created additional protections under the Horizon Europe Framework Programme (HEFP), with the goal of developing, promoting, and advancing science. The program is divided into three pillars with the European Research Council (ERC), a premier funding organization for research, falling under that umbrella [22]. HEFP regulations outline the ethical principles for conducting research and establish the requirement for ethical assessment and clearance prior to starting the project. Similar to the IRB, the ERC Executive Agency is responsible for carrying out the ethics review process.

International ethics guidelines have also been set forth by the Council for International Organizations of Medical Sciences (CIOMS) and the World Health Organization (WHO) [23]. CIOMS outlines 25 guidelines that should be upheld in ethical reviews of research, with a specific focus on protections of human subjects. These guidelines cover a wide spectrum of topics, including ones discussed at the regional level such as informed consent, research with special populations such as children, vulnerable persons, and pregnant women, and the requirement for an

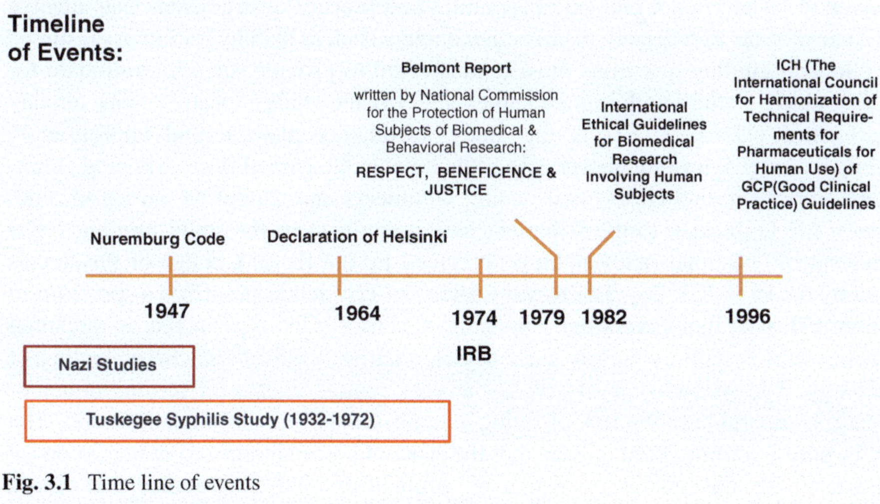

Fig. 3.1 Time line of events

ethical review committee. Other topics discussed include the collection, storage, and use of biological materials and health data, compensations for research related harm, and public accountability.

Ethical Aspects

There are different ethical requirements if a study has been designed to assess the safety or the efficacy of a cosmetic product. First, a cosmetic product should be cleared for safety before its efficacy is being evaluated. Efficacy testing is subsequently performed to support marketing claims and can only be carried out ethically when there is evidence that the product does not cause local or systemic adverse responses. Evaluation of safety and efficacy in the same test can be considered as unethical as there are opportunities to test safety only without using human volunteers. However, if an adverse reaction is generated unintentionally in an efficacy trial, it should be recorded and treated as complementary information for the safety profile of the product prior to its release on the market.

During safety evaluations, the main concern is avoiding skin irritation and sensitization (allergic contact dermatitis), and considering systemic toxicity from percutaneous absorption or from accidental or reasonably foreseeable oral intake [24, 25]. This evaluation should not only include the ingredients itself, but also consider parameters such as method and frequency of application, duration of contact, and application to sun exposed areas. EU guidelines recommend in vitro and/or human volunteers for both skin compatibility testing and local tolerance testing.

For efficacy testing, the goal is to assess the performance of the cosmetic product. EU guidelines set forth two experimental approaches on human volunteers: sensorial tests and instrumental tests. Sensorial tests involve assessing product performance based on observation, touch, and olfaction, either by the consumers themselves or by physician clinical observation and scoring. Instrumental tests involve the use of tools to precisely measure parameters such as skin hydration or elasticity.

Several guiding questions must be answered to provide scientific rationale for undertaking a study with human subjects: (1) Is the study repeating work already performed elsewhere; (2) Is the study adequately planned and appropriately designed to give a valid answer; (3) Is the knowledge gained from exposing volunteers important enough to justify using volunteers and cannot be gained in other ways; (4) Is the risk to the volunteer as a participant in the study minimal? The concept of "minimal risk"has been described by the Royal College of Physicians and by the FDA [21, 26]. The Royal College of Physicians describes a spectrum of "minimal risk" that covers two opposing scenarios. One type of risk is the small chance of a reaction which is itself trivial, such as a mild headache or feeling of lethargy. The second type of risk is the very remote chance of serious injury or death, comparable to the risk of flying as a passenger on a scheduled aircraft. The FDA notes, "minimal risk means that the risks of harm anticipated in the proposed research are not greater, considering probability and magnitude, than those ordinarily encountered in daily life or during the performance of routine physical or psychological examinations or tests." Risk during cosmetics testing must be limited and similar to the daily risks encountered by volunteers.

When cosmetics are tested for compatibility on human subjects in vivo, the endpoints measured are usually non-permanent dermatological conditions such as varying degrees of erythema, edema and dryness. In sensitization trials, however, it can happen that a healthy human volunteer with no history of previous sensitization becomes sensitized. Therefore, in some countries, testing laboratories do not consider it ethical to willfully sensitize healthy volunteers. The risk imposed on the human volunteer, namely to generate a permanent adverse health effect, is considered too high. However, other countries allow for predictive allergic patch testing on human beings to detect allergens and eliminate them from formulations. In this case, the risk of inducing a sensitization reaction in a healthy volunteer is considered very remote when compared to the benefit that ensues for the whole consumer population from such a study. A typical example of a predictive sensitization test is the human repeated insult patch test, which is commonly used in cosmetics testing laboratories. Depending on the applied framework, the risk of generating an allergic response, including its photodynamic or photosensitizing variants and cross-allergies, in a non-sensitized human volunteer, cannot be outweighed by the information derived from conducting such a test.

The evaluation of a product's safety in a human volunteer must be justified on a case-by-case basis. Some basic criteria, however, must be fulfilled and can be summarized as follows: an ethically performed human test should comply with the ethical recommendations included in the Declaration of Helsinki and its subsequent revisions. The volunteers should be selected in accordance with a well-designed study protocol and with the inclusion/exclusion criteria defined in the protocol. Only fully informed human volunteers, signing a written informed consent form prior to the study, should participate in the study. The informed consent form should explain the purpose and nature of the study, as well as any foreseeable risk or benefit which may result from participation in the study. Relevant safety information on the test material is necessary before the test starts. Previous experience with the test formulation and its individual ingredients, as well as the quality of the toxicological data available, will determine the eventual risk to which the subjects will be exposed. The test should be conducted by a trained and qualified investigator. The study should be submitted to an IRB or ERC when appropriate, especially if unusual risks to participants are involved. Appropriate medical coverage in the event of unexpected/adverse reactions should have been foreseen; and, finally, the human volunteers should be compensated for their time and inconvenience, but the reward must not be so large as to incite them to participate in the study. Research subjects should also be informed that they have the freedom to withdraw from the research (autonomy) at any time with the reassurance of no retaliation.

Conclusion

Both national and international regulations have been established to safeguard production and distribution of cosmetic products to the population. A core principle behind these regulations is to ensure that the products are safe for human use. The means of assuring that safety varies, with certain nations having stricter regulations regarding the methods of product testing that are acceptable. The EU has banned all animal testing for cosmetic products while the US only encourages the use of alternative methods but does not place a specific ban. This has led to an increased need for alternative testing methods for cometic products. One alternative is the use of human volunteers for product testing. However, there are increased ethical concerns for the volunteers participating in these studies.

History has shown that guidelines need to be established to protect the human volunteers to ensure their ethical treatment. As new research practices have developed, so have these guidelines. The FDA, ERC, and other organizations have set forth regulatory guidelines for any human subject's research that must be followed, complimented by recommendations from other bodies. For cosmetic testing, the safety of the individual components should be tested prior to efficacy testing to mitigate harmful reactions in human volunteers. In addition, the benefit of using a human subject and the information gained from doing such must be sufficiently greater than if other testing methods were used. The safety and well-being of the subject should always take precedent over the interests of science.

Although there is a movement to have more unified guidelines, with the development of CIOMS, these guidelines are for general research practices and not for cosmetics testing specifically. There is still a large discrepancy between cosmetic regulations among the EU, U.S., and other nations. Without international consensus, it remains difficult to set forth ethical recommendations that would be universally acceptable to compliment regulatory policy.

References

1. Federal Food, Drug, and Cosmetic Act, 21 U.S.C § 361 (2022).
2. U.S. Food and Drug Administration. Cosmetics Science & Research. Accessed July 30, 2024. www.fda.gov
3. U.S. Food and Drug Administration. Modernization of Cosmetic Regulation Act of 2022 (MoCRA). Accessed July 30, 2024. www.fda.gov
4. Guidance for industry: safety of nanomaterials in cosmetic products. Center for Food Safety and Applied Nutrition; 2014.
5. Regulation (EC) No 1223/2009 of the European Parliament and of the Council of 30 November 2009 on Cosmetic Products.
6. International Cooperation on Cosmetics Regulation (ICCR) - Standard Operating Procedures; 2024.

7. Lee M, Hwang JH, Lim KM. Alternatives to in vivo draize rabbit eye and skin irritation tests with a focus on 3D reconstructed human cornea-like epithelium and epidermis models. Toxicol Res. 2017;33(3):191–203. https://doi.org/10.5487/TR.2017.33.3.191.
8. European Centre for the Validation of Alternative Methods (ECVAM): its role and contribution, In Conference proceedings: alternatives to animal testing: new approaches in the development and control of biologicals. Strasbourg (France), EDQM, Council of Europe, 2008, JRC44990.
9. ICCVAM Authorization Act, 42 U.S.C § 2851-3 (2000).
10. Catalyzing the development and use of novel alternative methods. National Institutes of Health; 2023.
11. Basketter DA, York M, McFadden JP, Robinson MK. Determination of skin irritation potential in the human 4-h patch test. Contact Derm. 2004;51(1):1–4. https://doi.org/10.1111/j.0105-1873.2004.00385.x.
12. Basketter DA, Whittle E, Chamberlain M. Identification of irritation and corrosion hazards to skin: an alternative strategy to animal testing. Food Chem Toxicol. 1994;32(6):539–42. https://doi.org/10.1016/0278-6915(94)90111-2.
13. Basketter DA, Chamberlain M, Griffiths HA, Rowson M, Whittle E, York M. The classification of skin irritants by human patch test. Food Chem Toxicol. 1997;35(8):845–52. https://doi.org/10.1016/S0278-6915(97)00053-7.
14. DHSS (Department of Health and Social Security, UK). Report No. 27 on Health and Social Subjects. Guidelines for the Testing of Chemicals for Toxicity; 1982. p. 1–57.
15. Garcia C, Chesne C. In vitro approaches for cosmetic product development and claim substantiation. Cosmet Toilet Manuf Worldw. 1994:267–8.
16. The Nuremberg Code (1947). BMJ. 1996;313(7070):1448–1448. https://doi.org/10.1136/bmj.313.7070.1448.
17. World Medical Association Declaration of Helsinki: ethical principles for medical research involving human subjects. JAMA. 2013;310(20):2191. https://doi.org/10.1001/jama.2013.281053.
18. Good clinical practice for trials on medicinal products in the European Community: CPMP working party on efficacy of medicinal products. Pharmacol Toxicol. 1990;67(4):361–73. https://doi.org/10.1111/j.1600-0773.1990.tb00847.x.
19. Belmont report: ethical principles and guidelines for the protection of human subjects of research. National Commission for the Protection of Human Subjects of Biomedical and Behavioral Research; 1979.
20. 45 CFR Part 46. Department of Health and Human Services.
21. Title 21 of the CFR. Food and Drug Administration, Department of Health and Human Services.
22. Regulation (EU) 2021/695 of the European Parliament and of the Council of 28 April 2021 Establishing Horizon Europe—the Framework Programme for Research and Innovation, Laying down Its Rules for Participation and Dissemination, and Repealing Regulations (EU) No 1290/2013 and (EU) No 1291/2013.
23. International ethical guidelines for health-related research involving humans, 4th ed. Council for International Organizations of Medical Sciences (CIOMS); 2016.
24. Guidelines for the safety assessment of a cosmetic product. Cosmetics Europe; 2004.
25. Guidelines for the evaluation of the efficacy of cosmetics products. Cosmetics Europe; 2008.
26. Research on healthy volunteers. A report of the Royal College of Physicians. J R Coll Physicians Lond. 1986;20(4):243–57.

Chapter 4
Methods for Antiperspirant and Deodorant Efficacy Evaluations

Meike Streker

Introduction

The evaluation of deodorants and antiperspirants represents a central aspect of dermatological and cosmetic research. A primary focus lies on the regulation of sweat secretion, which serves a vital function in the thermoregulation of the human body [1].

The axillary region (axilla), due to its anatomical and physiological characteristics, such as a high density of eccrine and apocrine sweat glands, sebaceous glands, and hair follicles, constitutes a key area for the application and assessment of such products. While eccrine glands primarily contribute to thermal regulation, apocrine glands secrete a protein- and lipid-rich fluid which, through bacterial decomposition, leads to the formation of characteristic body odors [2]. These odors mainly arise from microbial transformation of the secretions into volatile organic compounds (VOCs), including short-chain fatty acids, thioalcohols, and steroidal derivatives [3, 4]. Furthermore, visible underarm wetness and unpleasant odor can significantly impair individuals' subjective well-being, social interactions, and self-image, thereby explaining the high demand for effective products for sweat and odor control [5]. The global market for antiperspirants and deodorants accordingly reports annual revenues in the billions. According to the IKW (German Cosmetic, Toiletry, Perfumery and Detergent Association), deodorants alone generated a turnover of € 959 million in Germany in 2023, marking a 21.2% increase compared to the previous year's report [6]. Various test methods are currently available for assessing the efficacy of these products. Among the classical approaches is the gravimetric test, which quantifies the amount of sweat produced under standardized heat

M. Streker (✉)
Cosmetic Scientist, Königsberger Straße 54, Ellerau, Germany
e-mail: mail@meikestreker.de; https://www.meikestreker.de/

P. Elsner et al. (eds.), *Cosmetics*, https://doi.org/10.1007/978-3-032-14644-1_4

stress conditions, thereby enabling conclusions regarding the sweat-reducing effect of a given product. More recent developments, such as electrochemical or colorimetric sensors, allow for more practical, and in some cases continuous, monitoring of sweat parameters. Particularly promising are colorimetric sensors based on polydiacetylenes (PDA), which selectively respond to specific sweat components.

This chapter provides a comprehensive overview of both established and innovative methods for the objective and subjective evaluation of the efficacy and safety of antiperspirants and deodorants.

Mechanisms of Action of Antiperspirants and Deodorants

Antiperspirants reduce eccrine sweat secretion primarily by temporarily occluding the sweat gland ducts. The main active ingredients are aluminum salts such as aluminum chloride ($AlCl_3$), aluminum chlorohydrate (ACH), and aluminum-zirconium complexes, which form stable precipitates with mucosal components and damage the acrosyringium [7, 8]. Reller and Luedders already described this principle in 1977 as the "gel plug theory," based on the pH-dependent precipitation of acidic aluminum salts [9]. Yuan et al. later confirmed this mechanism experimentally using bovine serum albumin (BSA) as a model protein [10]. Additionally, aluminum salts exhibit astringent and mildly antiseptic effects, which reduce bacterial colonization and thus odor formation [11].

Deodorants, on the other hand, primarily target body odor without reducing the amount of sweat. They act by inhibiting odor-producing microorganisms, masking odors with fragrances, or neutralizing volatile compounds. In general, body odor arises from the bacterial decomposition of sweat components, particularly in the axillary region, where species such as *Corynebacterium*, *Staphylococcus*, and others produce volatile organic compounds (VOCs) including aldehydes, sulfur-containing compounds (e.g., 3M3SH), and carboxylic acids (e.g., HMHA) [12–16].

Ethical and Regulatory Requirements for Testing Antiperspirants and Deodorants

Studies involving antiperspirants and deodorants in human subjects are subject to strict ethical standards. Prerequisites include the voluntary and informed consent of participants, as well as, in most cases, a favorable ethics committee vote. These requirements apply equally to basic and applied research. The foundation of these ethical obligations lies in the Declaration of Helsinki by the World Medical Association (1964), along with the "International Ethical Guidelines for Biomedical Research Involving Human Subjects" developed by CIOMS in collaboration with the WHO, most recently revised comprehensively in 2002 [17, 18]. These documents establish both general ethical principles and specific guidelines to ensure the safety, dignity, and informed participation of human subjects. Adherence to these standards is essential for the acceptance of cosmetic studies.

From a regulatory perspective, the authorization of cosmetic products such as deodorants and antiperspirants within the European Union is governed by Regulation (EC) No. 1223/2009 [19]. This regulation mandates a comprehensive safety assessment, the compilation of a Product Information File (PIF), and proper product labeling. Since 2013, the use of animal testing for cosmetic products and ingredients has been prohibited, necessitating the use of alternative methods such as in vitro assays or Human Repeat Insult Patch Tests. Claims made in advertising must be substantiated by scientific evidence, in accordance with guidelines from Cosmetics Europe. Prior to market entry, registration via the Cosmetic Products Notification Portal (CPNP) is mandatory [20, 21].

Methods for Antiperspirant and Deodorant Efficacy Evaluations

Gravimetric Method (Measurement of Sweat Volume)

The gravimetric measurement method is suitable for the quantitative determination of secreted sweat. In its 2003 publication, the European Expert Group on Efficacy Measurement of Cosmetics and Other Topical Products (EEMCO) identified it as one of the most reliable, objective, and standardized methods for evaluating antiperspirants [22]. It is based on the quantitative assessment of the amount of fluid secreted by eccrine sweat glands under controlled conditions. Central to this method is the determination of Sweat Weight Reduction (SWR), which refers to the percentage reduction in sweat production compared to an untreated control area [8, 23–26]. The SWR is calculated by comparing the treated side to the untreated side. The method is considered objective, reproducible, and independent of subjective influences. Due to these characteristics, EEMCO has recognized it as the gold standard for the quantitative evaluation of antiperspirant efficacy. It yields reliable data and thus serves as a key instrument in both clinical and cosmetic research. A standardized experimental setup is essential for the objective and reproducible measurement of the sweat-reducing effect of antiperspirants. Studies are typically conducted in a climate chamber with constant environmental conditions (temperature: 38 ± 1 °C; relative humidity: 40 ± 5%) [27]. Before the thermal stress phase begins, participants are acclimatized to room temperature in a climate-controlled resting room. The heat stress phase generally lasts 30–40 min and is intended to uniformly and physiologically activate the eccrine sweat glands [28]. A split-body design is commonly used for product application, in which the test product is applied to one side of the body, while the opposite side remains untreated or receives a placebo. This intra-individual study design allows for direct comparability of sweat production under identical physiological conditions. The quantification of sweat is performed using pre-weighed, dried absorbent materials (e.g., pads or cotton compresses) placed in the axilla for a defined duration (typically 20 min). The difference between the initial and final weight of the compresses corresponds to the amount of sweat produced [29]. Despite its widespread use, the gravimetric method has several limitations. Sweat production is subject to significant intra- and interindividual variability, which can be influenced by genetic predisposition, hormonal factors, time of day, stress level, hydration status, and habitual physical activity. The presence or absence of a habituation effect due to repeated thermal exposure may also distort the results. Another critical factor is the accuracy of sweat collection. Incomplete skin contacts of the pads, premature evaporation, and mechanical artifacts due to movement can lead to measurement errors. Moreover, it is important to note that this method measures only the final product of sweat secretion and provides no information on the location, mechanism, or temporal dynamics of sweat inhibition.

To improve comparability and reproducibility, standardized testing protocols have been developed, such as those outlined by the FDA in the Final Monograph for Antiperspirant Drug Products for Over-the-Counter Human Use. These protocols provide specific guidelines regarding the test population (e.g., number of participants, inclusion criteria), climate chamber conditions, application regimen, and statistical analysis [30]. In modern research, the gravimetric method is increasingly combined with imaging techniques or biochemical analyses to gain a more comprehensive understanding of antiperspirant mechanisms and their interaction with skin physiology. Despite modern alternatives, gravimetric sweat measurement remains a fundamental component of objective efficacy testing for antiperspirants.

Minor's Sweat Test—A Qualitative Evaluation

Minor's test (also known as the iodine-starch test) is an established diagnostic method for the qualitative detection of localized sudomotor activity. Originally developed to visualize focal hyperhidrosis, this method has since become a validated tool in clinical research and product development for assessing the efficacy of antiperspirant agents [26, 27, 31, 32]. The procedure is based on a chemical color reaction between Lugol's iodine solution and starch, which results in a deep blue to black-violet discoloration upon contact with sweat [33]. Various formulations for Lugol's solution are reported in the literature, differing in the concentrations of iodine and potassium iodide used; however, all share a common 2:1 molar ratio of potassium iodide to iodine [34]. This visual reaction enables differentiated assessment of sweat-active skin areas under standardized test conditions. In the context of efficacy testing for antiperspirants, Minor's test is applied in controlled in vivo studies to evaluate the topographical distribution and intensity of sweat production before and after application of the test product. The procedure follows several standardized steps: following thorough cleansing and drying of the target area (typically axillary, palmar, plantar, or frontal regions), Lugol's iodine solution is applied, followed by a dry application of a starch preparation (e.g., cornstarch). After adequate drying and optional stimulation (e.g., physical exertion, thermal provocation), the endogenous sweat reacts with the starch-iodine complex, resulting in a characteristic color change. The intensity of the discoloration correlates with the local sweat volume [35].

For scientific evaluation, the test areas are typically documented photographically and analyzed using computer-assisted image processing techniques, allowing surface-based quantification of discoloration. The resulting data can be used to calculate the *Sweat Reduction Rate* (SRR), thereby complementing quantitative methods such as gravimetric analysis [36, 37]. Although Minor's test exhibits high sensitivity for detecting localized sweat activity, its utility in evaluating deodorants—whose primary mechanisms involve microbial modulation or odor masking—is limited. Nevertheless, the method can be employed to detect potential secondary anhidrotic effects of such formulations.

The limitations of the method include the absence of absolute quantification, subjective interpretation of the color changes, and susceptibility to confounding factors such as skin moisture, pH, or residues from application media. Despite these constraints, Minor's test, when used in conjunction with standardized protocols and modern image analysis systems, remains a relevant instrumental approach for the preclinical and clinical evaluation of antiperspirant products. Its application significantly contributes to the objectification of efficacy claims and supports scientifically sound product development and regulatory approval in the field of cosmetic and medical skin care.

Sensory Evaluation (Sniff Test)

Sensory evaluation, commonly referred to as the "sniff test," represents an essential component in the efficacy assessment of deodorants and antiperspirants. In contrast to gravimetric quantification of sweat volume, this method focuses on the olfactory assessment of perceived body odor intensity and subjective product acceptability. Evaluations are conducted both by trained expert panels (sensory assessors) and by the test subjects themselves. This approach is utilized in both product development and clinical research to evaluate product performance. In controlled studies, standardized test methods are used to ensure reproducible and comparable assessments of body odor. A widely established approach involves the use of standardized odor scales, such as those outlined in ASTM E1207 (American Society for Testing and Materials) or ISO 4120 [38, 39]. These scales typically range from 0 ("no perceptible odor") to 10 ("extremely strong, unpleasant body odor") (see Table 4.1). Assessments are conducted by trained raters under controlled environmental conditions (e.g., climate-controlled test chambers), with subjects having applied the test product and been exposed to defined physical or thermal stress scenarios [40]. A washout period of 10–14 days is recommended prior to testing. To minimize bias and inter-subjective variability, evaluations are generally conducted in a

Table 4.1 Example sniff test (according to ASTM E1207-14)

Score	Odor description
0	No perceivable odor
1	Very faint odor
2	Faint but detectable odor
3	Moderate odor
4	Strong, unpleasant odor
5	Extremely strong, very unpleasant odor

Modified according to [38]

double-blind design. Odor samples—commonly obtained by collecting axillary sweat on textile pads—are anonymized and presented in standardized glass containers ("sniff jars") to ensure consistent olfactory perception. Multiple evaluations by a panel of at least 3–6 experts per sample increase the validity of results [41]. Alternatively, direct axillary odor assessment can be conducted on-site by trained evaluators.

Despite standardized methodology, olfactory assessment remains subject to individual perception, cultural differences, and external influences such as diet or microbiome composition. Nevertheless, sensory testing is crucial for the practical evaluation of personal care products. These tests complement objective gravimetric and analytical techniques and are gaining importance in regulatory studies, especially for evaluating new formulations and market authorizations. In combination with microbiological, chemical, and physiological data, sensory methods enable a comprehensive performance assessment of deodorants and antiperspirants.

Microbiological Methods

The pivotal role of the axillary microbiome in the formation of body odor is well-documented, particularly with respect to the involvement of *Corynebacterium* and *Staphylococcus* species in the enzymatic conversion of sweat-borne precursors into odorous volatile organic compounds (VOCs) [42]. To assess the antimicrobial efficacy of deodorant products, common in vitro methods include the determination of the *Zone of Inhibition* (ZOI) and the *Minimum Inhibitory Concentration* (MIC). The qualitative Kirby-Bauer assay measures the ZOI by evaluating the bacteria-free region surrounding a drug-impregnated disc on an inoculated agar plate, while the MIC is determined via broth dilution assay as the lowest concentration inhibiting visible microbial growth [43, 44]. Interpretation of results is based on the standards provided by the Clinical and Laboratory Standards Institute (CLSI). Since these assays operate under constant concentrations and static conditions, they do not fully reflect the dynamic environment of the skin. As such, technological innovations like the SnO_2-based gas sensor system developed by Fujimoto et al. (1996) have been established to quantify VOC emissions before and after product application [45]. This method is considered a standardized, cost-effective, and highly sensitive alternative, and has since undergone significant refinement.

A central technique for taxonomic analysis of microbial communities is 16S rRNA gene sequencing, which leverages both conserved and variable regions of the 16S rRNA gene [46]. Samples from axillary skin are typically collected via swabbing or tape-stripping. The extracted DNA is then amplified using PCR and sequenced on platforms such as the Illumina MiSeq. Bacteria with ≥97% sequence similarity are grouped into operational taxonomic units (OTUs), whose relative abundance and diversity are classified at the phylum and genus levels (e.g., *Actinobacteria*, *Staphylococcus*, *Corynebacterium*) [47]. Owing to its high resolution and comprehensive reference databases, this technique is considered the gold standard for microbial community analysis. Microbiological methods provide objective, mechanistically grounded data on antimicrobial efficacy and microbiome-modulating effects of topical products. They complement sensory and gravimetric methods and are an integral component of modern efficacy studies in light of increasing regulatory and consumer expectations.

Analytical Methods for VOC Detection

The analysis of volatile organic compounds (VOCs) serves as an objective approach for evaluating body odor and has thus become an established method in assessing the efficacy of deodorants and antiperspirants. VOCs are primarily generated via microbial conversion of sweat-associated precursors—such as long-chain fatty acids, amino acids, and steroids—into odor-active molecules including 3-methyl-2-hexenoic acid, sulfur compounds, and short-chain carboxylic acids [48]. Highly sensitive techniques have been established for the qualitative and quantitative analysis of these compounds, including gas chromatography–mass spectrometry (GC-MS), headspace analysis, and proton transfer reaction time-of-flight mass spectrometry (PTR-ToF-MS) [49, 50]. GC-MS is considered the gold standard for the specific detection of VOCs in the ppt to ppb range, typically performed post-application of the product and standardized stress exposure, using solid-phase microextraction (SPME) [51]. Headspace analysis allows for contamination-minimized VOC detection in the gas phase from skin or textile samples, making it ideal for complex matrices such as axillary pads [52]. PTR-ToF-MS enables real-time measurements without the need for sample preparation. Based on proton transfer reactions and high-resolution time-of-flight detection, it is particularly suited for dynamic in situ analysis of VOC emissions [53]. These analytical techniques not only provide objective data on changes in odor-active fractions but also offer mechanistic insights into action principles such as bacterial inhibition, enzyme suppression, or pH modulation. Due to their scientific rigor, such methods are integral components of regulatory-compliant study protocols.

Wear Trials under Real-Life Conditions

In addition to established in vitro and in vivo methods for evaluating the efficacy of deodorants and antiperspirants, recent research efforts increasingly focus on developing innovative model platforms to better understand the underlying molecular mechanisms of these agents. In 2017, Bretagne et al. introduced a microfluidic T-junction system that functionally mimics the narrow, channel-like geometry of human eccrine sweat ducts [54]. The study aimed to analyze the influence of protein components on gel plug formation, a central mechanism of antiperspirant efficacy. It demonstrated that proteins such as bovine serum albumin play a critical role in the formation of a water-insoluble gel plug, which mechanically occludes sweat ducts. This process occurs in two phases: initially, a membrane structure forms at the contact site between aluminum chlorohydrate and sweat (nucleation), followed by volumetric expansion via protein adsorption (growth phase).

Such microfluidic systems offer a controlled, functional preclinical model environment for analyzing the protein-binding and gel-forming capabilities of antiperspirants. However, it is important to note that the continuous application of active ingredients under experimental conditions does not fully replicate the intermittent, real-world application patterns, a factor that must be considered when interpreting results.

Self-Assessment by Study Participants

In addition to objective expert assessments, subjective self-evaluation by study participants is a central element in evaluating the efficacy of deodorants and antiperspirants. These patient-centered instruments complement objective measures and provide valuable insights into individual perceptions of product performance in everyday settings. In practice, visual analog scales (VAS) or numerical rating scales are commonly used, allowing subjects to rate body odor intensity on a standardized scale. These tools are widely applied in both controlled clinical trials and home-use tests (HUTs). Self-assessments also capture skin tolerability data, enabling participants to report sensations such as burning, dryness, or itching, which yield critical information regarding the dermatological safety of products. It should be noted, however, that subjective ratings may be influenced by individual differences in odor perception and psychosocial factors. Therefore, combining self-assessments with objective measurement methods is recommended for a comprehensive evaluation of antiperspirant efficacy and tolerability. Relevant instruments in this context include the Hyperhidrosis Disease Severity Scale (HDSS) and the Hyperhidrosis Quality of Life Index (HidroQoL©).

The HDSS is a disease-specific, time-efficient, and user-friendly diagnostic tool that qualitatively assesses the severity of hyperhidrosis based on its impact on daily activities [55]. It is also suitable for evaluating antiperspirant effectiveness. Patients are asked to choose the statement that best reflects their individual experience with sweating in the affected body region. The statements are numerically coded, allowing for classification of disease severity (see Table 4.2) [56]. An improvement of one point on the HDSS is associated with approximately a 50% reduction in sweat production; a two-point improvement corresponds to a reduction of about 80% [57]. The validity and reliability of the HDSS have been confirmed in scientific studies [58].

Table 4.2 HDSS is a four-point scale of the severity of excessive sweating

HDSS score	Patient statement	Severity level
1	My sweating is never noticeable and never interferes with my daily activities.	No or mild hyperhidrosis
2	My sweating is tolerable but sometimes interferes with my daily activities.	Moderate hyperhidrosis
3	My sweating is barely tolerable and frequently interferes with my daily activities.	Severe hyperhidrosis
4	My sweating is intolerable and always interferes with my daily activities.	Very severe hyperhidrosis

Modified according to [58]

The HidroQoL© is gaining increasing relevance for assessing treatment effects in clinical trials and real-world observational studies [59, 60]. It allows for a nuanced assessment of therapy-related quality of life and was specifically designed to quantify the psychosocial and functional impact of hyperhidrosis. The questionnaire includes 18 items distributed across two main domains: psychosocial aspects (e.g., emotional burden, self-esteem, social interaction) and functional limitations (e.g., clothing choices, physical activity, occupational impact). Developed using robust psychometric methods, the HidroQoL© exhibits high internal consistency (Cronbach's alpha >0.9) and strong test-retest reliability. Its validity has been demonstrated through significant correlations with other health-related quality of life instruments, such as the Dermatology Life Quality Index (DLQI), and its ability to differentiate between severity levels of hyperhidrosis [61].

Modern Techniques and AI-Driven Instruments

Emerging approaches to deodorant and antiperspirant evaluation are increasingly incorporating sensor technology, artificial intelligence (AI), and personalized diagnostics. While classical methods such as gravimetric measurements, questionnaires, and sensory panels are well-established, they are often labor-intensive and not well suited to real-life contexts. Innovations in materials science and digital technologies are driving significant advancements in this field.

Wearable sensor systems now enable continuous monitoring of physiological parameters such as sweat rate in daily life [62]. Advanced electrochemical sensors detect not only fluid volume but also specific analytes like electrolytes and metabolites [63, 64]. Despite their utility, limitations persist regarding sensitivity, calibration, and cost. An alternative solution involves colorimetric sensors based on "smart materials" that respond with visible color changes to specific sweat components and are designed for user-friendly, real-world applications. One such example is the SweatSENSE patch developed by Hand et al., a paper-based chemosensor that changes color from blue to red upon exposure to sweat constituents—but not to water [65]. In an in vivo study involving 52 participants, the system showed a significant reduction in sweat area following application of an antiperspirant compared to a control deodorant. This method enables non-invasive, real-time visual analysis without complex laboratory instruments. This development is complemented by AI-supported image analysis for objective quantification of color changes. Machine learning algorithms can correlate sensor data with parameters such as activity level or skin type. When combined with smartphone interfaces and cloud-based evaluation, these technologies offer a personalized, standardized assessment of product performance. Looking ahead, multifunctional sensor systems are being developed to simultaneously capture not only sweat volume but also chemical parameters (e.g., ammonia, VOCs), pH, temperature, and microbial profile. AI-driven pattern recognition enables precise characterization of skin and sweat physiology—relevant not only for product development but also for investigating pathophysiological conditions (e.g., hyperhidrosis, bromhidrosis). The combination of wearable sensors and AI represents a paradigm shift toward evidence-based, individualized evaluation of cosmetic products—applicable in both research and consumer practice.

Tolerability Testing of Deodorants and Antiperspirants

In addition to efficacy testing, the tolerability of deodorants and antiperspirants is a central criterion in clinical safety assessment. Despite their widespread use, deodorants in particular are among the most common triggers of contact eczema in the axillary region. Numerous clinical and epidemiological studies have identified fragrances as primary contact allergens [66–70]. However, assessing tolerability in the axillary area is particularly challenging. Unlike other topical cosmetic products, deodorants and antiperspirants pose specific challenges arising from the anatomical, physiological, and functional characteristics of the axilla. For example, the physiological pH level in intertriginous areas such as the underarm is higher than on flat skin surfaces [71]. Additionally, this pH is further modulated by sweat secretion, significantly complicating standardized pH-based measurements in this region. Another issue in objectively assessing tolerability is the preconditioning of the skin: shaving, epilation, or prior application of skincare products can alter the skin's barrier function and thus influence the irritative potential of the tested formulations. Mechanical factors such as respiratory movements may also introduce motion artifacts, limiting the standardization and reproducibility of test procedures in the axillary region. For these reasons, controlled clinical studies under standardized conditions are indispensable to ensure valid tolerability assessments. It is recommended to use combined testing strategies that incorporate both subjective reporting tools (e.g., symptom scores, self-reports) and objective biophysical measurement methods. Biophysical parameters such as transepidermal water loss (TEWL), pH measurement, and corneometry have been widely established in clinical studies to evaluate the impact of cosmetic products on the skin barrier (see Table 4.3) [25, 26, 31]. These provide objective, quantifiable metrics for detecting potential barrier disruptions caused by external substances.

Table 4.3 Skin physiological parameters and biophysical measuring instruments

Skin physiological parameter	Device
Determination of skin pH value	Skin-pH-Meter PH 900
Measurement of skin moisture	Corneometer CM 825
Determination of transepidermal water loss (TEWL)	Tewameter TM 210

To improve standardization and reproducibility in tolerability testing of deodorants, a modified test site design was proposed in a 2002 clinical study [72]. In this study design, the test preparation was applied both to the axilla and the volar forearm. While the axillary application reflected realistic use conditions, the forearm served as the preferred site for conducting standardized objective biophysical measurements due to its better reproducibility. The modern sensor-based real-time monitoring systems described in modern sensor-based real-time monitoring systems could provide future insights into the dynamic nature of skin reactions under real-world conditions [63–65].

Summary and Outlook

The evaluation of efficacy in antiperspirants and deodorants is currently undergoing a paradigm shift. Increasing emphasis is being placed on microbiome-friendly, skin-tolerant, and sustainable product concepts. Natural active ingredients, prebiotic and postbiotic strategies, as well as physical absorption mechanisms enable odor-reducing effects without significantly interfering with physiological sweat regulation or the skin microbiome. Digital technologies are fundamentally transforming study designs. Wearables, mobile apps, and AI-supported data analytics now enable continuous and real-life measurement of both objective and subjective efficacy parameters. Multimodal study designs yield differentiated insights into product performance, tolerability, and user acceptance under realistic conditions. Augmented by electronic noses and digital questionnaires, objective odor assessment is being expanded, and the user perspective is systematically integrated. These technologies not only enhance data quality but also enable the development of personalized, data-driven product solutions. Combined with advances in biotechnology, sensor technology, and 3D printing, novel application forms are emerging that align with the expectations of modern consumers. In the long term, efficacy assessment is expected to become increasingly interdisciplinary. Dermatology, microbiology, bioinformatics, and materials science are collaborating to investigate physiological and microbial processes of the skin. As a result, a new standard of cosmetic product development is evolving—scientifically grounded, regulatorily compliant, evidence-based, personalized, and future-oriented.

References

1. Buono MJ, Mc Kenzie BK, Kasch FW. Effects of ageing and physical training on the peripheral sweat production of the human eccrine sweat gland. Age Ageing. 1991;20(6):439–41.
2. Sato K. The physiology, pharmacology, and biochemistry of the eccrine sweat gland. Rev Physiol Biochem Pharmacol. 1977;79:51–131.
3. James AG. The axillary microbiome and its relationship with underarm odor. In: Skin microbiome handbook: from basic research to product development; 2020. p. 79–129.
4. Natsch A, Emter R. The specific biochemistry of human axilla odour formation viewed in an evolutionary context. Philos Trans R Soc Lond B Biol Sci. 2020;375(1800):20190269. https://doi.org/10.1098/rstb.2019.0269. Epub 2020 Apr 20
5. Parashar K, Adlam T, Potts G. The impact of myperhidrosis on quality of life: a review of the literature. Am J Clin Dermatol. 2023;24(2):187–98. https://doi.org/10.1007/s40257-022-00743-7. Epub 2023 Jan 9
6. https://www.ikw.org/jahresbericht/2023-2024/wirtschaft. Stand: Mai 2025.
7. McWilliams SA, Montgomery I, Jenkinson DM, Elder HY, Wilson SM, Sutton AM. Effects of topically-applied antiperspirant on sweat gland function. Br J Dermatol. 1987;117(5):617–26. https://doi.org/10.1111/j.1365-2133.1987.tb07494.x.
8. Streker M, Kerscher M. Antiperspirantien bei der Behandlung der fokalen Hyperhidrose [Antiperspirants for the therapy of focal hyperhidrosis]. Hautarzt. 2012;63(6):452–5. German. https://doi.org/10.1007/s00105-012-2330-2.
9. Reller Luedders HHWL. Pharmacologic and toxicologic effects of topically applied agents on the eccrine sweat glands. In: Dermatotoxicology and pharmacology. New York: Wiley; 1977. p. 1–54.
10. Yuan S, Vaughn J, Pappas I, Fitzgerald M, Masters Pan JGL. Optimal aluminum/zirconium: protein interactions for predicting antiperspirant efficacy using zeta potential measurements. J Cosmet Sci. 2015;66(2):95–111.
11. Hölzle E, Neubert U. Antimicrobial effects of an antiperspirant formulation containing aqueous aluminum chloride hexahydrate. Arch Dermatol Res. 1982;272(3–4):321–9. https://doi.org/10.1007/BF00509063.
12. Kanlayavattanakul M, Lourith N. Body malodours and their topical treatment agents. Int J Cosmet Sci. 2011;33(4):298–311. https://doi.org/10.1111/j.1468-2494.2011.00649.x. Epub 2011 Mar 15
13. Callewaert C, Kerckhof, Granitsiotis FM, Van Gele MSM, Van de Wiele T, Boon N. Characterization of Staphylococcus and Corynebacterium clusters in the human axillary region. PLoS One. 2013;8(8):e70538. https://doi.org/10.1371/journal.pone.0070538.
14. Haze S, Gozu Y, Nakamura S, Kohno Y, Sawano K, Ohta H, Yamazaki K. 2-Nonenal newly found in human body odor tends to increase with aging. J Invest Dermatol. 2001;116(4):520–4. https://doi.org/10.1046/j.0022-202x.2001.01287.x.
15. Natsch A, Schmid J, Flachsmann F. Identification of odoriferous sulfanylalkanols in human axilla secretions and their formation through cleavage of cysteine precursors by a C-S lyase isolated from axilla bacteria. Chem Biodivers. 2004;1(7):1058–72. https://doi.org/10.1002/cbdv.200490079.
16. Stewart JC. Tomatoes cause under-arm odour. Med Hypotheses. 2014;82(5):518–21. https://doi.org/10.1016/j.mehy.2014.02.001. Epub 2014 Feb 13
17. https://www.wma.net/policies-post/wma-declaration-of-helsinki/. Stand: Mai 2025.
18. Council for International Organizations of Medical Sciences. International ethical guidelines for biomedical research involving human subjects, vol. 182. Bull Med Ethics; 2002. p. 17–23.
19. Verordnung (EG) Nr. 1223/2009 des Europäischen Parlaments und des Rates vom 30. November 2009 über kosmetische Mittel (Neufassung) (Text von Bedeutung für den EWR).
20. https://www.cosmeticseurope.eu/files/3714/6407/8024/Guidelines_for_the_Safety_Assessment_of_a_Cosmetic_Product_-_2004.pdf. Stand: Mai 2025.
21. https://webgate.ec.europa.eu/cpnp/. Stand. Mai 2025.

22. Piérard Elsner G, Elsner P, Marks R, Masson P, Paye M, EEMCO Group. EEMCO guidance for the efficacy assessment of antiperspirants and deodorants. Skin Pharmacol Appl Ski Physiol. 2003;16(5):324–42. https://doi.org/10.1159/000072072.
23. Heckmann M, Ceballos-Baumann AO, Plewig G, Hyperhidrosis Study Group. Botulinum toxin A for axillary hyperhidrosis (excessive sweating). N Engl J Med. 2001;344(7):488–93. https://doi.org/10.1056/NEJM200102153440704.
24. Heckmann M. Evidence-based medicine and the treatment of hyperhidrosis. J Am Acad Dermatol. 2004;50(2):327–8; author reply 328. https://doi.org/10.1016/s0190-9622(03)02085-1.
25. Streker M, Reuther T, Hagen L, Kerscher M. Hyperhidrosis plantaris - a randomized, half-side trial for efficacy and safety of an antiperspirant containing different concentrations of aluminium chloride. J Dtsch Dermatol Ges. 2012;10(2):115–9. https://doi.org/10.1111/j.1610-0387.2011.07750.x. Epub 2011 Aug 16
26. Streker M, Reuther T, Verst S, Kerscher M. Hyperhidrosis axillaris--Effektivität und Verträglichkeit eines aluminiumchloridhaltigen Antiperspirants. Prospektive Evaluation an 20 Patienten mit idiopathischer Hyperhidrosis axillaris. Hautarzt. 2010;61(2):139–44. German. https://doi.org/10.1007/s00105-009-1841-y.
27. Hund M, Kinkelin I, Naumann M, Hamm H. Definition of axillary hyperhidrosis by gravimetric assessment. Arch Dermatol. 2002;138(4):539–41. https://doi.org/10.1001/archderm.138.4.539.
28. Stefaniak TJ, Proczko M. Gravimetry in sweating assessment in primary hyperhidrosis and healthy individuals. Clin Auton Res. 2013;23(4):197–200. https://doi.org/10.1007/s10286-013-0201-2. Epub 2013 Jun 13
29. Verbraecken J, Van de Heyning P, De Backer W, Van Gaal L. Body surface area in normal-weight, overweight, and obese adults. A comparison study. Metabolism. 2006;55(4):515–24. https://doi.org/10.1016/j.metabol.2005.11.004.
30. Food and Drug Administration, HHS. Antiperspirant drug products for over-the-counter human use; final monograph. Final rule. Fed Regist. 2003;68(110):34273–93.
31. Romero FR, Haddad GR, Miot HA, Cataneo DC. Palmar hyperhidrosis: clinical, pathophysiological, diagnostic and therapeutic aspects. An Bras Dermatol. 2016;91(6):716–25. https://doi.org/10.1590/abd1806-4841.20165358.
32. Lütgerath C, Weiß C, Faulhaber J, Karsai S. Vergleich eines neuen Aluminiumlactat-basierten mit einem Aluminiumchlorid-basierten Antitranspirant bei übermäßigem axillären und inguinalen Schwitzen: Erste randomisierte kontrollierte Studie. J Dtsch Dermatol Ges. 2022;20(12):1589–602. https://doi.org/10.1111/ddg.14898_g.
33. Minor V. Ein neues Verfahren zu der klinischen Untersuchung der Schweissabsonderung. Dtsch Z Nervenheilk. 1928;101:302–8.
34. Deutsches Arzneibuch 6. Ausg., Neudruck 1951, S.796 Reagenzien. Stuttgart: Deutscher Apotheker-Verlag; 1951.
35. Hexsel D, Rodrigues Soirefmann TCM, Zechmeister-Prado D. Recommendations for performing and evaluating the results of the minor test according to a sweating intensity visual scale. Dermatol Surg. 2010;36(1):120–2. https://doi.org/10.1111/j.1524-4725.2009.01364.x. Epub 2009 Nov 23
36. Rzany B, Bechara Feise FGK, Heckmann M, Rapprich S, Wörle B. Aktualisierung der S1-Leitlinie zur Definition und Therapie der primären Hyperhidrose. J Dtsch Dermatol Ges. 2018;16(7):945–53. https://doi.org/10.1111/ddg.13579_g.
37. Swaile DF, Elstun LT, Benzing KW. Clinical studies of sweat rate reduction by an over-the-counter soft-solid antiperspirant and comparison with a prescription antiperspirant product in male panelists. Br J Dermatol. 2012;166(Suppl 1):22–6. https://doi.org/10.1111/j.1365-2133.2011.10786.x.
38. Standard Guide for Sensory Evaluation of Axillary Deodorancy ASTM E1207–14. American Society for Testing Materials; n.d. https://www.astm.org/Standards/E1207.htm.
39. Sensory analysis - Methodology - Triangle test (ISO 4120:2021); German version EN ISO 4120:2021.

40. Maxeiner B, Ennen J, Rützel-Grünberg S, Traupe B, Wittern Schmucker KPR, Keyhani R. Design and application of a screening and training protocol for odour testers in the field of personal care products. Int J Cosmet Sci. 2009;31(3):193–9. https://doi.org/10.1111/j.1468-2494.2009.00494.x.
41. Teerasumran P, Velliou E, Bai S, Cai Q. Deodorants and antiperspirants: new trends in their active agents and testing methods. Int J Cosmet Sci. 2023;45(4):426–43. https://doi.org/10.1111/ics.12852. Epub 2023 Mar 21
42. Dumas ER, Michaud AE, Bergeron C, Lafrance JL, Mortillo S, Gafner S. Deodorant effects of a supercritical hops extract: antibacterial activity against Corynebacterium xerosis and Staphylococcus epidermidis and efficacy testing of a hops/zinc ricinoleate stick in humans through the sensory evaluation of axillary deodorancy. J Cosmet Dermatol. 2009;8(3):197–204. https://doi.org/10.1111/j.1473-2165.2009.00449.x.
43. Kirby WM, Yoshihara GM, Sundstedt KS, Warren JH. Clinical usefulness of a single disc method for antibiotic sensitivity testing. Antibiot Annu. 1956;1956-1957:892–7.
44. Ackerman BH, Dello Buono FA. In vitro testing of antibiotics. Pharmacotherapy. 1996;16(2):201–17.
45. Fujimoto C, Hayakawa Y, Ono A. Evaluation of the efficiency of deodorants by semiconductor gas sensors. Sens Actuators B Chem. 1996;32:191–4.
46. Langille ZMGJ, Caporaso MJGDD, Knights D, Reyes Clemente JA, Burkepile JC, Vega Thurber DE, Knight RLR, Beiko, Huttenhower RGC. Predictive functional profiling of microbial communities using 16S rRNA marker gene sequences. Nat Biotechnol. 2013;31(9):814–21. https://doi.org/10.1038/nbt.2676. Epub 2013 Aug 25
47. Johnson JS, Spakowicz DJ, Hong BY, Petersen LM, Demkowicz P, Chen L, Leopold SR, Hanson BM, Agresta HO, Gerstein M, Sodergren E, Weinstock GM. Evaluation of 16S rRNA gene sequencing for species and strain-level microbiome analysis. Nat Commun. 2019;10(1):5029. https://doi.org/10.1038/s41467-019-13036-1.
48. Peters R, Veenstra R, Heutinck K, Baas A, Munniks S, Knotter J. Human scent characterization: a review. Forensic Sci Int. 2023;349:111743.
49. Roquencourt C, Grassin-Delyle S, Thévenot EA. ptairMS: real-time processing and analysis of PTR-TOF-MS data for biomarker discovery in exhaled breath. Bioinformatics. 2022;38(7):1930–7. https://doi.org/10.1093/bioinformatics/btac031.
50. Boudard E, Fisson L, Moumane N, Dugay J, Vial J, Thiébaut D. Study of sampling phases for body odor sampling prior to analysis by TD-GC×GC/ToFMS. Anal Bioanal Chem. 2025;417(14):3177–90. https://doi.org/10.1007/s00216-025-05857-5.
51. Brattoli M, Cisternino E, Dambruoso PR, de Gennaro G, Giungato P, Mazzone A, Palmisani J, Tutino M. Gas chromatography analysis with olfactometric detection (GC-O) as a useful methodology for chemical characterization of odorous compounds. Sensors (Basel). 2013;13(12):16759–800.
52. Medrano Cantu A, Cantu A, Aviles-Rosa EO, Hall NJ, Maughan MN, Gadberry JD, Prada-Tiedemann PA. Chemical characterization of human body odor headspace components. Separations. 2024;11(3):85. https://doi.org/10.3390/separations11030085.
53. Obermeier J, Trefz P, Happ J, Schubert Staude JKH, Fischer Miekisch DCW. Exhaled volatile substances mirror clinical conditions in pediatric chronic kidney disease. PLoS One. 2017;12(6):e0178745. https://doi.org/10.1371/journal.pone.0178745.
54. Bretagne A, Cotot F, Arnaud-Roux M, Sztucki M, Cabane B, Galey JB. The mechanism of eccrine sweat pore plugging by aluminium salts using microfluidics combined with small angle X-ray scattering. Soft Matter. 2017;13(20):3812–21. https://doi.org/10.1039/c6sm02510b.
55. Kowalski JW, Eadie N, Dagget S, Lai PY. Validity and reliability of the hyperhidrosis disease severity scale (HDSS). J Am Acad Dermatol. 2004;50(3):51.
56. A comprehensive approach to the recognition, diagnosis, and severity-based treatment of focal hyperhidrosis: recommendations of the Canadian hyperhidrosis advisory committee. Dermatologic Surg. 2007;33:908–23.
57. Stashak AB, Brewer JD. Management of hyperhidrosis. Clin Cosmet Investig Dermatol. 2014;7:285–99. https://doi.org/10.2147/CCID.S53119.

58. Şener S, Karakoç Y. Effects of direct current administration on hyperhidrosis disease severity scale in patients with axillary hyperhidrosis. Biomed Res Int. 2019;2019:3232015. https://doi.org/10.1155/2019/3232015.
59. Kamudoni P, Mueller B, Salek MS. The development and validation of a disease-specific quality of life measure in hyperhidrosis: the Hyperhidrosis Quality of Life Index (HidroQOL©). Qual Life Res. 2015;24(4):1017–27. https://doi.org/10.1007/s11136-014-0825-2. Epub 2014 Nov 1
60. Gabes M, Jourdan C, Schramm K, Masur C, Abels C, Kamudoni P, Salek S, Apfelbacher C. Hyperhidrosis Quality of Life Index (HidroQoL©): further validation and clinical application in patients with axillary hyperhidrosis using data from a phase III randomized controlled trial. Br J Dermatol. 2021;184(3):473–81. https://doi.org/10.1111/bjd.19300. Epub 2020 Sep 1
61. Grieshaber D, MacKenzie R, Vörös J, Reimhult E. Electrochemical biosensors - sensor principles and architectures. Sensors (Basel). 2008;8(3):1400–58. https://doi.org/10.3390/s80314000.
62. Lobo DP, Wemyss AM, Smith DJ, Straube A, Betteridge KB, Salmon AH, Foster RR, Elhegni HE, Satchell SC, Little HA, Pacheco-Gómez R, Simmons MJ, Hicks MR, Bates DO, Rodger A, Dafforn TR, Arkill KP. Direct detection and measurement of wall shear stress using a filamentous bio-nanoparticle. Nano Res. 2015;8(10):3307–15. https://doi.org/10.1007/s12274-015-0831-x.
63. Yang Y, Xing S, Fang Z, Li R, Koo H, Pan T. Wearable microfluidics: fabric-based digital droplet flowmetry for perspiration analysis. Lab Chip. 2017;17(5):926–35. https://doi.org/10.1039/c6lc01522k.
64. Hand, Efstathiou RAS, Wemyss Grypioti AMM, Kirby G, Barlow T, Tinley Ford EMJ, Jamieson A, Reynolds J, Miller J, Bates S, Khoshdel E, Haddleton DM. A simple approach to determining the efficacy of antiperspirants using paper-based colorimetric paper sensors: SweatSENSE††Electronic supplementary information (ESI). RSC Appl Polym. 2024;2(1):98–104. https://doi.org/10.1039/d3lp00214d.
65. Koh A, Kang D, Xue Y, Lee S, Pielak RM, Kim J, Hwang T, Min S, Banks A, Bastien P, Manco MC, Wang L, Ammann KR, Jang KI, Won P, Han S, Ghaffari R, Paik U, Slepian MJ, Balooch G, Huang Y, Rogers JA. A soft, wearable microfluidic device for the capture, storage, and colorimetric sensing of sweat. Sci Transl Med. 2016;8(366):366ra165. https://doi.org/10.1126/scitranslmed.aaf2593.
66. Adams RM, Maibach HI. A five-year study of cosmetic reactions. J Am Acad Dermatol. 1985;13(6):1062–9. https://doi.org/10.1016/s0190-9622(85)70258-7.
67. de Groot AC, Frosch PJ. Adverse reactions to fragrances. A clinical review. Contact Dermatitis. 1997;36(2):57–86. https://doi.org/10.1111/j.1600-0536.1997.tb00418.x.
68. Reeder MJ. Allergic contact dermatitis to fragrances. Dermatol Clin. 2020;38(3):371–7. https://doi.org/10.1016/j.det.2020.02.009. Epub 2020 May 4
69. Johansen JD, Rastogi SC, Bruze M, Andersen KE, Frosch P, Dreier B, Lepoittevin JP, White I, Menné T. Deodorants: a clinical provocation study in fragrance-sensitive individuals. Contact Dermatitis. 1998;39(4):161–5. https://doi.org/10.1111/j.1600-0536.1998.tb05887.x.
70. Heisterberg MV, Menné T, Andersen KE, Avnstorp C, Kristensen B, Kristensen O, Kaaber K, Laurberg G, Henrik Nielsen N, Sommerlund M, Thormann J, Veien NK, Vissing S, Johansen JD. Deodorants are the leading cause of allergic contact dermatitis to fragrance ingredients. Contact Dermat. 2011;64(5):258–64. https://doi.org/10.1111/j.1600-0536.2011.01889.x.
71. Stenzaly-Achtert S, Schölermann A, Schreiber J, Diec Rippke KHF, Bielfeldt S. Axillary pH and influence of deodorants. Skin Res Technol. 2000;6(2):87–91. https://doi.org/10.1034/j.1600-0846.2000.006002087.x.
72. Keil D, Jung EG, Bayerl C. Zur Problematik der Verträglichkeitstestung bei Deodorantien. Aktuelle Dermatol. 2002;28(3):83–9. https://doi.org/10.1055/s-2002-25236.

Chapter 5
Sun Protection Products: What Happens ON and IN the Skin?

Christian Surber, Uli Osterwalder, and Howard Maibach

The Essence of the Sunscreen Product

Figure 5.1 shows the fundamental parts of a sunscreen product. Up to 10 different filters absorb or scatter UV-radiation. The type of filters or filter combination determines the protection spectrum (e.g., broad-spectrum), and the filter concentrations determine the level of protection (e.g., SPF). The vehicle ingredients perform a number of functions that are important to the physicochemical (solubilization, stability) and cosmetic (spreadability, skin feel) product properties in the primary container, during and after application onto skin [1, 2].

The Sunscreen Product ON the Skin

After spreading the sunscreen product, all volatile ingredients in the product evaporate and turn the product into a highly viscous layer of about 1–3 μm on the skin [3]. In this superficial layer, the filters are present in dissolved or undissolved (particulate) form and absorb or scatter radiation. The protective effect primarily takes place

C. Surber (✉)
Department of Dermatology, University Hospital, Zurich, Switzerland

Department of Dermatology, University Hospital, Basel, Switzerland
e-mail: christian.surber@unibas.ch

U. Osterwalder
SPF GmbH, Basel, Switzerland

H. Maibach
Department of Dermatology, University of California San Francisco,
San Francisco, CA, USA

P. Elsner et al. (eds.), *Cosmetics*, https://doi.org/10.1007/978-3-032-14644-1_5

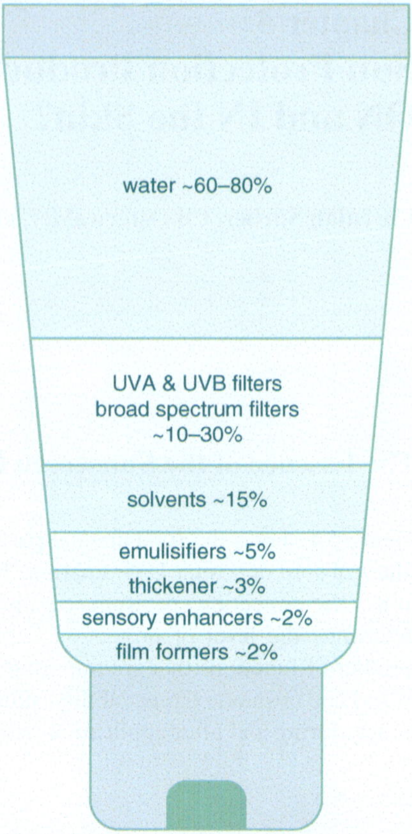

Fig. 5.1 Fundamental parts of a sunscreen product

in this superficial layer. Small proportions of dissolved filters may penetrate into the stratum corneum forming a "reservoir" with repeated application and may subsequently penetrate into deeper layers of the skin (Fig. 5.2). The potential for a filter to permeate through skin primarily depends on its physicochemical properties. Filters that are highly lipophilic accumulate in the stratum corneum and will not penetrate into deeper, more hydrophilic layers. Particulate filters, including nanoparticles, are too big to enter the stratum corneum. Furthermore, they become "trapped" in the viscous superficial layer on the skin [4, 5]. The properties of the vehicle ingredients determine the residence time (e.g., water resistance) on the skin, the skin feel and the appearance of the skin. Lipophilic products tend to be more water resistant but may feel sticky or appear glossy. Although the determination of water resistance is ISO standardized, this criterion may give consumers a false sense of security and prevent them from re-applying sunscreen product after contact with water and sweating [6]. Additionally, many consumers are unaware that in Europe, unlike in the US and Australia, water resistance products only ensure half the sun protection factor (SPF) indicated on the packaging. Globally, some regulatory bodies and consumer protection organizations have started to recommend re-applying sunscreen

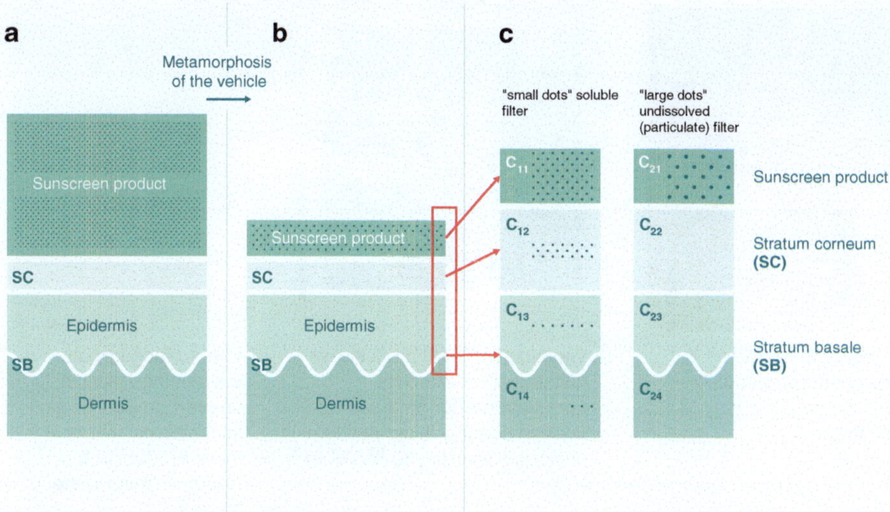

Fig. 5.2 (**a**) Sunscreen product on the skin immediately after application. (**b**) Sunscreen products on the skin after all volatile ingredients have evaporated. The product turns into a superficial highly viscous layer of about 1–3 μm. The phenomenon—coined as "metamorphosis of the vehicle"—is often described as the product "is well absorbed" or "dries up well" [8]. (**c**) (C_{11}) Dissolved sunscreen filters (molecular disperse) in the superficial product film. (C_{12}) Lipophilic sunscreen filters may partition into the stratum corneum. Multi-day applications result in saturation filters in stratum corneum (SC). (C_{13}) Less lipophilic sunscreen filters may reach deeper parts of the epidermis in minute amounts. (C_{14}) For a few sunscreen filters systemic absorption has been observed. (C_{21}) Undissolved sunscreen (particulate) filters in the superficial product film. The undissolved filters are "trapped" in the superficial viscous film on the skin's surface and are not able to partition into the stratum corneum. (C_{22}) Undissolved sunscreen (particulate) filters do not penetrate into the stratum corneum (SC). (C_{23}) Undissolved sunscreen (particulate) filters do not penetrate into deeper parts of the epidermis. (C_{24}) Undissolved sunscreen (particulate) filters do not permeate skin and are systemically not available via skin [5]

products after every contact with water and sweating, as well as every 2 hours. In some regions, the criterion is less advertised. The recommendations are reasonable, but experimental evidence is lacking.

Product Effectiveness ON the Skin

The product effectiveness depends primarily on the thickness and the completeness of coverage (homogeneity) of the product layer on the skin after all volatile ingredients have evaporated (metamorphosis of the vehicle) (Fig. 5.2) [7]. Inadequate thickness and incomplete coverage are obvious reasons for the repeatedly reported ineffectiveness of sunscreen products (protection failure). It is well documented that consumers apply far less than the recommended product amount that would be necessary to achieve the claimed protection [8]. The incompleteness of coverage at the

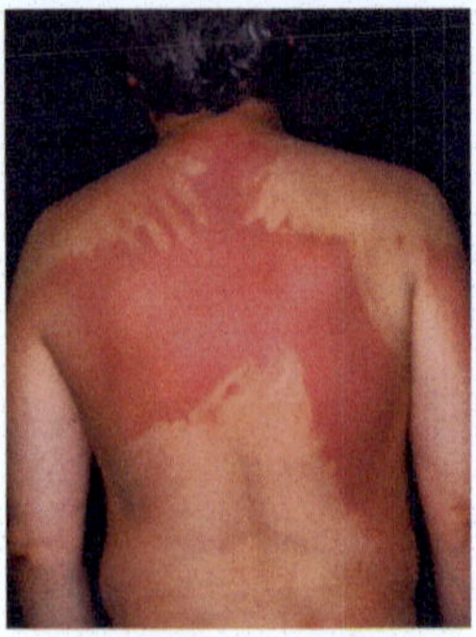

Help of third parties is required for complete coverage (Courtesy to P. Itin)

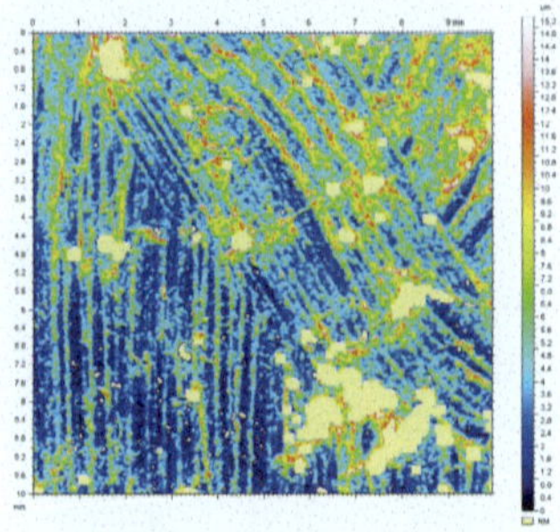

Visualization of film thickness distribution of a model formulation after application. The uneven coating thickness is obvious (Courtesy to M.Sohn)

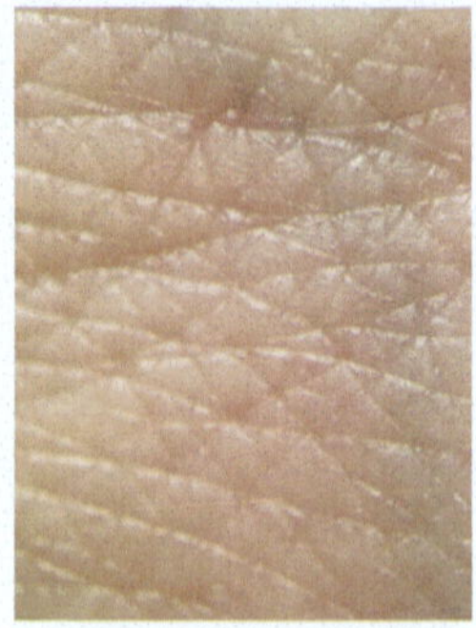

The surface structure of the skin can lead to uneven product layer thicknesses. There is more product in the "valleys" than on the "plateau".

Fig. 5.3 Completeness of product coverage on the skin—macro level (left) and micro level (middle, right)—is essential for sun protection effectiveness

macro level is known to many from their own experience or observation. Less well known is the incompleteness of coverage at the micro level (Fig. 5.3) [3]. The product amount applied and hence the thickness of the layer and the completeness of the coverage (macro level) is in the hands of the consumer and can only be improved through information and training. The completeness of coverage at the micro level depends on the physicochemical properties of the vehicle ingredients and thus resides with the manufacturer of the sunscreen product. Good product spreadability may indicate more complete micro coverage. However, there is still little data publicly available on this aspect.

Product Effectiveness IN the Skin

The effectiveness of sunscreen products in preventing skin cancers is repeatedly debated and occasionally questioned [9]. The doubts come from older studies that were conducted with products, filters and combinations thereof that are no longer used. Furthermore, the long-term studies were accompanied by numerous confounding factors, such as lack of information on adherence (also those described above) and quality of protection provided by the products (filter stability or level of protection). The sometimes-ambiguous results have led some to conclude that sunscreen products fail to prevent skin cancers. Analyzing the materials and methods of the original studies, one must conclude that the number of confounding factors is very large and their effects on the results are hardly discussed nor assessed. What is particularly disturbing is the often-inadequate description of the sunscreen products itself. The characterization by the SPF only is insufficient and provides limited information about the protection range. As has only recently become known from newer studies, the reliability of in vivo SPF measurement is low [10]. The authors suggest having the SPF determined in three to four different laboratories in order to obtain a reliable (true) value. The above-mentioned studies do not provide any information about the entire UV-protection range (e.g., UVA) nor the reliability of the protection characterization. One may conclude that the studies used to determine the skin cancer preventive effectiveness of sunscreen products do not meet today's standards for efficacy/effectiveness studies and should therefore no longer be used in discussions of this matter.

Product Efficacy IN the Skin

Considering the physical properties of filters alone or in formulations, the effect of radiation reduction can be well characterized experimentally both in cell cultures and in animal and human models [11, 12]. The preventive effect of radiation reduction using filters has also been impressively demonstrated clinically in a number of photo sensitive dermatoses (Fig. 5.4) [13]. The effect of UVA radiation reduction, which is often forgotten in the discussion about the effect of sunscreen products, can also be compellingly demonstrated [14]. Against this background, there is no reason to doubt the efficacy of sunscreen products.

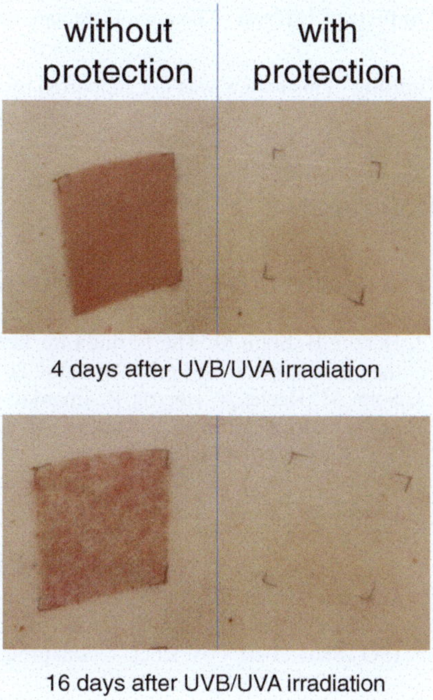

Fig. 5.4 Preventive effect of radiation reduction in a prospective, open-label study in patients with cutaneous lupus erythematosus [13]

Conclusion and Outlook

The long-term studies conducted around the turn of the millennium have not provided the hoped-for clarity regarding the skin cancer preventive effect and thus the effectiveness of topical sunscreen products. This is not primarily due to the sunscreen products itself, but to the study design (e.g., duration), the countless confounding factors (e.g., improper application, inadequate adhesion) and the etiology of the various skin cancers. It is unlikely that similar studies will be conducted with sunscreen products in the future, as product formulations are frequently changed or are approved as cosmetics (Europe). By contrast, the efficacy of sunscreen products is very well documented under controlled conditions. It is relatively easy—logistically and economically—to conduct such studies, and most importantly, it also allows to demonstrate improved efficacy of new developments.

There is no doubt that the public needs to re-think how to behave in the sun. The desire for a healthy tan and the still popular beach vacations would have to give way to other goals and activities. Nevertheless, the application of sunscreen products can definitely be improved. Finding a product that people like to wear, apply in sufficient quantities (e.g., twice before exposition), and that they do not forget to reapply after contact with water and sweating, and at least re-apply every 2 h, would be a huge step forward.

It must be made clear to the public that of all the measures—shade, clothing and use of sunscreen products—the latter remains the least effective! In absence of shade and clothing it is the best.

Conflicts of Interest The authors declare no personal or financial conflicts of interest.

Funding This review was not supported by any sponsor.

References

1. Osterwalder U, Sohn M, Herzog B. Global state of sunscreens. Photodermatol Photoimmunol Photomed. 2014;30(2-3):62–80. https://doi.org/10.1111/phpp.12112.
2. Herzog B, Sohn M. The formula for best sunscreen performance: beer-Lambert's law under the microscope. Curr Probl Dermatol. 2021;55:133–43. https://doi.org/10.1159/000517663.
3. Sohn M, Hêche A, Herzog B, Imanidis G. Film thickness frequency distribution of different vehicles determines sunscreen efficacy. J Biomed Opt. 2014;19(11):115005. https://doi.org/10.1117/1.JBO.19.11.115005.
4. Surber C, Plautz J, Sohn M, Maibach HI. Percutaneous absorption of sunscreen filters: review of issues and challenges. Curr Probl Dermatol. 2021;55:188–202. https://doi.org/10.1159/000517595.
5. Surber C, Plautz J, Osterwalder U. Nano ist groß! : Fakten und Mythen über nanopartikuläre UV-Filter [Nano is big! : Facts and myths about nanoparticulate UV filters]. Hautarzt. 2022;73(4):266–74. German. https://doi.org/10.1007/s00105-022-04954-1.
6. ISO 18861:2020. Cosmetics — Sun protection test methods — Percentage of water resistance.

7. Bimczok R, Gers-Barlag H, Mundt C, Klette E, Bielfeldt S, Rudolph T, Pflucker F, Heinrich U, Tronnier H, Johncock W, Klebon B, Westenfelder H, Flosser-Muller H, Jenni K, Kockott D, Lademann J, Herzog B, Rohr M. Influence of applied quantity of sunscreen products on the sun protection factor--a multicenter study organized by the DGK Task Force Sun Protection. Skin Pharmacol Physiol. 2007;20(1):57–64. https://doi.org/10.1159/000096173.
8. Surber C, Knie U. Metamorphosis of vehicles: mechanisms and opportunities. Curr Probl Dermatol. 2018;54:152–65. https://doi.org/10.1159/000489529.
9. Silva ESD, Tavares R, Paulitsch FDS, Zhang L. Use of sunscreen and risk of melanoma and non-melanoma skin cancer: a systematic review and meta-analysis. Eur J Dermatol. 2018;28(2):186–201. https://doi.org/10.1684/ejd.2018.3251.
10. Miksa S, Lutz D, Guy C, Delamour E. Sunscreen sun protection factor claim based on in vivo interlaboratory variability. Int J Cosmet Sci. 2016;38(6):541–9. https://doi.org/10.1111/ics.12333.
11. Narbutt J, Philipsen PA, Harrison GI, Morgan KA, Lawrence KP, Baczynska KA, Grys K, Rogowski-Tylman M, Olejniczak-Staruch I, Tewari A, Bell M, O'Connor C, Wulf HC, Lesiak A, Young AR. Sunscreen applied at ≥ 2 mg cm-2 during a sunny holiday prevents erythema, a biomarker of ultraviolet radiation-induced DNA damage and suppression of acquired immunity. Br J Dermatol. 2019;180(3):604–14. https://doi.org/10.1111/bjd.17277.
12. Olsen CM, Wilson LF, Green AC, Biswas N, Loyalka J, Whiteman DC. Prevention of DNA damage in human skin by topical sunscreens. Photodermatol Photoimmunol Photomed. 2017;33(3):135–42. https://doi.org/10.1111/phpp.12298.
13. Patsinakidis N, Wenzel J, Landmann A, Koch R, Gerß J, Luger TA, Metze D, Surber C, Kuhn A. Suppression of UV-induced damage by a liposomal sunscreen: a prospective, open-label study in patients with cutaneous lupus erythematosus and healthy controls. Exp Dermatol. 2012;21(12):958–61. https://doi.org/10.1111/exd.12035.
14. Schleyer V, Weber O, Yazdi A, Benedix F, Dietz K, Röcken M, Berneburg M. Prevention of polymorphic light eruption with a sunscreen of very high protection level against UVB and UVA radiation under standardized photodiagnostic conditions. Acta Derm Venereol. 2008;88(6):555–60. https://doi.org/10.2340/00015555-0509.

Chapter 6
Sunless Tanning Products

Stanley B. Levy

Introduction

Improvements in the formulation and aesthetics of sunless or self-tanning products have resulted in them being a viable alternative to UV tanning. Public awareness as to the hazards of both natural and artificial UV tanning has facilitated self-tanners becoming a significant component of the overall suncare market. 10 to over 20% of adolescent and young adults in both the United States and Australia reported using these products [2, 5, 9]. Individual users were also more likely to have sunburned consistent with higher use of these products in lighter skin types. Other studies suggest exclusive users of sunless tanners were more likely to practice overall sun protection [25, 41] and decrease their use of UVL tanning beds [39, 40]. A randomized trial at the beach for skin cancer prevention promoting sunless tanning reduced sunbathing and sunburns [33]. A larger, nationally representative, cross-sectional study would suggest that improved behaviours may not be associated with sunless tanning [10].

Dihydroxyacetone (DHA), a keto-sugar, is the active ingredient in sunless or self-tanners, and responsible for darkening the skin by staining. DHA is classified in the *International Cosmetic Ingredient Dictionary and Handbook* as a colorant or a colorless dye. Other similar sugars such as erythrulose and glyceraldehyede are occasionally used. Products containing DHA should not be confused with bronzers intended to produce a darker coloration of skin with use of water-soluble colorants or dyes. Other agents that have been used to enhance skin pigmentation with and without UV stimulation have varying degrees of success and toxicity (Table 6.1). They will not be discussed in detail here [6, 31].

S. B. Levy (✉)
Department of Dermatology, Duke University, Durham, NC, USA

P. Elsner et al. (eds.), *Cosmetics*, https://doi.org/10.1007/978-3-032-14644-1_6

Table 6.1 Tanning product types

Product type	Active ingredient
Sunless or self-tanner	Dihydroxyacetone
Bronzer	Dyes
Tanning simulator	Melanins
Tanning preparation	UVB sunscreens
Tan accelerator	Tyrosine
Tanning promoter	5-Methoxypsoralen
Tanning pill	Canthaxanthin
Hormone	Synthetic analogues α-MSH

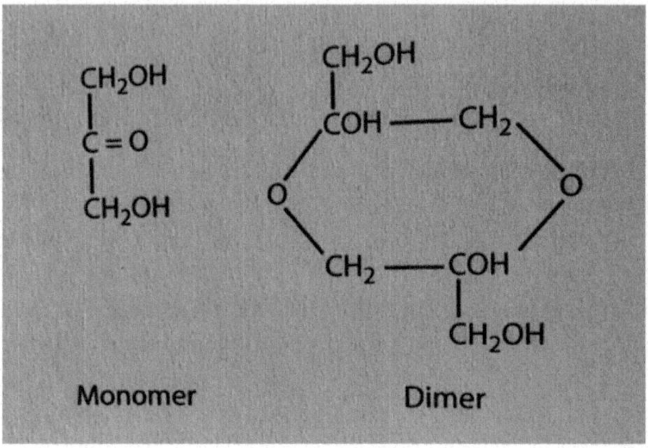

Fig. 6.1 Chemical structure of dihydroxyacetone

Chemistry

Dihydroxyacetone (C3H6O3) is a white, crystalline hygroscopic powder. This 3-carbon sugar forms a dimer in freshly prepared aqueous solution (Fig. 6.1). With heating to effect a solution in alcohol, ether, or acetone it reverts to the monomer. The monomeric form is less stable but more important in the browning reaction leading to the skin color change [24]. DHA is stable between pH 4 to 6, but above pH 7 efficacy is lost with the formation of brown- colored compounds. A buffered mixture at pH 5 is most stable. Heating above 38 °C for long periods of time will also affect stability. DHA needs to be stored in a cool, dry place, ideally 4 °C and low atmospheric humidity [1]. Glyceraldehyde, the isomer of DHA, is also present in solution. Glyceraldehyde may degrade into formaldehyde and formic acid. In acidic solution (pH 4), this isomerization and therefore these latter undesirable ingredients are minimized. Commercially available formulations generally contain 2.5%–10% DHA (Fig. 6.1).

The Maillard or browning reaction has been defined as the reaction of an amino group of amino acids, peptides, or proteins with the glycosidic hydroxyl group of sugars. DHA in the context of this reaction may be considered a 3-carbon sugar, reacting with free amino groups available as amino acids, peptides, and proteins supplied by the keratin to form products or chromophores referred to as melanoidins [44]. Melanoidins have some physicochemical properties similar to naturally occurring melanin [27]. Electron spin resonance has shown that free radicals are produced in vivo by the Maillard reaction [23]. A recent study documented a DHA-induced specific cutaneous stress response distinct from solar UV induced tanning [34].

Mechanism of Action

The site of action of DHA is the stratum corneum [17]. Tape stripping of the skin quickly removes the color [26], as does mechanical rubbing. Deeper staining in areas with thicker stratum corneum and no staining of mucous membranes lacking a stratum corneum is also consistent with this being the site of action. DHA may be used as a substitute for dansyl chloride as a measure of stratum corneum turnover time. Microscopic studies of stripped stratum corneum and hair reveal irregular pigment masses in the keratin layers [36] consistent with melanoidins. These melanoidins are formed via the Maillard reaction with DHA as a sugar reacting with the amino groups supplied by the keratin.

Application

Following application of a typical DHA containing self-tanning lotion, color change may be observed within an hour [22]. The color change can be seen under Wood's light (black light) within 20 min. Maximal darkening may take 8–24 h to develop. Individuals can make several successive applications every few hours to achieve their desired depth of coloration. Coloration may last as long as 5–7 days with a single application. Depending on anatomical location, the same shade can be maintained with repeat applications every 1–4 days. The face requires fewer applications but more frequent reapplication to maintain the tint than the extremities. Depth of coloration varies with the thickness and compactness of the stratum corneum. Palms and soles stain most deeply necessitating washing of hands after application to avoid staining. Hair and nails will pigment but not mucous membranes lacking a stratum corneum or keratin layer. Rough hyperkeratotic skin over the knees, elbows, and ankles will shade more unevenly as will older skin with keratoses and mottled pigmentation. Coloration will also persist longer in these areas.

As in the formulation, the pH of the skin before application may have effects on the tonality [24]. Alkaline residues from soaps or detergents will interfere with the reaction between DHA and the amino acids on the skin surface, resulting in a less natural (more yellow) appearing tint. Wiping the skin surface with a hydroalcoholic,

Table 6.2 Application instructions for self-tanners

Prepare skin with mechanical exfoliation
Spot test
Wipe skin with hydroalcoholic acidic toner
Apply carefully and evenly
Apply less to thicker skin
Allow to dry
Reapply regularly
Remember sun protection

acidic toner just prior to DHA application may improve results. Ex-vitro epidermal studies suggest that skin hydration [29] and relative humidity [30] influence the development of coloration.

Careful application is key to using these sunless tanning products (Table 6.2). The skin may be prepared with a mild form of exfoliation. Even application is required, with lighter application around elbows, knees, and ankles to avoid excessive darkening in these areas. Care also needs to be taken around the hairline where lighter hair may darken. Hands need to be washed immediately after use to avoid darkening of the palms, fingers, and nails. Skill and experience are necessary with using these products to produce the most satisfactory result.

Spray-on tanning formulations may provide more even application. Larger air-operator assisted delivery units are available for airbrushing on by a technician [38]. Tanning booths using sprays are commonplace in spas and salons. This form of application does however introduce the potential hazard of inhalation of sprayed material.

Some formulations include colorants as used in bronzers, including dyes and caramel, to achieve an immediate effect. Similarly tinting with iron oxides or titanium can provide immediate coloration and allow the user to more easily visualize the evenness of application. Metal oxides may, however, induce degradation of DHA [7]. Vitamins, botanical extracts, antioxidants [28], anti-irritants, and even alpha hydroxy acids may be added to broaden the manufacturer's claims with a given product. The addition of sunscreen ingredients to self-tanners warrants a more detailed discussion.

Sunscreen Activity

DHA itself has at most a modest effect on SPF [12], providing perhaps SPF 3 or 4 protection. SPF increases with DHA concentration and number of applications [12]. Low level SPF persists for several days, decreasing with loss of coloration. The brown shade obtained on the skin does absorb in the low end of the visible spectrum with overlap into long UVA and may provide some UVA I protection [19]. Melanoidins can act as free-radical scavengers as they demonstrate an electron spin resonance signal [23]. Superficial skin coloration induced by frequent topical application of DHA in high concentrations delays skin cancer development in hairless mice irradiated with moderate UV doses [35].

Individuals using DHA-containing tanning products need to be cautioned that despite visible darkening of their skin, these products provide minimal sun protection. Confusion may be compounded by the addition of UV filters to the formulation providing significant sun protection. The stated SPF for the product is applicable for a few hours after application, but not for the days during which the skin coloration may remain perceptible. Care should be taken with lasers utilizing wavelengths in the 400–700 nm range for a week after application, as increased absorption has been noted with DHA [18].

Indications

Even with recent improvement in DHA formulations, the color achieved remains dependent on skin type. Individuals of medium complexion with skin phototypes II or III [14], as opposed to those who are lighter or darker, will obtain a more pleasing tint. Individuals with underlying golden skin tones will achieve better results than individuals with a rosy, sallow, or olive complexion. Older consumers with roughened, hyperkeratotic skin or mottled pigmentation with freckling may be less pleased with results.

Dermatologists regularly recommend these products for tanning as a safe alternative to UV exposure. They may be utilized to camouflage some skin irregularities such as leg spider veins. Light to medium complected patients with vitiligo who show increased contrast with the vitiliginous areas with natural or unavoidable tanning in their normal skin may also benefit [37, 42]. DHA provides some protection for individuals with certain photosensitivity disorders [16]. Protection of uninvolved skin by DHA during psoralen-UVA (PUVA) treatment allows higher UVA exposures to be tolerated, with fewer treatments resulting in faster clearing, known as Turbo-PUVA [43].

Safety

The visible color change associated with the use of artificial tanning products may suggest to some users that these products are hazardous. Based on the chemistry of DHA and its toxicologic profile, it can be considered relatively nontoxic with occasional use. It reacts quickly in the stratum corneum, minimizing systemic absorption. The phosphate of DHA is found naturally as one of the intermediates in the Krebs cycle. Additional studies may be warranted focusing on concentration and frequency of use [32]. Toxicity based on inhalation in closed spray-on tanning booths is unknown.

Contact dermatitis to DHA has only rarely been reported [45]. As with other topical products with active ingredients, such as sunscreens, much the reported sensitivity is secondary to other ingredients in the vehicle [4]. Adverse reactions are more likely to occur based on irritation and not true allergy. Ultimately all claims related to product safety are based on testing the final formulation.

Although not approved by regulatory agencies, some of the alternative agents for increasing skin pigmentation (Table 6.1) are available to individuals. Tanning pills containing carotenoids such as canthaxanthin have been reported to cause retinopathy, urticaria, hepatitis, and aplastic anemia [3]. More recently, injections of analogues of melanocyte-stimulating hormone may be gaining in popularity [21]. Of potential benefit to individuals with photosensitive disorders, synthetic analogues of α-MSH may drive proliferation of neoplastic melanocytic cells in the nevi of predisposed individuals [8]. New analogues may be on the horizon [20].

Conclusion

Increasing awareness as to the hazards of UV light should fuel ongoing interest in self-tanning products. It is incumbent upon dermatologists to be familiar with this category. The benign toxicologic profile of DHA reinforces the notion that these products represent a safe alternative to a UV-induced tan. The results obtained are dependent on the specific formulation, individual application technique, and the consumer's skin type. Greater experience in formulation combined with increasing sophistication on the part of consumers has led to increased satisfaction with the use of these products.

Users need to be clearly informed that these products do not offer significant protection against UVB. If formulated with standard sunscreens, individuals should be cautioned that the duration of UV protection is more short-lived than the perceived change in skin color.

References

1. Aretz C, Buczys R, Buchholz, Driller H. Degradation reactions of dihydroxyacetone. Euro Cosmet. 1999;6:32–6.
2. Beckmann KR, Kirke BA, McCaul KA, et al. Use of fake tanning lotions in the South Australian population. Med J Aust. 2001;174(2):75–8. https://doi.org/10.5694/j.1326-5377.2001.tb143158.x. PMID: 11245507.
3. Bluhm R, Branch R, Johnston P. Aplastic anemia associated with canthaxanthin ingested for tanning purposes. JAMA. 1990;264:1141–2. PMID: 2117075.

4. Bovenschen HJ, Korver JEM, Van der Valk PGM. Contact dermatitis to self-tanning products. Contact Derm. 2009;60:290–1. https://doi.org/10.1111/j.1600-0536.2009.01523.x. PMID: 19397623.
5. Brooks K, Brooks D, Dajani Z, et al. Use of artificial tanning products among young adults. J Am Acad Dermatol. 2006;54(6):1060–10606. https://doi.org/10.1016/j.jaad.2006.01.014. PMID: 16713463.
6. Brown DA. Skin pigmentation enhancers. *J*. Photochem Photobiol. 2001;63:148–61. https://doi.org/10.1016/s1011-1344(01)00212-3. PMID: 11684462.
7. Chaudhuri RK. Dihydroxyactone: Chemistry and and applications in self-tanning products. In: Schlossman ML, editors. The chemistry and manufacture of cosmetics. Volume III. Carol Stream, IL: Allured Publishing, 2002; pp. 383–402.
8. Carderones A, Grichnik JM. Melanocyte-stimulating hormone-induced eruptive nevi. Arch derm 2009;145:441–4.
9. Cokkinides VE, Bandi P, Weinstock MA, Ward E. Use of sunless tanning products among U.S. adolescents aged 11 to 18 years. Arch Dermatol. 2010;146(9):987–92. https://doi.org/10.1001/archdermatol.2010.220. PMID: 20855697.
10. Dodds M, Arron ST, Linos E, et al. Characteristics and skin cancer Behaviors of adult sunless Tanner in the United States. JAMA Dermatol. 2018;154(9):1066–71. https://doi.org/10.1001/jamadermatol.2018.2054. PMID: 30046802 PMCID: PMC6143043.
11. Fabrikant J, Khasha T, Brown SM. A review and update on melanocyte stimulating hormone therapy: afamelanotide. J Drugs Dermatol. 2013;12(7):775–9. https://doi.org/10.1111/j.1600-0781.2004.00118.x. PMID: 15379873.
12. Faurschou A, Wulf HC. Durability of the sun protection factor provided by dihydroxyacetone. Photodermatol Photoimmunol Photomed. 2004;20:239–42. https://doi.org/10.1111/j.1600-0781.2004.00118.x. PMID: 15379873.
13. Faurschou A, Janjua NR, Wulf HC. Sun protection effect of dihydroxyacetone. Arch Dermatol. 2004;140:886–7. https://doi.org/10.1001/archderm.140.7.886. PMID: 15262709.
14. Fitzpatrick TB. The validity and practicality of sun reactive skin types I through IV. Arch Dermatol. 1988;124:869–71. https://doi.org/10.1001/archderm.124.6.869. PMID: 3377516.
15. Forest SE, Grothaus JT, Ertel KD, Rader C, Plante J. Flourescence spectral imaging of dihydroxyacetone on skin in vivo. Photochem Photobiol. 2003;77:524–30. https://doi.org/10.1562/0031-8655(2003)077<0524:fsiodo>2.0.co;2. PMID: 12812295.
16. Fusaro RM, Johnson JA. Photoprotection of patients sensitive to short and/or long ultraviolet light with dihydroxyacetone/naphthoquinone. Dermatologica. 1974;148:224–7. PMID: 4853627.
17. Goldman L, Barkoff J, Blaney D, Nakai T, Suskind R. The skin coloring agent dihydroxyacetone. Gen Pract. 1960;12:96–8. https://doi.org/10.1038/jid.1960.100. PMID: 13706563.
18. Graves MS, Lloyd AA, Ross EV. Defining the absorption spectrum of the skin after application of a popular sunless tanner, dihydroxyacetone, using reflectance photospectrometry. J Drugs Dermatol. 2016;15(11):11459–60. PMID: 28095563.
19. Johnson JA, Fusaro RM. Protection against long ultraviolet radiation: topical browning agents and a new outlook. Dermatologica. 1987;175:53–7. https://doi.org/10.1159/000248786. PMID: 3653458.
20. Koikov L, Starner RJ, Swope VB, et al. Development of hMC1R selective small agonists for sunless tanning and prevention of genotoxicity of UV in melanocytes. J Invest Dermatol. 2021;141:1819–29. https://doi.org/10.1016/j.jid.2020.11.034. PMID: 33609553 PMCID: PMC9009400.
21. Langan EA, Nie Z, Rhodes LE. Melanotropic peptides: more than just 'Barbie drugs' and 'suntan jabs'? Br J Dermatol. 2013;163:451–5. https://doi.org/10.1111/j.1365-2133.2010.09891.x. PMID: 2054568.
22. Levy SB. Dihydroxyacetone-containing sunless or self-tanning lotions. J Am Acad Dermatol. 1992;27:989–93. https://doi.org/10.1016/0190-9622(92)70300-5. PMID: 1479107.

23. Lloyd RV, Fong AJ, Sayre RM. In vivo formation of Maillard reaction free radicals in mouse skin. J Invest Dermatol. 2001;117:740–2. https://doi.org/10.1046/j.0022-202x.2001.01448.x. PMID: 11564185.
24. Maes DH, Marenus KD. Self-tanning products. In: Baran R, Maibach HI, editors. Textbook of cosmetic dermatology. 3rd ed. Boca Raton: Taylor & Francis; 2005. p. 225–7.
25. Mahler HI, Kulik JA, Harrell J, et al. Effects of UV photographs, photoaging information, and use of sunless tanning lotion on sun protection behaviors. Arch Dermatol. 2005;141(3):373–80. https://doi.org/10.1001/archderm.141.3.373. PMID: 15781679.
26. Maibach HI, Kligman AM. Dihydroxyacetone: a suntan-simulating agent. Arch Dermatol. 1960;82:505–7.
27. Meybeck A. A spectroscopic study of the reaction products of dihydroxyacetone with amino acids. J Soc Cosmet Chem. 1977;28:25–35. https://doi.org/10.1001/archderm.141.3.373. PMID: 1578167.
28. Muizzuddin N, Marenus KD, Maes DH. Tonality of suntan vs sunless tanning with dihydroxyacetone. Skin Res Technol. 2000;6(4):199–204. https://doi.org/10.1034/j.1600-0846.2000.006004199.x. PMID: 11428958.
29. Nguyen BC, Kochevar IE. Influence of hydration on dihydroxyacetone-induced pigmentation of stratum corneum. J Invest Dermatol. 2003a;120:655–61. https://doi.org/10.1046/j.1523-1747.2003.12089. PMID: 12648231.
30. Nguyen BC, Kochevar IE. Factors influencing sunless tanning with dihydroxyacetone. Br J Dermatol. 2003b;149:332–40. https://doi.org/10.1046/j.1365-2133.2003.05434.x. PMID: 12932240.
31. O'Leary RE, Dieh J, Levins PC. Update on tanning: more risks: fewer benefits. J Am Acad Dermatol. 2014;70:562–8. https://doi.org/10.1016/j.jaad.2013.11.004. PMID: 24388421.
32. Owji S, Teklehaimanot F, Maghfour J, Lim HW. Properties and safety of topical dihydroxyacetone in sunless tanning products: a review. Photodermatol Photoimmunol Photomed. 2023;39:567–72. https://doi.org/10.1111/phpp.12913. PMID: 37697919.
33. Pagoto SL, Schneider KL, Oleski J, et al. The sunless study: a beach randomized trial of a skin cancer prevention intervention promoting sunless tanning. Arch Dermatol. 2010;146(9):979–84. https://doi.org/10.1001/archdermatol.2010.203. PMID: 20855696 PMCID: PMC3221310.
34. Perer J, Jandova J, Fimbres J, et al. The sunless tanning agent dihydroxyacetone induces stress response gene expression and signaling in cultures human keratinocytes and reconstructed epidermis. Redux Biol. 2020;36:101594. https://doi.org/10.1016/j.redox.2020.101594. PMID: 32506039. PMCID: PMC7276426.
35. Petersen AB, Na R, Wulf HC. Sunless skin tanning with dihydroxyacetone delays broad spectrum ultraviolet photocarcinogenesis in hairless mice. Mutat Res. 2003;542:129–38. https://doi.org/10.1016/j.mrgentox.2003.09.003. PMID: 14644361.
36. Purcetti G, Leblanc RM. A sunscreen tanning compromise: 3D visualization of the actions of titanium dioxide particles and dihydroxyacetone on human epidermis. Photochem Photobiol. 2000;71:426–30. https://doi.org/10.1562/0031-8655(2000)071<0426:astcvo>2.0.co;2. PMID: 10824593.
37. Rajatanavin N, Suwanachote S, Kulkolllakarn S. Dihydroxy-acetone: a safe camouflaging option in vitiligo. Int J Dermatol. 2008;47:402–6. https://doi.org/10.1111/j.1365-4632.2008.03356.x. PMID: 18377610.
38. Rogers CJ. Spray-on tanning. Aesthet Surg J. 2005;25:413–5. https://doi.org/10.1016/j.asj.2005.04.003. PMID: 19338841.
39. Sahn RE, McIlwain MJ, Mager KH, et al. A cross-sectional study examining the correlation between sunless tanning product use and tanning belief and behaviors. Arch Dermatol. 2012;148(4):448–54. https://doi.org/10.1001/archdermatol.2011.2072. PMID: 22184716.
40. Sheehan DJ, Lesher JL. The effect of sunless tanning on behavior in the sun: a pilot study. South Med J. 2005;98(12):11922–5. https://doi.org/10.1097/01.smj.0000189988.12031.ac. PMID: 16440919.

41. Stryker JE, Yaroch AL, Moser RP, et al. Prevalence of sunless tanning product use and related behaviors among adults in the United States: results from a national survey. J Am Acad Dermatol. 2007;56(3):387–90. https://doi.org/10.1016/j.jaad.2006.08.051. PMID: 17097362.
42. Suga Y, Ikejima A, Matsuba S, Ogawa H. Medical pearl: DHA application for camouflaging segmental vitiligo and piebald lesions. J Am Acad Dermatol. 2002;47:436–8. https://doi.org/10.1067/mjd.2002.119670. PMID: 12196756.
43. Taylor CR, Kwagsukstith C, Wimberly J, Kollias N, Anderson RR. Turbo-PUVA: dihydroxyacetone-enhanced photochemo-therapy for psoriasis: a pilot study. Arch Dermatol. 1999;135:540–4. https://doi.org/10.1001/archderm.135.5.540. PMID: 10328194.
44. Turner J, O'Loughlin DA, Green P, McDonald TO, Hamill KJ. In search of the perfect tan: chemical activity, biological effects, business considerations, and consumer implications of dihydroxyacetone sunless tanning products. J Cosmet Dermatol. 2023;1:79–88. https://doi.org/10.1111/jocd.14968. PMID: 35384270 PMCID: PMC10083914.
45. Zokaie S, Singh S, Wakelin SH. Allergic contact dermatitis caused by dihydroxyacetone—optimal concentration and vehicle for patch testing. Contact Derm. 2011;64:291–2. https://doi.org/10.1111/j.1600-0536.2010.01870.x. PMID: 21480916.

Chapter 7
Efficacy of Skin Protective Creams

Christoph Skudlik

Introduction

The main area of application of skin protective creams is the prevention of irritant contact dermatitis, which occurs more frequently in workplaces with repetitive exposure to potential irritants and wet work [49]. In contrast, the prevention of allergic contact dermatitis where sensitization has already occurred is not an indication for skin protective creams [49]. Terms such as "barrier cream"or "invisible glove", which are often used synonymously with the term "skin protective cream", should be avoided as they could give consumers misconceptions about the area of application and effectiveness of such products.

Effectiveness of Skin Protective Creams

The effectiveness of a skin protective cream is generally linked to the overall formulation and not to individual ingredients. The current state of scientific knowledge basically permits different galenic systems for the formulation of occupational skin protective creams (e.g. W/O, O/W, amphiphilic and multiple emulsions, suspension ointments, hydrogels and oleogels) [58]. However, the effectiveness of a skin protective cream cannot be assessed on the basis of a theoretical consideration of the

C. Skudlik (✉)
Institute for Interdisciplinary Dermatologic Prevention and Rehabilitation (iDerm), Osnabrück University, Osnabrück, Germany

Lower-Saxonian Institute of Occupational Dermatology (NIB), Osnabrück, Germany

BG Trauma Hospital Hamburg, Dermatology, Osnabrück and Hamburg, Germany
e-mail: cskudlik@uos.de

P. Elsner et al. (eds.), *Cosmetics*, https://doi.org/10.1007/978-3-032-14644-1_7

respective galenic system or the pH value. The frequent assumption that hydrophilic skin protective creams (e.g. O/W emulsions) are always particularly effective when used with lipophilic substances and lipophilic skin protective creams (e.g. W/O emulsions) are always particularly effective when used with aqueous substances can be regarded as scientifically refuted [18, 28, 29]. Some claims of skin protective creams (e.g. "liquid glove") could neither be verified in studies nor in practical application. Claims should therefore be critically scrutinized.

The spectrum of action of a skin protective cream or the effectiveness of a formulation can be enhanced by the use of special ingredients [54], for example perfluoropolyether [38], aluminum chlorohydrate [7] and synthetic tanning agents [7], the latter two of which are recommended above all under the idea of attenuating the swelling of the horny layer through sweat. The use of such ingredients therefore only makes sense in skin protection products, but not in skin care products that are used after work [14].

Some ingredients typically used in skin care products are unsuitable for use in skin protective creams applied before and during work. For example, urea promotes penetration into the skin, which is why the application of urea-containing topicals before work is not recommended and such products should only be applied to the skin after work [14, 36]. Another example of unsuitable components in skin protection products are substances that have the potential to sensitize even in rinse-off products: For example, sodium cocoamphopropionate was additionally introduced as a cleaning component ("dirt remover") in a skin protection product advertised as a "universal skin protection cream with dirt remover" that was used comparatively frequently in the metal industry in Germany. Allergic contact eczema to this leave-on product was observed, which could ultimately be attributed to this surfactant [47].

As randomized controlled studies or intervention studies under workplace conditions are not feasible for every preparation and every specific exposure due to organizational and methodological difficulties and the resources required [9, 54], model experiments under idealized conditions are used to prove the efficacy of skin protective creams. Here, the efficacy is quantified by assessing the reduction of an irritative effect on the skin by means of visual evaluation and very often by bioengineering techniques, that means skin physiological measurement methods. These methods have meanwhile gained great importance in the assessment of barrier impairments and for the quantification of inflammatory reactions on the skin organ [12, 19] and are used for standardized testing of the efficacy of skin protection products [3, 6, 16, 46]. Nowadays, efficacy is generally evaluated using validated repetitive irritation models in the context of human in-vivo-procedures, as they mimic the natural conditions under which irritant contact dermatitis develops. The test results from previously used in-vitro and ex-vivo procedures are only of an indicative nature and therefore have a very limited informative value for assessing the efficacy of skin protective creams. The informative value of the results of model irritation tests is also limited by the fact that in the working environment there is often complex exposure to a large number of both hydrophilic and lipophilic occupational substances, which can be harmful to the skin alone and/or in combination [17, 25, 54].

By using repetitive irritation models, some of which were carried out using a multicenter approach using a multicenter approach, it could be shown that repetitive application in vivo of diluted irritants is sufficient to be able to comparatively investigate the efficacy of skin protective creams [42, 45, 56, 57].

So-called standard irritants are usually used to test efficacy. These substances show different physico-chemical characteristics, penetration pathways, binding and damage patterns within the epidermal barrier of the skin [10, 11, 13, 48, 59–63]. Therefore, the results against special irritants cannot be transferred to other irritants [40]. A general claim of protection is therefore generally not justified.

For example, a standardized test procedure for testing against hydrophilic irritants was developed in Germany [40, 42]. The test procedure is based on a 5-day human in-vivo evaluation model to test the efficacy of skin protective creams for various representative exposure situations. A total of 3 relevant categories of aqueous irritants were identified, which are of particular importance in the development of irritant contact dermatitis in the working environment. These were hydrophilic irritants with an alkaline pH value, an acidic pH value, or surfactants. The procedure tests the effectiveness of skin protective creams against sodium lauryl sulphate—an anionic detergent—as a model substance for water-soluble skin-irritating substances. The effectiveness of the Skin Protective Cream is assessed clinically by means of a visual score using the scoring system of the European Society of Contact Dermatitis (ESCD). This is a sum score that includes the clinical characteristics of erythema, roughness, scaling, oedema and fissures. Using skin-physiological test procedures, the skin barrier function is also determined by measuring the transepidermal water loss (TEWL), skin hydration is determined using chromametry and skin redness is measured using chromametry. If the effectiveness of a Skin Protective Cream is proven, it receives a test mark ("effectiveness tested") from the German Social Accident Insurance, which may be affixed to the product. Skin protective creams that have been awarded this test mark have proven their effectiveness against modeling irritants and offer protection against aqueous substances such as soaps. Comparable test methods for testing a protective effect against lipophilic irritants do not exist and a comparable effectiveness to that of hydrophilic irritants has not yet been proven for skin protective creams [41].

Skin Protective Creams as Part of an Integrative Skin Protection Concept

Strictly speaking, the term "skin protective creams"refers to products for external use that are primarily intended to protect the skin from irritation at the workplace [49, 54, 58]. Suitable products should be used as part of a concept for integrative skin protection at the workplace before starting work and during work. In this context, skin protection products are combined with so-called mild skin cleansers, which are intended to gently remove dirt and aggressive substances from the skin, and with skin care products, i.e. products that promote regeneration.i.e. products that can contribute to the regeneration of the epidermal skin barrier [32, 43, 49, 55]. This concept of integrative skin protection is also referred to as the "3-pillar model".

A recent Cochrane review with meta-analysis of randomized controlled trials on the primary prevention of irritant hand eczema showed that the regular use of skin care products, alone (RR 0.71; 95% CI 0.46–1.09) or in combination with skin protective creams (RR 0.68; 95% CI 0.33–1.42), showed a trend towards risk reduction, although this effect did not reach statistical significance.

Similar results were obtained from the evaluations of skin protection training measures, which were also not statistically significant (RR 0.76, 95% CI 0.54–1.08). Overall, the published evidence on skin protection and care products or educational interventions is not sufficient to be able to reliably assess the effectiveness of primary prevention measures [4]. In the secondary prevention of contact eczema of the hands, however, it has been shown that intensive skin protection training measures have lasting positive effects, e.g. in the healthcare sector, hairdressers and in food and cleaning professions. The measures were more effective in mild to moderate cases of hand eczema than in severe cases, which underlines the importance of early intervention in the early stages of the disease [24, 35, 50, 52, 65].

Skin protective creams should be applied to dry and clean skin [49]. The application times should be taken into account in the respective work processes. The question of the sufficient and optimal application frequency cannot be answered in general terms and has not been sufficiently scientifically investigated to date. Rather, it should be based on the risks at the workplace, the galenics of the Skin Protective Cream and individual factors. Manufacturers recommend applying skin protective creams before every exposure to skin-irritating noxae and after every work break or even after a certain period of time (e.g. half a work shift), provided there are no activity-related impediments. In contrast, skin care products can be applied during longer breaks and after work [22]. This concept has become established in practice [49] and is recommended internationally [22]. Small pack sizes are advantageous for the individual care of employees. They can be carried by employees to different work locations, making it easier to reapply cream during work or during breaks.

The protective effect of skin protective creams depends, among other things, on the application quantity of the product. The so-called Finger Tip Unit (FTU) can provide an indication of the sufficient application quantity, whereby the use of one FTU per hand is considered sensible. According to the definition, an FTU describes the amount of cream that an adult can apply to the index finger from the tip of the fingertip to the first crook of the finger; one FTU corresponds to 0.5 g of the cream, i.e. the amount required for application to two palms [64].

Limitations of the Use of Skin Protective Creams

Human studies have shown that skin protective creams used for the purpose of attenuating irritation can also lead to an increase in irritation [18]. It is conceivable that this could be due to an irritant effect of the Skin Protective Cream itself—depending on the composition—or that these phenomena occur via the path of increased penetration or increased binding of the noxious agent within the skin.

In animal models, for example, it was shown that the use of a skin protective cream can increase irritation caused by cooling lubricants [21]. One study also found that one of the test preparations increased irritation to toluene [56]. In a randomized double-blind study with repetitive irritation tests on test subjects, also found an increase in irritation with two of six skin protection products tested against the lipophilic irritant n-octane and with a skin protective cream against cumene [41], so that the use of skin protective creams when handling solvents appears to be problematic. The results of the irritation enhancement correlate with in vitro diffusion cell studies, which demonstrated increased penetration by skin protection in connection with solvents. In addition, a recent experimental study has shown that some skin protective creams, when applied prior to glove occlusion, appeared to increase skin sensitivity compared to glove occlusion without skin protection [20].

The importance of the pH value of skin protective creams has been investigated in several studies [2, 27, 34]. Apparently, W/O emulsions with acidic pH values in the range of 3 and 4 show barrier-regenerating effects. The effects of more alkaline O/W emulsions (pH 8) are controversial in this respect. They could lead to increased skin sensitivity to the model detergent [27]. A possible disruption of the barrier function by leave-on products with relatively high pH values was observed [44]. Other studies, however, did not find any benefit of an acidic emulsion on the regeneration of the irritated skin barrier [8].

The distribution of a foreign substance into the stratum corneum can also be influenced by the vehicle used. Additives such as emulsifiers are held responsible for promoting the penetration of hazardous substances through skin protection products [15, 28, 30, 31], which are also used in transdermal therapeutic systems to deliver sufficient drug through the skin [37, 53]. Whether an inhibition of penetration can be explained by an additional physico-chemical barrier appears questionable.

Skin protective creams should therefore only be used to protect the skin from irritation and not to protect against the percutaneous absorption of systemically toxic substances. If protective measures against skin- and/or systemically toxic substances are indicated, these should be implemented through organizational and technical changes to work processes or the wearing of suitable protective clothing.

Experimental studies have also shown that the penetration of hydrophilic and lipophilic solvents is not reduced by human skin treated with skin protective creams [29, 33], but is generally promoted [23, 28–31, 51]. Furthermore, there are indications that skin protective creams can influence the absorption of high molecular weight allergens from latex gloves, although there are contradictory results here [1, 5].

For the practical use of skin protective creams, it is important to note that in the case of an allergy to an occupational substance, the benefit for the prevention of allergic contact dermatitis must be critically assessed [39]. The efficacy of commercially available skin protective creams to prevent allergic contact dermatitis, although being extensively tested, falls short, as recently described by Kim and Maibach [26]. In particular, skin protective creams do not protect against corrosive, toxic, mutagenic or carcinogenic substances. Technical and organizational measures as well as chemical-tight protective gloves are therefore indispensable for all the exposures mentioned [43, 49].

Conclusions

The preferred area of application for skin protective creams is the prevention of irritant contact dermatitis.

Skin protective creams are generally used in an integrative skin protection concept together with skin care products and skin cleansing products ("3-pillar model").

The effectiveness of a Skin Protective Cream is linked to the overall formulation and not to individual ingredients. Standard irritants are used to test the effectiveness.

Skin protective creams never offer universal skin protection; in particular, they are not preferentially indicated for protection against allergens, and corrosive, toxic, mutagenic or carcinogenic substances.

References

1. Allmers H. Wearing test with 2 different types of latex gloves with and without the use of a skin protection cream. Contact Derm. 2001;44(1):30–3.
2. Angelova-Fischer I, Fischer TW, Abels C, et al. Accelerated barrier recovery and enhancement of the barrier integrity and properties by topical application of a pH 4 vs. a pH 5·8 water-in-oil emulsion in aged skin. Br J Dermatol. 2018;179(2):471–7.
3. Aramaki J, Effendy I, Happle R, et al. Which bioengineering assay is appropriate for irritant patch testing with sodium lauryl sulfate? Contact Derm. 2001;45(5):286–90.
4. Bauer A, Rönsch H, Elsner P, et al. Interventions for preventing occupational irritant hand dermatitis. Cochrane Database Syst Rev. 2018;4(4):Cd004414.
5. Baur X, Chen Z, Allmers H, et al. Results of wearing test with two different latex gloves with and without the use of skin-protection cream. Allergy. 1998;53(4):441–4.
6. Berardesca E, Lévêque JL, Masson P. EEMCO guidance for the measurement of skin microcirculation. Skin Pharmacol Appl Ski Physiol. 2002;15(6):442–56.
7. Berndt U, Wigger-Alberti W, Gabard B, et al. Vergleich einer Hautschutzcreme und ihrer Grundlage bezüglich Wirksamkeit gegen das berufsbedingte irritative Handekzem bei Krankenschwester. Dermatol Beruf Umwelt. 2001;49:77–80.

8. Buraczewska I, Lodén M. Treatment of surfactant-damaged skin in humans with creams of different pH values. Pharmacology. 2005;73(1):1–7.
9. Coenraads PJ, Diepgen TL. Problems with trials and intervention studies on barrier creams and emollients at the workplace. Int Arch Occup Environ Health. 2003;76(5):362–6.
10. Fartasch M. Human barrier formation and reaction to irritation. In: Elsner P, Maibach H, editors. Irritant dermatitis new clinical and experimental aspects. Basel: Karger; 1995. p. 95–103.
11. Fartasch M. Ultrastructure of the epidermal barrier after irritation. Microsc Res Tech. 1997;37(3):193–9.
12. Fartasch M, Hüner A, Tepe A, et al. Hautphysiologische Untersuchungsmethoden in der Berufsdermatologie. Allergologic. 1993;16:25–34.
13. Fartasch M, Schnetz E, Diepgen TL. Characterization of detergent-induced barrier alterations—effect of barrier cream on irritation. J Investig Dermatol Symp Proc. 1998;3(2):121–7.
14. Fartasch M, Diepgen TL, Drexler H, et al. S1 guideline on occupational skin products: protective creams, skin cleansers, skin care products (ICD 10: L23, L24)-short version. J Dtsch Dermatol Ges. 2015;13(6):594–606.
15. Fischer T, Rystedt I. Skin protection against ionized cobalt and sodium lauryl sulphate with barrier creams. Contact Derm. 1983;9(2):125–30.
16. Fluhr JW, Kuss O, Diepgen T, et al. Testing for irritation with a multifactorial approach: comparison of eight non-invasive measuring techniques on five different irritation types. Br J Dermatol. 2001;145(5):696–703.
17. Fluhr JW, Akengin A, Bornkessel A, et al. Additive impairment of the barrier function by mechanical irritation, occlusion and sodium lauryl sulphate in vivo. Br J Dermatol. 2005;153(1):125–31.
18. Frosch PJ, Schulze-Dirks A, Hoffmann M, Axthelm I. Efficacy of skin barrier creams (II). Ineffectiveness of a popular "skin protector" against various irritants in the repetitive irritation test in the Guinea pig. Contact Derm. 1993;29(2):74–7.
19. Gabard B, Schliemann-Willers S. Effizienter Hautschutz durch neue Hautschutzpräparate. SÖFW-J. 2002;128:2–7.
20. Gina M, Wichert K, Kutz G, et al. Applying skin protective cream and the wearing of gloves? A randomized controlled experimental study. Contact Derm. 2023;88(5):372–82.
21. Goh CL. Cutting oil dermatitis on Guinea pig skin (I). Cutting oil dermatitis and barrier cream. Contact Derm. 1991;24(1):16–21.
22. Hines J, Wilkinson SM, John SM, et al. The three moments of skin cream application: an evidence-based proposal for use of skin creams in the prevention of irritant contact dermatitis in the workplace. J Eur Acad Dermatol Venereol. 2017;31(1):53–64.
23. Hui X, Maibach H. In vitro human skin percutaneous penetration: does a second topical application effect flux of first application? J Dermatolog Treat. 2022;33(2):916–21.
24. Ibler KS, Jemec GB, Diepgen TL, et al. Skin care education and individual counselling versus treatment as usual in healthcare workers with hand eczema: randomised clinical trial. BMJ. 2012;345:e7822.
25. Kappes UP, Göritz N, Wigger-Alberti W, et al. Tandem application of sodiumlauryl sulfate and n-propanol does not lead to enhancement of cumulative skin irritation. Acta Derm Venereol. 2001;81(6):403–5.
26. Kim P, Maibach H. Innovation in prevention of poison oak contact dermatitis. Arch Dermatol Res. 2024;316(8):596.
27. Kim E, Kim S, Nam GW, et al. The alkaline pH-adapted skin barrier is disrupted severely by SLS-induced irritation. Int J Cosmet Sci. 2009;31(4):263–9.
28. Korinth G, Geh S, Schaller KH, et al. In vitro evaluation of the efficacy of skin barrier creams and protective gloves on percutaneous absorption of industrial solvents. Int Arch Occup Environ Health. 2003;76(5):382–6.
29. Korinth G, Wellner T, Luersen L, et al. Beschleunigung der dermalen Penetration von Kühlschmierstoffen und kanzerogenen Arbeitsstoffen durch Hautschutzcremes. Arbeitsmed Sozialmed Umweltmed. 2006;41(3):106.

30. Korinth G, Weiss T, Penkert S, et al. Percutaneous absorption of aromatic amines in rubber industry workers: impact of impaired skin and skin barrier creams. Occup Environ Med. 2007;64(6):366–72166.
31. Korinth G, Lüersen L, Schaller KH, et al. Enhancement of percutaneous penetration of aniline and o-toluidine in vitro using skin barrier creams. Toxicol In Vitro. 2008;22(3):812–8.
32. Kresken J, Klotz A. Occupational skin-protection products—a review. Int Arch Occup Environ Health. 2003;76(5):355–8.
33. Lodén M. The effect of 4 barrier creams on the absorption of water, benzene, and formaldehyde into excised human skin. Contact Derm. 1986;14(5):292–6.
34. Lukić M, Pantelić I, Savić SD. Towards optimal pH of the skin and topical formulations: from the current state of the art to tailored products. Cosmetics. 2021;8(3):69.
35. Mollerup A, Veien NK, Johansen JD. Effectiveness of the Healthy Skin Clinic—a randomized clinical trial of nurse-led patient counselling in hand eczema. Contact Derm. 2014;71(4):202–14.
36. Mueller J, Oliveira JSL, Barker R, et al. The effect of urea and taurine as hydrophilic penetration enhancers on stratum corneum lipid models. Biochim Biophys Acta Biomembr. 2016;1858:2006–18.
37. Pont AR, Charron AR, Brand RM. Active ingredients in sunscreens act as topical penetration enhancers for the herbicide 2,4-dichlorophenoxyacetic acid. Toxicol Appl Pharmacol. 2004;195(3):348–54.
38. Schliemann S. Limitations of skin protection. Curr Probl Dermatol. 2007;34:171–7.
39. Schliemann S, Wigger-Alberti W, Elsner P. Prevention of allergy by protective skin creams: possibilities and limits. Schweiz Med Wochenschr. 1999;129(26):996–1001.
40. Schliemann S, Elsner P, Scheidt R. In-vivo-Evaluationsmodelle zur Überprüfung der Wirkung von Hautschutzexterna: Bestimmung der schützenden Wirksamkeit und Vergleichbarkeit, FP275. Abschlußbericht. 2013. Available from https://www.dguv.de/projektdatenbank/0275/abschlussberichtfp275final03.pdf. Accessed 13 June 2025.
41. Schliemann S, Kleesz P, Elsner P. Protective creams fail to prevent solvent-induced cumulative skin irritation—results of a randomized double-blind study. Contact Derm. 2013;69(6):363–71.
42. Schliemann S, Müller M, Stadeler M, et al. Doppelblinde, randomisierte repetitive In-vivo-Wirksamkeitsstudie zu kommerziellen Hautschutzprodukten gegen Natriumlaurylsulfat (SLS). J Dtsch Dermatol Ges. 2021;19(4):545–53.
43. Schliemann-Willers S, Elsner P. Occupational skin protection. J Dtsch Dermatol Ges. 2005;3(2):120–33, quiz 34–6.
44. Schmid-Wendtner M, Korting HC. pH and skin care. ABW Wissenschaftsverlag; 2007.
45. Schnetz E, Diepgen TL, Elsner P, et al. Multicentre study for the development of an in vivo model to evaluate the influence of topical formulations on irritation. Contact Derm. 2000;42(6):336–43.
46. Shah JH, Zhai H, Maibach HI. Comparative evaporimetry in man. Skin Res Technol. 2005;11(3):205–8.
47. Skudlik C, Markthaler M, John SM. Occupational contact allergy to sodium cocoamphopropionate in a skin protection cream. Contact Derm. 2018;78:295–6.
48. Soltanipoor M, Kezic S, Sluiter JK, et al. Effectiveness of askin care programme for the prevention of contact dermatitis in healthcare workers (the healthy hands project): a single-centre, cluster randomized controlled trial. Contact Derm. 2019;80(6):365–73.
49. Symanzik C, John SM, Skudlik C, et al. Hautmittel (Hautschutz, Hautpflege und Hautreinigung) im Betrieb [skin products (skin protection, skin care and skin cleansing) at the workplace]. In: Skudlik C, Schön MP, John SM, editors. Berufsdermatologie. Berlin/Heidelberg: Springer; 2023. p. 167–88.
50. Tauber M, Lourari S, Bérard E, et al. Positive change in hand care habits using therapeutic patient education in chronic hand eczema. Contact Derm. 2020;82(1):10–7.
51. Van der Bijl P, Gareis A, Lee H, et al. Effects of two barrier creams on the diffusion of benzo(a) pyrene across human skin. SADJ. 2002;57(2):49–52.

52. Weisshaar E, Radulescu M, Soder S, et al. Secondary individual prevention of occupational skin diseases in health care workers, cleaners and kitchen employees: aims, experiences and descriptive results. Int Arch Occup Environ Health. 2007;80(6):477–84.
53. Wellner T, Göen T, Drexler H. Systemische Therapie durch dermale Applikation: Transdermale Therapeutische Systeme. Dermatol Beruf Umwelt. 2006;54:13–8.
54. Wigger-Alberti W. Möglichkeiten und Grenzen von Hautschutzmitteln. Dermatol Beruf Umwelt. 2005;53:158–66.
55. Wigger-Alberti W, Elsner P. Preventive measures in contact dermatitis. Clin Dermatol. 1997;15(4):661–5.
56. Wigger-Alberti W, Rougier A, Richard A, et al. Efficacy of protective creams in a modified repeated irritation test. Methodological aspects. Acta Derm Venereol. 1998;78(4):270–3.
57. Wigger-Alberti W, Caduff L, Burg G, et al. Experimentally induced chronic irritant contact dermatitis to evaluate the efficacy of protective creams in vivo. J Am Acad Dermatol. 1999;40(4):590–6.
58. Wigger-Alberti W, Diepgen T, Elsner P, et al. Berufliche Hautschutzmittel. Gemeinsame Leitlinie der Arbeitsgemeinschaft für Berufs- und Umweltdermatologie (ABD) in der Deutschen Dermatologischen Gesellschaft (DDG) und der Gesellschaft für Dermopharmazie e.V. (GD). Dermatol Beruf Umwelt. 2003;51:15–21.
59. Willis CM, Stephens CJ, Wilkinson JD. Epidermal damage induced by irritants in man: a light and electron microscopic study. J Invest Dermatol. 1989;93(5):695–9.
60. Willis CM, Stephens CJ, Wilkinson JD. Selective expression of immune-associated surface antigens by keratinocytes in irritant contact dermatitis. J Invest Dermatol. 1991;96(4):505–11.
61. Willis CM, Stephens CJ, Wilkinson JD. Differential effects of the structurally unrelated chemical irritants on the density of proliferating keratinocytes in 48 h patch test reactions. J Invest Dermatol. 1992;99(4):449.
62. Willis CM, Stephens CJ, Wilkinson JD. Differential patterns of epidermal leukocyte infiltration in patch test reactions to structurally unrelated chemical irritants. J Invest Dermatol. 1993;101(3):364–70.
63. Wilmer JL, Burleson FG, Kayama F, et al. Cytokine induction in human epidermal keratinocytes exposed to contact irritants and its relation to chemical-induced inflammation in mouse skin. J Invest Dermatol. 1994;102(6):915–22.
64. Wohlrab J, Staubach P, Augustin M, et al. S2k guidelines for the use of topical preparations on the skin. J Dtsch Dermatol Ges. 2018;16(3):376–92.
65. Wulfhorst B, Bock M, Gediga G. Sustainability of an interdisciplinary secondary prevention program for hairdressers. Int Arch Occup Environ Health. 2010;83(2):165–71.

Chapter 8
Anti-cellulite

Enzo Berardesca

Introduction

Cellulite, a common skin condition characterized by a "orange peel"or "cottage cheese" appearance, affects a large percentage of post-pubertal women, regardless of body weight. While not a harmful medical condition, it can be a source of aesthetic concern for many individuals. Cellulite results from a complex interaction of hormonal, genetic, vascular, and structural factors, leading to the enlargement of fat cells (adipocytes) and fibrosis of the subcutaneous connective tissue, which pulls the skin downwards, creating the typical dimples [1, 2].

Over the years, research has led to the development of a multitude of treatments aimed at improving the appearance of cellulite. This document explores the different categories of anti-cellulite treatments available, discussing their mechanisms of action, efficacy, and important considerations [3].

Classification of Anti-cellulite Treatments

Anti-cellulite treatments can be broadly classified into several categories:

E. Berardesca (✉)
Dr. Phillip Frost Department of Dermatology and Cutaneous Surgery, Miller School of Medicine, University of Miami, Miami, FL, USA

P. Elsner et al. (eds.), *Cosmetics*, https://doi.org/10.1007/978-3-032-14644-1_8

Topical Treatments (Creams and Lotions)

Topical products are often the first line of approach for those seeking to reduce cellulite. They contain active ingredients that aim to improve circulation, reduce fat accumulation, and strengthen skin structure.

- **Caffeine:** Acts as a diuretic and stimulant, promoting lipolysis (fat breakdown) and improving fluid drainage.
- **Retinoids (Vitamin A):** Stimulate collagen production, improving skin elasticity and thickness, which can make cellulite dimples less noticeable [4].
- **Botanical Extracts:** Ingredients like ginkgo biloba, Centella asiatica (gotu kola), and ivy are often included for their anti-inflammatory, antioxidant, and microcirculation-enhancing properties [5].
- **Aminophylline:** A derivative of theophylline believed to mobilize fat deposits.

Efficacy: Topical treatments generally offer modest and temporary improvements. They require consistent application, and results can vary significantly among individuals. They are most effective for mild cellulite.

Mechanical Treatments and Massages

These treatments rely on physical action to manipulate subcutaneous tissue, improve lymphatic drainage, and break down fat accumulations [6].

- **Endermologie (Lipomassage):** Uses a motorized device with rollers and suction to massage the skin and underlying tissue. It is believed to improve circulation, lymphatic drainage, and the breakdown of fibrous adhesions.
- **Circulatory Massage and Manual Lymphatic Drainage:** Specific massage techniques aimed at stimulating blood and lymphatic flow, reducing swelling, and improving skin appearance.
- **Cupping:** Although less studied for cellulite, some alternative practices use cupping to improve circulation and fascial release.

Efficacy: Can lead to temporary improvements in skin appearance, primarily through reduced swelling and improved circulation. Multiple and regular sessions are necessary to maintain results.

Energy-Based Treatments

These technologies use various forms of energy to heat tissue, stimulate collagen production, break down fat cells, or improve circulation [7, 8].

- **Radiofrequency (RF):** RF devices heat the subcutaneous tissue, stimulating the contraction of existing collagen and the production of new collagen, which can tighten the skin and reduce the appearance of cellulite. Some RF systems combine energy with massage or suction.
- **Laser and Infrared Light:** Low-energy lasers or infrared light can be used to heat tissue, stimulate collagen production, and improve circulation. Some laser devices are minimally invasive and are inserted under the skin to melt fat and break fibrous septae [6].
- **Acoustic Waves (Shockwave Therapy):** These high-energy waves are applied to the skin to break down fibrous septae and stimulate collagen production, improving skin elasticity and reducing dimples.
- **Ultrasound (Cavitation):** High-intensity focused ultrasound (HIFU) or low-frequency ultrasound can be used to selectively break down fat cells.
- **Cryotherapy (CoolSculpting):** While not a direct treatment for cellulite, cryolipolysis (fat freezing) can reduce localized fat deposits, which may indirectly improve the appearance of cellulite if fat is a significant contributing factor.

Efficacy: Energy-based treatments can offer more lasting results than topicals and massages, with visible improvements after a course of sessions. Results vary depending on the type of technology, the number of sessions, and individual response [9, 10].

Injectable Treatments

These treatments involve injecting substances directly into the cellulite-affected tissue [11].

- **Enzymes (Collagenase):** Recently, an injectable collagenase-based treatment (e.g., QWO) has been approved, which works by breaking down the fibrous septae that cause cellulite dimples.
- **Mesotherapy:** Involves injecting a mixture of vitamins, minerals, enzymes, and medications into the mesoderm (middle layer of the skin). The efficacy and safety of mesotherapy for cellulite are still debated and it is not widely approved by health authorities.

Efficacy: Injectable treatments, particularly collagenase, have shown promising results in reducing cellulite dimples. Mesotherapy has less proven efficacy and higher risks.

Minimally Invasive Surgical Interventions

These treatments aim to sever the fibrous septae that cause the dimples.

- **Subcision (Cellfina):** A minimally invasive technique where a small instrument is inserted under the skin to sever the fibrous septae that pull the skin down, releasing the dimples [12].
- **Laser Liposuction (SmartLipo):** While primarily for fat reduction, laser-assisted liposuction can also help tighten the skin and improve the appearance of cellulite in some cases.

Efficacy: Subcision has proven to be very effective in reducing cellulite dimples with long-lasting results. Liposuction can be useful for fat reduction but has a variable impact on cellulite itself.

Important Considerations

- **No Definitive Cure:** It is crucial to understand that there is no definitive "cure" for cellulite. Most treatments offer temporary or lasting improvements, but the condition can recur or require maintenance sessions.
- **Combined Approach:** Often, the most effective approach to cellulite is a combination of treatments, along with a healthy lifestyle that includes a balanced diet, regular exercise, and adequate hydration.
- **Realistic Expectations:** It is important to have realistic expectations regarding the results. The severity of cellulite, individual response to treatment, and consistency in maintenance play a crucial role.
- **Professional Consultation:** Before undergoing any treatment, it is advisable to consult a qualified dermatologist or aesthetic physician. They can assess the type and severity of cellulite, discuss the most appropriate treatment options, and inform about potential risks and side effects.
- **Costs:** The costs of anti-cellulite treatments can vary significantly depending on the type of procedure, the number of sessions required, and the clinic.

Conclusion

Cellulite is a multifactorial condition that requires a personalized approach to treatment. From the simple use of topical creams to more advanced energy-based or minimally invasive procedures, a wide range of options is available. The choice of the most suitable treatment depends on individual factors, the severity of cellulite, and the patient's expectations. A holistic approach combining professional treatments with a healthy lifestyle is often key to achieving the best results and maintaining lasting improvement in skin appearance. Research continues to explore new and more effective ways to address this common aesthetic concern.

References

1. Rossi ABR, Vergnanini F. Cellulite: a review of its etiology and treatment. J Cosmet Dermatol. 2000;1(2):70–6.
2. Hexsel D, Mazzuco R. Cellulite: a review of its anatomy, physiology, and treatment. Dermatologic Surg. 2011;37(1):1–14.
3. Seidenari S, Bassoli S, Flori ML, Rigano L, Sparavigna A, Vesnaver R, Berardesca E. Methods for the assessment of the efficacy of products and slimming treatments for cellulite according to the Italian Interdisciplinary Group for the standardization of efficacy tests on cosmetic products. G ItalDermatol Venereol. 2013;148(2):217–23.
4. Bertin C, Zunino H, Pittet JC, et al. A double-blind evaluation of the activity of an anti-cellulite product containing retinol, caffeine, and ruscogenine by a combination of several non-invasive methods. Int J Cosmet Sci. 2001;52:199–210.
5. Buscaglia DA, Conte ET. The treatment of cellulite with methylxanthine and herbal extract based cream: an ultrasonographic analysis. Cosmet Dermatol. 1996;9:30–10.
6. Bayrakci Tunay V, Akbayrak T, Bakar Y, et al. Effects of mechanical massage, manual lymphatic drainage and connective tissue manipulation techniques on fat mass in women with cellulite. J Eur Acad Dermatol Venereol. 2010;24(2):138–42.
7. Alster TS, Tehrani M. Treatment of cellulite with optical devices: an overview with practical considerations. Lasers Surg Med. 2006;38(8):727–30.
8. Goldberg DJ, Fazeli A, Berlin AL. Clinical, laboratory, and MRI analysis of cellulite treatment with a unipolar radiofrequency device. Dermatologic Surg. 2008;34(2):204–9.
9. Goldberg DJ. Laser and light procedures in cosmetic dermatology. Saunders Elsevier; 2008.
10. Manuskiatti W, Wachirakaphan C, Lektrakul N, et al. Circumference reduction and cellulite treatment with a TriPollar radiofrequency device: a pilot study. J Eur Acad Dermatol Venereol. 2009;23:820.
11. Smalls LK, Hicks J, Shrestha R, Vasilenko A, Storozhuk O. Effect of a novel injectable collagenase clostridium histolyticum for the treatment of cellulite. Dermatologic Surg. 2015;41(Suppl 1):S15–23.
12. Hexsel DM, Mazzuco R. Subcision: a treatment for cellulite. Int J Dermatol. 2000;39(7):539–44.

Chapter 9
Racial Differences in Skin Function: Related to Claim Support

E. Berardesca and H. Maibach

Understanding Racial Skin Differences for Claim Support

The study of racial variability in skin function is an area of increasing importance for advancing skin care, preventing dermatological conditions, and optimizing treatment strategies. While all humans belong to the same species, distinct physical differences exist among human populations. These variations, which have emerged during the later stages of evolution, are attributable to a complex interplay of both genetic and environmental factors [1]. Understanding and quantifying these inherent differences are paramount for developing effective dermatological and cosmetic interventions.

A key feature that characterizes race is skin color, which raises fundamental questions regarding whether deeply pigmented skin (black or brown) responds differently to chemical and environmental insults compared to fair skin.* This inquiry extends to the efficacy of general skin care regimens, and whether certain racial groups face a different risk of developing skin diseases after exposure to similar challenges. The complexity of this issue necessitates a comprehensive approach, where the interpretation of pathophysiological phenomena must consider not only the anatomical and functional characteristics of various ethnic groups but also the influence of socioeconomic, hygienic, and nutritional factors [1].

The ultimate objective of this scientific inquiry is to move towards refined claim support and the development of more appropriate formulations for race-based skin care. A "one-size-fits-all" approach to skin care and product claims is inherently

E. Berardesca
Dr. Phillip Frost Department of Dermatology and Cutaneous Surgery, Miller School of Medicine, University of Miami, Miami, FL, USA

H. Maibach (✉)
Department of Dermatology, University of California, San Francisco, CA, USA
e-mail: Howard.Maibach@ucsf.edu

P. Elsner et al. (eds.), *Cosmetics*, https://doi.org/10.1007/978-3-032-14644-1_9

insufficient given the inherent biological variability across racial groups. A thorough understanding of these differences is critical for substantiating product claims with scientific rigor, ensuring both efficacy and safety across diverse populations.

Barrier Function and Stratum Corneum Characteristics

The stratum corneum, the outermost layer of the skin, serves as the primary barrier against environmental insults and regulates transepidermal water loss. While its thickness is reported to be equal in Black and White skin, deeper structural and compositional analyses reveal significant racial distinctions that bear important implications for product development and claims.

Structural and Compositional Differences

Studies have demonstrated that the stratum corneum in Black individuals contains a greater number of cell layers and exhibits increased resistance to removal by cellophane tape stripping compared to that of Caucasians. This observation suggests a heightened intercellular cohesion within Black skin, contributing to its increased resilience against physical disruption. Furthermore, considerable variance in these values has been noted among Black subjects, contrasting with the more homogeneous data observed in white subjects. Interestingly, no direct correlation has been established between the degree of pigmentation and the number of cell layers [2, 3].

The lipid content of the stratum corneum also varies racially, with higher values consistently observed in Black individuals [4] This elevated lipid content is a contributing factor to the increased intercellular cohesion, as evidenced by studies showing that delipidized stratum corneum specimens from both races exhibit equal weight, implying that the initial weight difference was primarily due to lipids. Complementing these findings, the mean electrical resistance of adult Black skin has been measured at twice that of adult white skin, further supporting the notion of increased cohesion or effective thickness of the stratum corneum in Black individuals [5].

Corneocyte Desquamation and Ceramide Profiles

Investigations into corneocyte surface area and spontaneous desquamation have revealed nuanced differences. While no significant variations in corneocyte surface area were found among Black, white, and Oriental skin, a notable increase in spontaneous desquamation (up to 2.5 times) was observed in Black individuals. This suggests that while the individual cell size may be similar, the rate at which these cells are shed differs, potentially linked to a distinct composition of the intercellular cement within the stratum corneum [6].

Further biochemical analyses have identified significant racial disparities in ceramide levels within the stratum corneum. The lowest levels of ceramides have been reported in Black individuals, followed by Caucasians, Hispanics, and Asians. In these experiments, ceramide levels demonstrated an inverse correlation with transepidermal water loss (TEWL) and a direct correlation with skin water content, potentially offering an explanation for some of the controversial findings in the literature regarding skin sensitivity [7].

The data presented in Table 9.1 directly contrasts a key functional aspect, desquamation, with a structural one, corneocyte size, across different racial groups. The significant difference in desquamation, being 2.5 times higher in Black individuals while the corneocyte surface area remains similar, indicates a dynamic process rather than simply static structural differences. This provides evidence for distinct epidermal turnover characteristics, which can influence how products penetrate the skin, the need for exfoliation, and overall skin texture claims. It visually supports the hypothesis of differing intercellular cement composition as a factor in these observed differences.

Transepidermal Water Loss (TEWL) and Permeability Variations

Evaluations of TEWL, a measure of barrier function, have revealed varied results depending on the testing conditions. However, in vitro studies, which bypass environmental and physiological influences, indicated that Black skin consistently had a significantly higher mean TEWL than white skin, with a significant correlation between skin temperature and increased TEWL in both groups [8–10].

Table 9.1 Racial differences in corneocyte surface area and spontaneous desquamation

	Mean surface area ($\mu m^2 \pm SE$)	Desquamation ($N°/cm^2 \pm SE$)
Black	911 ± 20	26,500 ± 4900
White	899 ± 22	11,800 ± 1700
Oriental	909 ± 24	10,400 ± 2100

Modified from Ref. [6]
Spontaneous desquamation is significantly increased in Black ($P < 0.001$)

Barrier Recovery Dynamics

Following induced barrier damage, such as tape stripping, darker skin has been observed to recover faster. While Reed et al. noted differences in barrier recovery between subjects with skin type II/III and skin type IV, they found no significant differences between Caucasians in general and Asians [9].

Implications for Claims

The observed differences in stratum corneum structure, lipid content, and barrier recovery necessitate a nuanced approach to product claims. Claims related to "skin hydration," "barrier repair," or "strengthening the skin barrier" must be carefully considered. While Black skin demonstrates increased cohesion and lipid content, suggesting a robust barrier, the lower ceramide levels and higher TEWL after stripping indicate specific vulnerabilities or distinct hydration dynamics. Products targeting hydration or barrier repair may therefore require different formulations or active ingredient concentrations to achieve optimal efficacy across racial groups. The increased resistance to stripping and higher electrical resistance in Black skin suggest a more resilient physical barrier, which could support claims related to enhanced protection against external insults. Furthermore, these unique barrier properties, including increased cell layers and lipid content, can significantly influence percutaneous penetration, making race-specific testing essential for claims of "active delivery" or "deep absorption."

Reactions to Light and Photoprotection

The interaction of skin with light, particularly ultraviolet (UV) radiation, exhibits profound racial differences, primarily due to variations in melanin content and distribution. These distinctions are critical for understanding inherent photoprotection and for substantiating claims related to sun care and anti-aging.

Light Penetration, Reflectance, and Epidermal Transmission

Despite structural differences in the stratum corneum, the total reflectance of light is remarkably similar, ranging between 4% and 7%, for both Black and white individuals. However, spectral remittance across the 300–800 nm wavelength range shows a two- to threefold difference in Black individuals. Caucasian epidermis demonstrates greater transparency to both ultraviolet and visible wavelengths; at

300 nm, a considerable increase in transmission through Caucasian epidermis has been observed. Light transmission through American Indian skin has been found to be intermediate between that of white and Black epidermis [11–14].

The Role of Melanin and Melanosome Characteristics

Measurements of the UVB protection factor and light transmission in the stratum corneum and epidermis highlight melanin's crucial role. The mean UVB protection factor for Black epidermis was 13.4, significantly higher than the 3.4 observed for white epidermis. Correspondingly, UVB transmission by Black epidermis was 7.4%, compared to 29.4% for white epidermis. This indicates that Black epidermis is inherently three to four times more photoprotective than white epidermis across all wavelengths [15].

The primary site of this light filtration appears to be the epidermis rather than the stratum corneum, with melanin in the malpighian layer being the main effector of photoprotection. Interestingly, when melanin in Black skin reaches the stratum corneum, it appears to lose much of its protective capabilities. The structural organization of melanosomes also contributes to these differences: in Black individuals, melanosomes are individually dispersed within the keratinocyte, while in most Caucasian and Oriental individuals, they are found in membrane-bound aggregates. A strong correlation exists between skin color and the degree of melanosome aggregation. The larger and more melanized melanosomes found in Black individuals are more efficient at adsorbing and scattering energy, thereby providing superior photoprotection [16, 17].

Implications for Claims

Claims for sun protection products must acknowledge the significantly higher inherent photoprotection of darker skin. While darker skin possesses a higher natural SPF, it remains susceptible to UV damage, particularly from UVA, and is prone to hyperpigmentation. Products for darker skin tones might therefore focus on broader spectrum protection or additional benefits such as antioxidant support. Given melanin's protective role, anti-aging claims for darker skin might emphasize the prevention of photo-induced changes beyond sunburn, such as maintaining skin elasticity and managing post-inflammatory hyperpigmentation, which is a common concern in darker skin. Claims about "natural protection" or "melanin's power" should specify that this protection is primarily epidermal and attributed to melanosome characteristics, rather than solely to the stratum corneum.

Percutaneous Penetration of Topical Agents

The efficacy of topically applied substances, whether pharmaceutical or cosmetic, is heavily reliant on their ability to penetrate the skin barrier. Racial differences in skin structure and function can significantly influence this process, impacting claims related to product delivery and therapeutic effect.

Variability in Absorption Patterns

In vitro penetration studies have yielded varied results. In vivo investigations further complicate the picture, showing different patterns of penetration depending on the specific molecules tested [18].

Regarding specific substances, tritiated diflorasone diacetate has been found to exhibit no discernible differences in pharmacokinetics between Black and white individuals. However, topical application of the local anesthetic EMLA demonstrated less efficacy in Black individuals [19, 20]. Furthermore, C-labeled dipyrithione showed 34% less absorption by Black individuals when applied in various vehicles to both stripped and unstripped skin [21].

Vascular Reactivity

Studies on methylnicotinate-induced vasodilatation, a measure of vascular reactivity, revealed statistically indistinguishable differences among racial groups in terms of time to peak response, area under the response-time curve, and time from response to 75% decay. Only the magnitude of the peak response showed significant differences, with increased levels observed in young white subjects. Overall, no important differences seem to exist between Black and white skin when tested with this chemical model. Similarly, percutaneous penetration of nicotine via transdermal tape did not significantly differ between Oriental and Caucasian individuals [22, 23].

Implications for Claims

Claims regarding the efficacy of topically applied drugs or cosmetic ingredients must explicitly consider racial differences in percutaneous penetration. The effectiveness of certain active ingredients may vary across racial groups, necessitating targeted formulations or dosage recommendations. For instance, a claim of "fast absorption" might hold true for one racial group but not another. The molecule-dependent nature of penetration suggests that formulators need to optimize vehicles and delivery systems specifically for different racial skin types to ensure consistent efficacy. For pharmaceutical products, varying penetration rates could imply the need for different dosing strategies or application frequencies based on race.

Conclusion: Advancing Race-Based Skincare and Claim Support

The comprehensive review of racial differences in skin function underscores a multifaceted biological reality. Variations are evident across numerous parameters, including barrier integrity, photoprotection, percutaneous penetration, biophysical properties, and unique responses to topically applied products. These distinctions are not merely superficial but involve fundamental structural, cellular, and physiological variations, influenced by a complex interplay of genetic, environmental, and socio-economic factors [24].

The existing data, while expanding, can sometimes be conflicting, highlighting the challenges in making broad generalizations. Nuanced interpretation is crucial, requiring careful consideration of methodological differences in studies, such as the distinction between in vivo and in vitro measurements or the type of irritation assessment employed.

To advance the field of dermatological and cosmetic science, several recommendations emerge:

1. Call for more Ethnic-Specific Research: there is an imperative need for further research to fully elucidate the various mechanisms underlying the different clinical expressions. Future studies should explicitly account for the intersection of race, sex, and other demographic factors to provide a more granular understanding of skin physiology.
2. Refined Claim Support: Claim substantiation must evolve beyond a "one-size-fits-all" approach. Product claims should be specific and validated for diverse ethnic groups, reflecting the differences of skin physiology and potential differences in product efficacy and safety outcomes.
3. Appropriate Formulations: The dermatological and cosmetic industries must commit to developing more appropriate, racially tailored formulations. These formulations should address the unique needs, responses, and concerns of different skin types, considering not just primary efficacy but also potential side effects such as post-inflammatory hyperpigmentation.

While much work remains, continued scientific inquiry is anticipated to lead to refined claim support and the development of more appropriate formulations for race-based skin care. This progress will ultimately benefit all individuals by ensuring that skincare solutions are truly effective and safe across the spectrum of human skin diversity.

References

1. Shriver MD. Ethnic variation as a key to the biology of human disease. Ann Intern Med. 1997;127:401–3.
2. Thomson ML. Relative efficiency of pigment and horny layer thickness in protecting the skin of European and Africans against solar ultraviolet radiation. J Physiol (Lond). 1955;127:236.
3. Weigand DA, Haygood C, Gaylor JR. Cell layers and density of Negro and Caucasians stratum corneum. J Invest Dermatol. 1974;62:563–5.
4. Rienertson RP, Wheatley VR. Studies on the chemical composition of human epidermal lipids. J Invest Dermatol. 1959;32:49–51.
5. Johnson LC, Corah NL. Racial differences in skin resistance. Science. 1963;139:766–9.
6. Corcuff P, Lotte C, Rougier A, Maibach H. Racial differences in corneocytes. Acta Derm Venereol. 1991;71:146–8.
7. Sugino K, Imokawa G, Maibach H. Ethnic difference of stratum corneum lipid in relation to stratum corneum function. J Invest Dermatol. 1993;100:597.
8. Kompaore F, Marty JP, Dupont C. In vivo evaluation of the stratum corneum barrier function in Blacks, Caucasians and Asians with two noninvasive methods. Skin Pharmacol. 1993;6:200–7.
9. Reed JT, Ghadially R, Elias PM. Effect of race, gender and skin type on epidermal permeability barrier function. J Invest Dermatol. 1994;102:537.
10. Wilson D, Berardesca E, Maibach HI. In vitro transepidermal water loss: differences between black and white human skin. Br J Dermatol. 1988;119:647–19.
11. Anderson R, Parrish J. The optics of human skin. J Invest Dermatol. 1981;77:13–7. *.
12. Pathak MA, Fitzpatrick TB. The role of natural photoprotective agents in human skin. In: Fitzpatrick TB, Pathak MA, Harber RC, et al., editors. Sunlight and man. Tokyo: University of Tokyo Press; 1974. p. 725–50. *.
13. Everett MA, Yeagers E, Sayre RM, et al. Penetration of epidermis by ultraviolet rays. Photochem Photobiol. 1966;5:533. *.
14. Kaidbey KH, Poh Agin P, Sayre RM, et al. Photoprotection by melanin-a comparison of black and Caucasian skin. Am Acad dermatol. 1979;1:249. *.
15. Szabo G, Gerald AB, Pathak MA. Racial differences in the fate of melanosomes in human epidermis. Nature. 1969;222:1081.
16. Hausser KW, Vahle W. Sunburn and suntanning. In: Urbach F, editor. The biologic effect of ultraviolet radiation, vol. 1. London: Pergamon Press; 1969. p. 3–21.
17. Olson RL, Gaylor J, Everett MA. Skin color, melanin and erythema. Arch Dermatol. 1973;108:541–4.
18. Berardesca E, Maibach HI. Physical antrolopgy and skin: a model for exploring skin function. In: Maibach HI, Lowe N, editors. Models in dermatology. 4th ed. Basel: Karger; 1989. p. 202–8.
19. Wickema-Sinha WJ, Shaw SR, Weber OJ. Percutaneous absorption and excretion of tritium-labelled diflorasone diacetate, a new topical corticosteroid in the rat, monkey and man. J Invest Dermatol. 1978;71:372–7.
20. Hymes JA, Spraker MK. Racial differences in the effectiveness of a topically applied mixture of local anesthetics. Reg Anesth. 1986;11:11–3.
21. Wedig JH, Maibach HI. Percutaneous penetration of dipyrithione in man: effect of skin color (race). Am Acad Dermatol. 1981;5:433–8.
22. Guy RH, Tur E, Bierke S, et al. Are there age and racial differences to methyl nicotinate-induced vasodilatation in human skin? J Am Acad Dermatol. 1985;12:1001.

23. Lin S, Ho H, Chien YW. Development of a new nicotine transdermal delivery system: in vitro kinetics studies and clinical pharmacokinetic evaluations in two ethnic groups. J Control Release. 1993;26:175–93.
24. Berardesca E, de Rigal J, Leveque JL, Maibach HI. In vivo biophysical characterization of skin physiological differences in races. Dermatologica. 1991;182:89–93. *.

Chapter 10
Skin Optical Detection Methods

K.-E. Peiponen and B. O. Asamoah

Introduction

Over the years, a variety of photonics-based devices have emerged for inspecting skin health and appearance [40, 56, 66]. While these devices are commonly used in medical settings, they also have significant applications in the realm of skin cosmetics. Advances in light sources like light-emitting diodes (LEDs) and lasers, along with sophisticated optical components and camera technologies, have paved the way for innovative sensor solutions that help in skin characterization.

By harnessing radiation sources that span from visible light to near-infrared (NIR) and even millimeter waves, we can probe various skin conditions effectively. Through the skin's natural ability to reflect, absorb, and scatter light, these technologies provide detailed information about skin properties such as gloss, color, hydration, protein levels, and thickness. They can even assist in diagnosing medical conditions.

In this chapter, we explore the measurement methods used by these photonics-based devices, particularly in the cosmetics industry. Given the overlapping use of these techniques in both cosmetics and dermatology, we will also extend the scope of applications to the dermatological field.

K.-E. Peiponen (✉) · B. O. Asamoah
Department of Physics and Mathematics, University of Eastern Finland, Joensuu, Finland
e-mail: kai.peiponen@uef.fi

P. Elsner et al. (eds.), *Cosmetics*, https://doi.org/10.1007/978-3-032-14644-1_10

Skin Optics

Human skin has a complex, inhomogeneous volume structure and surface roughness, serving various functions such as temperature regulation, waste removal and protection. Optically, it is both partly translucent and partly turbid [6, 45]. When ultraviolet-visible (UV-Vis) and NIR light interact with the skin, they undergo various optical phenomena at different skin layers, specifically the epidermis and dermis, due to the presence of chromophores and scatterers.

Incident radiation can experience specular reflection from the skin surface, absorption within the skin, or multiple scattering before either being absorbed or exiting the skin. Figure 10.1 illustrates these optical phenomena. Important optical properties of the skin include the absorption and scattering coefficients, as well as the effective refractive index, all of which depend on the wavelength of the probe radiation.

Additionally, the degree of polarization of both the incident and scattered or reflected light plays a significant role in the interaction with the skin, including skin treated with cosmetics. These interactions or phenomena significantly affect the detected light intensity, spectral fingerprints, and images of the skin, such as gloss

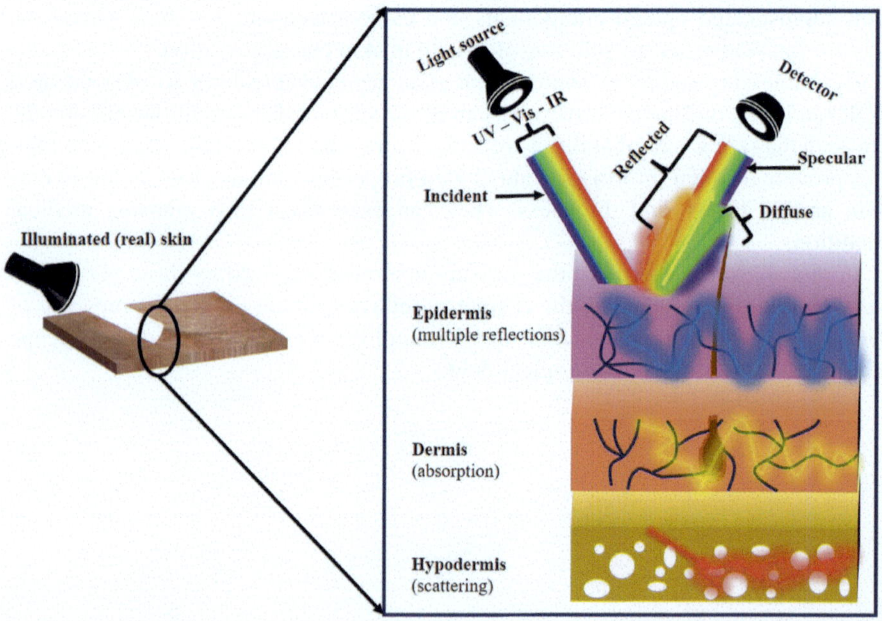

Fig. 10.1 Illuminated (real) skin (left) and schematics of the different phenomena of light interactions (right) illustrated in the different skin layers. Different light sources (LEDs, fluorescent, laser, thermal) can be used for the illumination. However, the phenomenon of light reflections (specular, diffuse, or multiple), absorptions, and scattering are likely to be present to a varying degree in all cases

and color [53]. For a coherent laser source illumination, the presence of skin roughness can lead to speckle pattern formation, which has been extensively used in the characterization of skin properties [84] . In the visible range, the skin's appearance and its perception, including color, are influenced by the human eye and lighting conditions. However, in the case of NIR, human perception is less important in the characterization as this kind of radiation is invisible to the eye. Sensitive detectors have been developed for applications in this part of the spectrum.

Skin Glossmetry

Specular gloss, as defined in Silvennoinen et al. [64] is a standardized parameter used to determine the quality of various industrial products. It involves measuring the intensity of light that is specularly reflected from a flat surface when illuminated by a collimated (or converging [51]) light source compared to a reference black glass standard. Depending on the material properties, which influence the measurement geometry, glossiness is typically classified into three regions: low (high angle of incidence), medium, and high (low angle of incidence, measured from the surface normal).

Skin gloss is classified within the low gloss regime [3, 23, 41], necessitating a sensitive measurement approach. The cosmetic industry requires precise skin gloss measurements to validate incremental variations introduced by skincare products. However, factors such as surface texture, curvature, and size significantly influence gloss measurements [64]. Moreover, given that human skin is not flat and is a complex optical structure, detecting gloss on such a relatively matte surface-like skin can be challenging.

Since the pioneering work of Lentner and Wienert [41, 82] in developing non-contact methods, gloss detection for human skin has significantly advanced, leading to the introduction of commercial skin glossmeters. These devices employ both contact and non-contact measurement modes to detect specular and diffuse reflections. For diffuse reflection, the detection angle differs from the light's angle of incidence. Gloss calculation primarily relies on the specular-to-diffuse ratio [10, 52]. Sometimes polarization imaging techniques [78] have also been used for the gloss calculation. The availability of these gloss devices has also enabled gloss measurements for other body areas, such as hair and lips.

Recently, other techniques with promising capabilities in the low gloss regime for skin have been developed. Ezerskaia et al. [23] developed a prototype glossmeter, which was compared to two different commercial skin glossmeters to evaluate its performance. The prototype used LEDs as a non-polarized white light source, detecting dynamic gloss after skin treatment with paraffin. The authors introduced two novel analysis methods based on the angle or slope of intensity variation from the specular-to-diffuse region and the number of pixels weighted at a cutoff threshold value normalized to its intensity. This prototype showed superior sensitivity in the low-gloss regime compared to traditional specular-to-diffuse ratio methods and detected time-dependent gloss changes after paraffin treatment.

A handheld skin glossmeter based on a diffractive-optical-element (DOE) [3] was also utilized to detect gloss profiles from dark to light skin tones in contact mode. This method allows the recording of gloss profiles to calculate average gloss and gloss variation. Single-point gloss measurements can determine difference in gloss, for instance, before and after applying tension to the skin or using skincare products. Unlike other methods that utilize diffuse reflection in gloss definition, the DOE allows spatial filtering of only specular reflection for gloss calculation. This handheld device uses a red semiconductor laser (narrow spectrum) as a light source since red light has lower absorption in the skin, enhancing light-tissue interaction [45]. With a light spot size of approximately 30 μm, the glossmeter enables local gloss determination, allowing gloss detection from small-sized objects like moles and even curved surfaces [39]. This DOE-based handheld glossmeter can also be used in non-contact measurement mode.

One of the notable deviations from traditional industrial gloss measurement methods is the variation in illumination angles. For example, the last two devices presented use 22° and 5° illumination angles, respectively.

Other Skin Characteristics Techniques

Skin Colorimetry

Gloss is just one of the four main attributes of surface appearance, along with color, texture, and translucency [47]. These factors all play a role in the overall appearance of the skin. The surface texture (roughness) and translucency of the skin can be measured using various photonics-based methods. Given its close correlation with gloss, skin color warrants a dedicated discussion, however.

The color of skin is primarily determined by the chromophores, melanin and hemoglobin, in this organ. Similar to gloss, skin color is crucial for assessing skin health and plays a significant role in both cosmetics and healthcare [21]. In objective skin color characterization, indices related to these chromophores [72] are typically measured using reflectance spectrophotometry or colorimetry [53], often within the popular CIELAB color space [76, 79] depending on the application [81]. Reflectance spectrophotometry measures the intensity of reflected light across specific wavelengths, whereas colorimetry considers human visual perception of color. While regular RGB (Red-Green-Blue) imaging devices can be used, sometimes, high-quality color-sensitive video cameras are also employed. In the CIELAB color space, where the L^* represents the lightness, the a^* and b^* represent the redness, and yellowness, respectively, the color differences is quantified as $\Delta E^* = [(\Delta L^*)^2 + (\Delta a^*)^2 + (\Delta b^*)^2]^{1/2}$.

Studies have demonstrated correlations between melanin and hemoglobin indices and skin color parameters [67], and the impact of color parameters on skin dullness [52]. Variations in skin color (and gloss) can be caused by skin defects like erythema (skin redness) and the application of skincare products [11], necessitating accurate measurement tools [17] for characterization. The repeatability and validity of skin color measurement tools have been thoroughly reviewed by [40].

A commercial portable spectral reflectometer, which measures both gloss and color coordinates, has been utilized to estimate the reflectance, transmittance, and absorbance of cosmetic foundation layers on skin, leveraging skin translucency [83].

Skin gloss and color can be considered as outward characteristics of the organ and these characteristics are fundamentally influenced by the subsurface constituents of the skin. To characterize such constituents and their contributions to the overall outlook of the skin, instruments such as a simple glossmeter is insufficient and other reliable methods based on spectroscopy are needed, therefore. The techniques used in these devices are the focus of the next section.

Near-Infrared Spectroscopy of Skin

Water content in the upper layers of the skin is crucial for its appearance and health [33, 63]. Controlling water content has, therefore, been a primary focus for cosmetics and skincare products aimed at improving skin health and appearance. Accurate devices for characterizing skin water content, retention, and the impact of skincare products rely heavily on their ability to detect water content reliably or its ratio to other substances in the skin. NIR spectroscopy is particularly suitable for this purpose, providing unique identifications of specific spectral fingerprints [32]. Typically, the diffuse reflection spectrum is measured over time after applying cream or oil on the skin. The reflection is diffuse due to the skin's turbidity.

Various measurement schemes are employed in NIR spectroscopy, including attenuated total internal reflection (ATR), Fourier transform (FT), ATR-FTIR, and NIR spectrophotometers with integrated fiber probes. In ATR, the measurement area consists of an internal reflection element (IRE) on which the sample is placed. Light is incident at a critical angle, enabling multiple reflections within the IRE. An evanescent field on the surface of the measurement area interacts with the sample to determine absorbance of the sample. Interferometric configurations in FTIR collect the interferogram generated from light interaction, which is then Fourier-transformed to obtain the spectrum. NIR spectrometers or spectrophotometers use optical fibers for illumination and collection of diffused light from the sample. Additionally, combined lasers of individual wavelengths in the NIR range are also used as light sources.

In the NIR spectral region (780–2500 nm), water exhibits specific spectral fingerprints at 970, 1200, 1450, and 1940 nm [6, 32]. These wavelengths are sensitive to NIR radiation and can distinguish different types of water in the skin [81], for example, water within or without the cell and water through the epidemis. They are hence used to detect skin hydration by cosmetic substances [34, 54, 56, 63]. NIR absorption near the 1940 nm band correlates well with skin dryness grades. Similarly, the area under the curve of the first derivative of the 1940 nm band correlates with skin water content, with relative humidity acting as a moisturizing effect. This demonstrated by [5], who demonstrated the effectiveness of near-infrared spectroscopy in assessing skin hydration. Kilpatrick-Liverman et al. [36] further explored the use of near-infrared spectroscopy to document skin water content as a function of product usage and changes in relative humidity. Additionally, [60] compared a near-infrared reflectance spectroscopy system and skin conductance measurements for in vivo estimation of skin hydration, highlighting the effectiveness of this method in assessing skin water content. Wavelengths at 1200, 1450, and 1780 nm are used to classify skin lesions [48] but they sometimes show alternating intensity behavior. Studies have noted that intensity at 1940 nm increases while intensity at 1450 nm decreases with regular moisturizer use, this intensity behavior reverses with disuse of the moisturizer [1, 2, 55]. The first derivative of broadbands corresponding to 1780 and 1940 nm are used to evaluate the long-term moisture retention capabilities of moisturizers. For estimating the volume fraction of water in simulated oily conditions, 1750 and 1779 nm laser-based sources provide strong correlations with traditional methods [22].

Despite NIR's popularity in skin characterization, it still faces some challenges. Results for water content quantification can be influenced by factors such as measurement geometry, probing light wavelength, fiber size, probing distance from the skin surface, and possible interference from other bands [1, 2, 56, 63, 81]. Addressing these challenges could further improve its popularity in many areas of applications. Future developments in skin moisture detection, particularly for cosmetic skin treatments, are leaning towards the use of miniature spectrometers [63]. This inevitably involves competition between benchtop and miniature devices and methods of analysis for the use of such devices.

Hyperspectral Skin Imaging

Hyperspectral imaging (HSI) combines the capabilities of spectral detection and imaging to provide both spatial and spectral information of an object under investigation. Each image pixel in HSI yields a diffuse reflection spectrum, resulting in a 3D dataset that requires more complex analysis compared to traditional spectroscopy. Illumination sources for HSI can include conventional light sources such as LEDs, thermal, fluorescent, and lasers, or even natural light. Typically, the imaging head moves in a straight light line to scan over the object, or the object itself moves under the probes. Standard hyperspectral cameras detect objects larger than 100 μm, and spectral cameras can operate across various wavelength ranges from Vis to NIR. For HSI spanning the entire Vis-NIR range, a combination of two cameras is often required.

When applied to the skin, HSI can also provide extensive information beyond gloss. For example, HSI can enable whole-face imaging for color evaluation with high repeatability and reproducibility after skin treatment with cosmetic foundation [9] and skin appearance in general [12, 14, 30, 35]. One of the challenges in the NIR range is accurately defining the thickness of various skin layers due to anatomical and racial differences. HSI, on the other hand, can estimate skin thickness to be approximately 100 μm [62, 75] and measure constituents within the skin, such as melanin, blood, oxygen saturation, bilirubin, and β-carotene [7, 13, 42, 62]. HSI can also measure the presence and distribution of lipids under the skin [28].

In cosmetics research, HSI enables quantitative evaluation of cosmetic product efficacy at specific wavelengths [49] and the effectiveness of permanent makeup removal by laser sources. It also evaluates color variation on the skin influenced by cosmetic foundation [9].

HSI has diagnostic capabilities as well. Custom-made HSI enhances sub-skin structures visibility compared to conventional microscopy [43] and facilitates screening of skin bruises. Employing polarization illumination and collection in HSI imaging helps distinguish skin disorders such as melanocytic nevus, vitiligo, and occlusions [73].

Traditionally, HSI's slow speed has been a disadvantage for real-time diagnostic needs. However, algorithm-based analysis of HSI has demonstrated the extraction of skin optical properties on a timescale of 3.5 ms per line of image data, indicating its potential for real-time applications [8].

While conventional HSI devices are costly for laboratory use, the concept is also evolving towards handheld devices [35]. A further step towards practical use is the development of smartphone-based HSI for skin inspection [27]. Additionally, integrating artificial intelligence for faster data extraction and analysis is becoming common in HSI [8, 32, 42] and improving the desirability of the method.

Skin Optical Coherence Tomography

Optical coherence tomography (OCT) is best known for its application in ophthalmology [18, 65] and has been extensively used in other medical fields [77]. The light source of the OCT system is a superluminescent diode that produces infrared (IR) radiation. A key component of the device is a Michelson interferometer. Interference between light scattered from the sample and the reference light produces depth-dependent axial, cross-sectional, or volumetric, respectively, 1D, 2D, or 3D images. The typical resolution of OCT ranges from 1 to 15 μm, allowing the examination of highly scattering biological tissues [19]. There are several types of OCT, differing in methods of illumination, detection, scanning, and domains of operation [77].

Due to its high resolution, OCT has recently been applied for rapid, real-time measurement of epidermal thickness across different body parts [44]. It also enables the evaluation parameters characterizing epidermal thickness in young and older individuals to understand the effects of aging [26, 50, 59], and to examine the morphology of skin pores and quantitatively assess sebum [37]. Additionally, OCT is used to analyze melanin content in the epidermis after cosmetic application [31].

To estimate hydration levels post-moisturizer application over several days, OCT was employed to measure the refractive index of the skin both in vivo and in vitro [38, 61, 68]. Hydration from moisturizers decrease the refractive index in the highly scattering skin medium. OCT can also be used to distinguish between different cosmetic creams and their penetration depths into the skin after application [26]. RGB LED sources enable full-color imaging of subsurface skin tissues with OCT, offering the potential for miniaturization into handheld devices using interferometric modules [25].

One commonly used device for characterizing skin surface texture and volume wrinkles is PRIMOS. However, it is usually prone to issues such as subject movement, orientation, and backscattering interference. Conversely, OCT provides more accurate information on surface roughness estimation [4, 29, 71, 74]. The same studies demonstrated OCT's effectiveness in quantifying the impact of cosmetics on wrinkles.

Lastly, OCT is also a key diagnostic tool in the medical industry [77, 80].

Raman Spectroscopy

Raman spectroscopy is a non-invasive technique that relies on the inelastic scattering of light by materials. Upon interaction, the frequency of the incident light is shifted by an amount proportional to the number of molecular vibrations present in the material. The frequency shift happens to be different for different materials. The collection of these frequency shifts and their intensities forms the Raman spectra, allowing for the distinct identification of material composition in various fields. Raman spectroscopy is often used alongside NIR spectroscopy as complementary devices. In dermatology and cosmetics, this technique is widely used for physiological and pathophysiological skin conditions for the skin [24, 46].

Similar to other spectroscopic techniques, Raman spectroscopy has been applied to study skin (in vivo and ex vivo) and other tissue compositions, as well as skin health [57]. Different concentrations of lipids and moisturizing factors have been measured with Raman spectroscopy, capable of probing skin up to ~100 μm due to the strong attenuation of the light source beyond this depth.

In cosmetics, the effectiveness of skincare products has been extensively studied using Raman spectroscopy. For example, enhanced Raman signals corresponding to OH stretching, proteins, and collagen have been identified after prolonged use of certain cosmetic products [70]. Using Raman spectroscopy, skin hydration and penetration depth can be examined for certain oils [15, 69]. It can reveal penetration depth for some oils up to 11 μm into the skin, but for certain vitamin derivatives, the depth can vary by age group [20]. Raman spectroscopy not only allows discrimination between existing products but also evaluates the effectiveness of newly developed products [16].

Future Outlook

Several methods for skin optical detection, particularly related to skin health, appearance, and water content, have been described above. These methods, as demonstrated, are already powerful and widely applicable in the cosmetic and skincare industries. However, further improvements can increase their capabilities particularly in addressing portability, standardization, and integration with emerging technologies.

In the context of skin gloss, the development of portable devices is crucial for personalized use in cosmetic applications. Standardizing skin gloss measurements across various tools can be achieved by calibrating portable glossmeters with standardized skin phantoms. This ensures consistency and reliability, fostering broader applicability in both research and industry. Where applicable, devices integrating together the measurement of common skin characteristics such as skin gloss and color can become more popular to thoroughly provide personalized device, especially.

For NIR spectroscopy, advancements in miniaturization represent a primary goal. While NIR techniques provide powerful insights into skin properties, the raw spectra obtained require robust statistical and analytical tools for meaningful interpretation skin-related conditions [35]. Standardizing these analytical tools is essential to ensure accuracy and comparability across studies. Furthermore, water vapor on the skin surface, which can influence the accuracy of spectral data [1, 2, 63] should be critically considered. For example, examining and defining a standard probe design that accounts for a consistent probing distance from the skin would address variability in spectral data and improve measurement reliability.

As the demand for environmentally sustainable cosmetic products grows, the need for sophisticated multi-sensor solutions and analytical methods for skin characterization increases [58]. One promising direction is the development of multi-sensor solutions based on existing photonics-powered solutions, which can potentially extend the capabilities. By leveraging such multi-sensor approaches, the limitations of individual methods can be mitigated, providing comprehensive and precise insights into skin properties. Additionally, advanced skin characterization technologies could play a critical role in validating sustainability claims and ensuring the development of eco-friendly skincare products.

References

1. Arimoto H, Egawa M. Non-contact skin moisture measurement based on near-infrared spectroscopy. Appl Spectrosc. 2004;58:1439.
2. Arimoto H, Egawa M, Yamada Y. Depth profile of diffuse reflectance near-infrared spectroscopy for measurement of water content in skin. Skin Res Technol. 2005;11:27–35.
3. Asamoah BO, Peiponen K-E. Scanning of skin gloss by a diffractive optical element-based handheld glossmeter. Opt Rev. 2018;25(6):694–700. https://doi.org/10.1007/s10043-018-0462-z.
4. Askaruly S, Ahn Y, Kim H, Vavilin A, Ban S, Kim PU, Kim S, Lee H, Jung W. Quantitative evaluation of skin surface roughness using optical coherence tomography in vivo. IEEE J Sel Top Quantum Electron. 2019;25(1):1–8. https://doi.org/10.1109/JSTQE.2018.2873489.
5. Attas M, Posthumus T, Schattka B, Sowa M, Mantsch H, Zhang S. Long-wavelength near-infrared spectroscopic imaging for in-vivo skin hydration measurements. Vib Spectrosc. 2002;28:37–43.
6. Bashkatov AN, Genina EA, Kochubey VI, Tuchin VV. Optical properties of human skin, subcutaneous and mucous tissues in the wavelength range from 400 to 2000 nm. J Phys D Appl Phys. 2005;38(15):2543–55. https://doi.org/10.1088/0022-3727/38/15/004.
7. Bish SF, Sharma M, Wang Y, Triesault NJ, Reichenberg JS, Zhang JXJ, Tunnell JW. Handheld diffuse reflectance spectral imaging (DRSi) for in-vivo characterization of skin. Biomed Opt Express. 2014;5(2):573. https://doi.org/10.1364/boe.5.000573.
8. Bjorgan A, Milanic M, Randeberg LL. Estimation of skin optical parameters for real-time hyperspectral imaging applications. J Biomed Opt. 2014;19(6):066003. https://doi.org/10.1117/1.jbo.19.6.066003.
9. Blaksley C, Udodaira K, Yoshida M, Nicolas A, Velleman D, Casolino M, Flament F. Repeatability and reproducibility of a hyperspectral imaging system for in vivo color evaluation. Skin Res Technol. 2022;28(4):544–55. https://doi.org/10.1111/srt.13160.
10. Budde W. Polarization effects in gloss measurements. Appl Opt. 1979;18(13):2252–7. https://doi.org/10.1364/AO.18.002252.
11. Caisey L, Grangeat F, Lemasson A, Talabot J, Voirin A. Skin color and makeup strategies of women from different ethnic groups. Int J Cosmet Sci. 2006;28(6):427–37. https://doi.org/10.1111/j.1467-2494.2006.00329.x.
12. Calin MA, Parasca SV, Calin MR, Petrescu E. An analysis of human dorsal hand skin texture using hyperspectral imaging technique for assessing the skin aging process. Appl Spectrosc. 2017;71(3):391–400. https://doi.org/10.1177/0003702816659667.
13. Chakravarty SK, Abbott AL. Non-invasive estimation of skin chromophores using hyperspectral imaging. Thesis, Virginia Polytechnic Institute and State University; 2024.
14. Chen TF, Baranoski GVG, Kimmel BW, Miranda E. Hyperspectral modeling of skin appearance. ACM Trans Graph. 2015;34(3):1–14. https://doi.org/10.1145/2701416.
15. Choe C, Lademann J, Darvin ME. Analysis of human and porcine skin in vivo/ex vivo for penetration of selected oils by confocal Raman microscopy. Skin Pharmacol Physiol. 2015;28(6):318–30. https://doi.org/10.1159/000439407.
16. Chrit L, Bastien P, Biatry B, Simonnet JT, Potter A, Minondo AM, Flament F, Bazin R, Sockalingum GD, Leroy F, Manfait M, Hadjur C. In vitro and in vivo confocal Raman study of human skin hydration: assessment of a new moisturizing agent pMPC. Biopolymers. 2007;85(4):359–69. https://doi.org/10.1002/bip.20644.
17. Clarys P, Alewaeters K, Lambrecht R, Barel AO. Skin color measurements: comparison between three instruments: the Chromameter A, the DermaSpectrometer A and the Mexameter A. Skin Res Technol. 2000;6:230–8.
18. de Carlo TE, Romano A, Waheed NK, Duker JS. A review of optical coherence tomography angiography (OCTA). Int J Retina Vitr. 2015;1(1):5. https://doi.org/10.1186/s40942-015-0005-8.
19. Drexler W, Fujimoto J. Introduction to optical coherence tomography. In: Drexler W, Fujimoto JG, editors. Optical coherence tomography: technology and applications. Springer; 2008. p. 40.

20. Essendoubi M, Gobinet C, Reynaud R, Angiboust JF, Manfait M, Piot O. Human skin penetration of hyaluronic acid of different molecular weights as probed by Raman spectroscopy. Skin Res Technol. 2016;22(1):55–62. https://doi.org/10.1111/srt.12228.
21. Everett JS, Budescu M, Sommers MS. Making sense of skin color in clinical care. Clin Nurs Res. 2012;21(4):495–516. https://doi.org/10.1177/1054773812446510.
22. Ezerskaia A, Pereira SF, Urbach HP, Verhagen R, Varghese B. Quantitative and simultaneous non-invasive measurement of skin hydration and sebum levels. Biomed Opt Express. 2016;7(6):2311. https://doi.org/10.1364/boe.7.002311.
23. Ezerskaia A, Ras A, Bloemen P, Pereira SF, Urbach HP, Varghese B. High sensitivity optical measurement of skin gloss. Biomed Opt Express. 2017;8(9):3981–92. https://doi.org/10.1364/BOE.8.003981.
24. Förster M, Bolzinger M-A, Montagnac G, Briançon S. Confocal Raman microspectroscopy for the skin. Eur J Dermatol. 2011;21(6):851–63.
25. Fujimoto JG, Pitris CP, Boppart SA, Brezinski ME, Lankenau E, Birngruber R, Engelhardt R, Gambichler T, Moussa G, Sand M, Sand D, Altmeyer P, Hoffmann K. Optical coherence tomography: an emerging technology for biomedical imaging and optical biopsy. J Am Acad Dermatol. 1998;254(15). http://www.tmt-mems.com/.
26. Han SH, Yoon CH, Conroy L, Vitkin IA. OCT monitoring of cosmetic creams in human skin in vivo. In: Photonic therapeutics and diagnostics VIII, vol. 8207. SPIE; 2012. p. 82070W. https://doi.org/10.1117/12.909504.
27. He Q, Wang R. Hyperspectral imaging enabled by an unmodified smartphone for analyzing skin morphological features and monitoring hemodynamics. Biomed Opt Express. 2020;11(2):895. https://doi.org/10.1364/boe.378470.
28. Ikawa T, Ishii K, Awazu K. Hyperspectral imaging of lipids using near-infrared super continuum light. In: Dössel O, Schlegel WC, editors. World congress on medical physics and biomedical engineering, Sept 7–12, Munich, Germany. Berlin/Heidelberg: Springer; 2009. p. 630–2.
29. Irani S, Turani Z, Fotouhi A, Daveluy S, Mehregan D, Chen W, Gelovani J, Nasiriavanaki M. The use of optical coherence tomography to analyze the efficacy of skin care products. In: Choi B, Zeng H, editors. Photonics in dermatology and plastic surgery 2018, vol. 10467. SPIE; 2018. p. 1046715. https://doi.org/10.1117/12.2291404.
30. Jagadeesha N, Trisal A, Tiwar VN. Skin tone assessment using hyperspectral reconstruction from RGB image. In: 2023 15th International conference on communication systems and networks (COMSNETS); 2023. p. 125–8. https://doi.org/10.1109/COMSNETS56262.2023.10041398.
31. Jdid R, Pedrazzani M, Lejeune F, Fischman S, Cazorla G, Forestier S, Khalifa YB. Skin dark spot mapping and evaluation of brightening product efficacy using line-field confocal optical coherence tomography (LC-OCT). Skin Res Technol. 2024;30(2):e13623. https://doi.org/10.1111/srt.13623.
32. Workman J, Weyer L. Practical guide and spectral atlas for interpretive near-infrared spectroscopy. 2nd ed. CRC Press; 2012. https://doi.org/10.1201/b11894.
33. Jiang Z-X, DeLaCruz J. Appearance benefits of skin moisturization. Skin Res Technol. 2011;17(1):51–5. https://doi.org/10.1111/j.1600-0846.2010.00462.x.
34. Martin, K. Cosmetic spectroscopy: a review of infrared and Raman studies of skin and hair. Internet J Vib Spectrosc. 1999;3(2). https://www.irdg.org/ijvs/ijvs-volume-3-edition-2/infrared-and-raman-studies-of-skin-and-hair-a-review-of-cosmetic-spectroscopy
35. Kern C, Speck U, Riesenberg R, Reble C, Khazaka G, Zieger M, Kaatz M, De Gregorio M, Fischer F. Mobile snapshot hyperspectral imaging device for skin evaluation using diffractive optical elements. Skin Res Technol. 2021;27(4):589–98. https://doi.org/10.1111/srt.12991.
36. Kilpatrick-Liverman L, Kazmi P, Wolff E, Polefka TG. The use of near-infrared spectroscopy in skin care applications. Skin Res Technol. 2006;12:162–9.
37. Kim H, Kang D, Seong D, Saleah SA, Luna JA, Kim Y, Kim H, Han S, Jeon M, Kim J. Skin pore imaging using spectral-domain optical coherence tomography: a case report. Biomed Eng Lett. 2023;13(4):729–37. https://doi.org/10.1007/s13534-023-00290-y.

38. Knüttel A, Bonev S, Knaak W. New method for evaluation of in vivo scattering and refractive index properties obtained with optical coherence tomography. J Biomed Opt. 2004;9(2):265. https://doi.org/10.1117/1.1647544.
39. Kuivalainen K, Oksman A, Peiponen K-E. Definition and measurement of statistical gloss parameters from curved objects. Appl Opt. 2010;49(27):5081–6. https://doi.org/10.1364/AO.49.005081.
40. Langeveld M, van de Lande LS, O'Sullivan E, van der Lei B, van Dongen JA. Skin measurement devices to assess skin quality: A systematic review on reliability and validity. Skin Res Technol. 2022;28(2):212–24. https://doi.org/10.1111/srt.13113.
41. Lentner A, Wienert V. A new method for assessing the gloss of human skin. Skin Pharmacol. 1996;9:184–9.
42. Li S. Human skin characterization and analysis based on hyperspectral reflectance using machine learning. Dissertation, Université de Lyon; 2021. https://theses.hal.science/tel-03412032.
43. Li Q, Sun Z, Wang Y, Liu H, Guo F, Zhu J. Histological skin morphology enhancement base on molecular hyperspectral imaging technology. Skin Res Technol. 2014;20(3):332–40. https://doi.org/10.1111/srt.12123.
44. Lin CH, Lukas BE, Rajabi-Estarabadi A, May JR, Pang Y, Puyana C, Tsoukas M, Avanaki K. Rapid measurement of epidermal thickness in OCT images of skin. Sci Rep. 2024;14(1):2230. https://doi.org/10.1038/s41598-023-47051-6.
45. Lister T, Wright PA, Chappell PH. Optical properties of human skin. J Biomed Opt. 2012;17(9):0909011. https://doi.org/10.1117/1.JBO.17.9.090901.
46. Lunter D, Klang V, Kocsis D, Varga-Medveczky Z, Berkó S, Erdő F. Novel aspects of Raman spectroscopy in skin research. Exp Dermatol. 2022;31(9):1311–29. https://doi.org/10.1111/exd.14645.
47. Marin Q, Honda T, Nakajima H, Okano Y, Cherel M, Prestat-Marquis E. Analysis of correlation and construction of a predictive model of skin transparency using parameters from digital images of the face. Skin Res Technol. 2022;28(4):582–95. https://doi.org/10.1111/srt.13161.
48. Mcintosh LM, Summers R, Jackson M, Mantsch HH, Mansfield JR, Howlett M, Crowson AN, Toole JWP. Towards non-invasive screening of skin lesions by near-infrared spectroscopy. J Invest Dermatol. 2001;116:175–81.
49. Nagaoka T, Kimura Y. Quantitative cosmetic evaluation of long-lasting foundation using multispectral imaging. Skin Res Technol. 2019;25(3):318–24. https://doi.org/10.1111/srt.12651.
50. Neerken S, Lucassen GW, Bisschop MA, Lenderink E, Nuijs T. Characterization of age-related effects in human skin: A comparative study that applies confocal laser scanning microscopy and optical coherence tomography. J Biomed Opt. 2004;9(2):274. https://doi.org/10.1117/1.1645795.
51. Noël M, Zwinkels J, Liu J. Optical characterization of a reference instrument for gloss measurements in both a collimated and a converging beam geometry. Appl Opt. 2006;45(16):3712–20. https://doi.org/10.1364/AO.45.003712.
52. Nurani AM, Kikuchi K, Iino M, Shirasugi Y, Sonoki A, Fujimura T, Hasegawa K, Shibata T. Development of a method for evaluating skin dullness: a mathematical model explaining dullness by the color, optical properties, and microtopography of the skin. Skin Res Technol. 2023;29(7):e13407. https://doi.org/10.1111/srt.13407.
53. Piérard GE. Continuing medical education EEMCO guidance for the assessment of skin colour 1. J Eur Acad Dermatol Venereol. 1998;10:1–11.
54. Qassem M, Kyriacou PA. In vivo optical investigation of short term skin water contact and moisturizer application using NIR spectroscopy. In: 35th Annual international conference of the IEEE Engineering in Medicine and Biology Society (EMBC); 2013. p. 2392–5. https://doi.org/10.1109/EMBC.2013.6610020.
55. Qassem M, Kyriacou PA. Reflectance near-infrared measurements for determining changes in skin barrier function and scattering in relation to moisturizer application. J Biomed Opt. 2015;20(9):095008. https://doi.org/10.1117/1.jbo.20.9.095008.

56. Qassem M, Kyriacou P. Review of modern techniques for the assessment of skin hydration. Cosmetics. 2019;6(1):19. https://doi.org/10.3390/cosmetics6010019.
57. Richters RJH, Falcone D, Uzunbajakava NE, Varghese B, Caspers PJ, Puppels GJ, Van Erp PEJ, Van De Kerkhof PCM. Sensitive skin: assessment of the skin barrier using confocal Raman microspectroscopy. Skin Pharmacol Physiol. 2017;30(1):1–12. https://doi.org/10.1159/000452152.
58. Rico F, Mazabel A, Egurrola G, Pulido J, Barrios N, Marquez R, García J. Meta-analysis and analytical methods in cosmetics formulation: a review. Cosmetics. 2024;11(1):1–45. https://doi.org/10.3390/cosmetics11010001.
59. Ruini C, Kendziora B, Ergun EZ, Sattler E, Gust C, French LE, Bağcı IS, Hartmann D. In vivo examination of healthy human skin after short-time treatment with moisturizers using confocal Raman spectroscopy and optical coherence tomography: preliminary observations. Skin Res Technol. 2022;28(1):119–32. https://doi.org/10.1111/srt.13101.
60. Saknite I, Zavorins A, Zablocka I, Kisis J, Spigulis J. Comparison of a near-infrared reflectance spectroscopy system and skin conductance measurements for in vivo estimation of skin hydration: a clinical study. J Biomed Photon Eng. 2017;3(1):010310. https://doi.org/10.18287/jbpe17.03.010310
61. Sand M, Gambichler T, Moussa G, Bechara FG, Sand D, Altmeyer P, Hoffmann K. Evaluation of the epidermal refractive index measured by optical coherence tomography. Skin Res Technol. 2005;12:114–8.
62. Seroul P, Hébert M, Jomier M. Hyperspectral imaging system for in-vivo quantification of skin pigments hyper-spectral imaging system for in-vivo quantification of skin pigments. In: Proceedings of the 28th IFSCC congress; 2014. p. 123–32. https://hal.science/hal-01080593.
63. Shen X, Lan S, Zhao Y, Xiong Y, Yang W, Du Y. Characterization of skin moisture and evaluation of cosmetic moisturizing properties using miniature near-infrared spectrometer. Infrared Phys Technol. 2023;132:104759. https://doi.org/10.1016/j.infrared.2023.104759.
64. Silvennoinen R, Peiponen K-E, Myller K. Specular gloss, vol. 53, no. 9. 1st ed. Elsevier; 2008.
65. Spaide RF, Fujimoto JG, Waheed NK, Sadda SR, Staurenghi G. Optical coherence tomography angiography. Prog Retin Eye Res. 2018;64:1–55. https://doi.org/10.1016/j.preteyeres.2017.11.003.
66. Taha BA, Addie AJ, Kadhim AC, Azzahran AS, Haider AJ, Chaudhary V, Arsad N. Photonics-powered augmented reality skin electronics for proactive healthcare: multifaceted opportunities. Mikrochim Acta. 2024;191(5):250. https://doi.org/10.1007/s00604-024-06314-3.
67. Takiwaki H. Measurement of skin color: practical application and theoretical considerations. J Med Investig. 1998;44:121–6.
68. Tearney GJ, Brezinski ME, Southern JF, Bouma BE, Hee MR, Fujimoto JG. Determination of the refractive index of highly scattering human tissue by optical coherence tomography. Opt Lett. 1995;20(21):2258–60. https://doi.org/10.1364/OL.20.002258.
69. Tippavajhala VK, de Oliveira Mendes T, Martin AA. In vivo human skin penetration study of sunscreens by confocal Raman spectroscopy. AAPS PharmSciTech. 2018;19(2):753–60. https://doi.org/10.1208/s12249-017-0852-8.
70. Tosato MG, dos Santos EP, de Souza Alves R, Raniero L, Menezes PFC, Kruger O, Praes CEO, Martin AA. In vivo Raman spectroscopy of biochemical changes in human skin by cosmetic application. In: Mahadevan-Jansen A, Petrich W, editors. Biomedical vibrational spectroscopy IV: advances in research and industry, vol. 7560. SPIE; 2010. p. 75600S. https://doi.org/10.1117/12.841209.
71. Trojahn C, Dobos G, Richter C, Blume-Peytavi U, Kottner J. Measuring skin aging using optical coherence tomography in vivo: a validation study. J Biomed Opt. 2015;20(4):045003. https://doi.org/10.1117/1.jbo.20.4.045003.
72. Tsumura N, Ojima N, Sato K, Shiraishi M, Shimizu H, Nabeshima H, Akazaki S, Hori K, Miyake Y. Image-based skin color and texture analysis/synthesis by extracting hemoglobin and melanin information in the skin. ACM Trans Graph. 2003;22:770–9.

73. Vasefi F, Mackinnon N, Saager RB, Durkin AJ, Chave R, Lindsley EH, Farkas DL. Polarization-sensitive hyperspectral imaging in vivo: a multimode dermoscope for skin analysis. Sci Rep. 2014;4:4924. https://doi.org/10.1038/srep04924.
74. Vasquez-Pinto LMC, Maldonado EP, Raele MP, Amaral MM, de Freitas AZ. Optical coherence tomography applied to tests of skin care products in humans—a case study. Skin Res Technol. 2015;21(1):90–3. https://doi.org/10.1111/srt.12161.
75. Vyas S, Meyerle J, Burlina P. Non-invasive estimation of skin thickness from hyperspectral imaging and validation using echography. Comput Biol Med. 2015;57:173–81. https://doi.org/10.1016/j.compbiomed.2014.12.010.
76. Wang M, Xiao K, Wuerger S, Cheung V, Luo MR. Measuring human skin colour. In: 23rd Color and imaging conference final program and proceedings. IS&T: Society for Imaging Science and Technology; 2015.
77. Wang Y, Liu S, Lou S, Zhang W, Cai H, Chen X. Application of optical coherence tomography in clinical diagnosis. J Xray Sci Technol. 2020;27(6):995–1006. https://doi.org/10.3233/XST-190559.
78. Wang J, Kuesten C, Mayne J, Majmudar G, Pappas TN. Human skin gloss perception based on texture statistics. IEEE Trans Image Process. 2021;30:3610–22. https://doi.org/10.1109/TIP.2021.3061276.
79. Weatherall IL, Coombs BD. Skin color measurements in terms of CIELAB color space values. J Invest Dermatol. 1992;99:468–73.
80. Welzel J, Lankenau E, Birngruber R, Engelhardt R. Optical coherence tomography of the human. J Am Acad Dermatol. 1997;37:958–63.
81. Wickett RP, Rluein LD, Babajanyan S. Noninvasive techniques to measure cutaneous effects of skin care products. Surfact Sci Ser. 2007;135:57–93.
82. Wienert V. Skin gloss metry. In: Elsner P, Maibach HI, Merk HF, editors. Cosmetics: controlled efficacy studies and regulation. Springer; 1999. p. 209–14. https://doi.org/10.1007/978-3-642-59869-2_17.
83. Yoshida K, Okiyama N. Estimation of reflectance, transmittance, and absorbance of cosmetic foundation layer on skin using translucency of skin. Opt Express. 2021;29(24):40038. https://doi.org/10.1364/oe.442219.
84. Zieger M, Kaatz M, Springer S, Riesenberg R, Wuttig A, Kanka M, Stanca S, Reble C, Khazaka G, Sieg R, De Gregorio M, Sattler M, Fischer F. Multi-wavelength, handheld laser speckle imaging for skin evaluation. Skin Res Technol. 2021;27(4):486–93. https://doi.org/10.1111/srt.12959.

Chapter 11
Nail Cosmetics: Safety and Regulation

Naeha Pathak and Shari R. Lipner

Introduction

Nails have many important functions, including protection, aiding in sensation, and serving cosmetic purposes [1]. Nail beautification involves a large variety of nail cosmetics, including nail polishes, hardeners, extensions, and artificial nails [1]. Nail beautification has evolved significantly over centuries, from colorants in ancient civilizations to specialized products that we use today. The earliest examples of nail coloring come from ancient Egypt and China, where natural ingredients, including flowers, henna, and egg whites were used [1, 2]. In China, red, silver, and gold colors for nails were reserved for royalty or those of high social status, while lighter shades were used by the general public [2]. Artificial nails originated around 600 BC and included gold and silver metals [2]. The popularity of nail cosmetics increased in the twentieth century with the development of modern nail polish. Modern day nail polish became commercially available in 1932, driven by Hollywood and the fashion industry [2]. Nail cosmetics are an integral part of the beauty industry today, with modern trends reflecting artistic expression. The nail cosmetic industry has broadened past simple nail polish to include gel nails, acrylic nails, nail art, and most recently, biodegradable nail products to increase sustainability. Current nail trends also appeal to individual people, favoring custom nail colors and designs that allow one to express one's own identity and personality. Furthermore, the influence of social media has helped nail cosmetics integrate into mainstream beauty culture. Because of the increase in popularity of nail cosmetics, it is imperative to understand the role of this industry on overall nail health.

N. Pathak
Icahn School of Medicine at Mount Sinai, New York, NY, USA

S. R. Lipner (✉)
Department of Dermatology, Weill Cornell Medicine, New York, NY, USA
e-mail: shl9032@med.cornell.edu

P. Elsner et al. (eds.), *Cosmetics*, https://doi.org/10.1007/978-3-032-14644-1_11

Anatomy and Physiology of Nails

An understanding of nail unit anatomy is essential to evaluate the effects of nail cosmetics on nail and skin health. The nail unit consists of several parts, with each playing an important role in nail health and function. The nail plate is the hard, visible part of the nail composed of keratin, providing protection for the underlying structures [3]. The nail matrix is located underneath the proximal nail fold and functions to produce new nail cells [3]. It is responsible for the regeneration and growth of the nail plate. Damage to the nail matrix can cause permanent damage to the nail plate [3]. The nail bed is composed of the skin underneath the nail plate [3]. It supplies nutrients to the nail and allows the nail to adhere to the digit [3]. The nail bed may also partially contribute to nail growth. The cuticle protects the nail matrix from pathogens [3]. The lunula is an opaque, half-moon shape of the nail, representing the distal end of the nail matrix [3].

Fingernails grow at an average rate of approximately 2–3 mm/month, whereas toenails grow slower at a rate of 1 mm/month [4]. Factors influencing nail growth include age, genetics, health status, smoking status, trauma or infections [4]. Poor nutrition, vitamin deficiencies, anemia, or other underlying health disorders, such as hypothyroidism or hyperthyroidism, can also affect nail growth rates [4].

The nails have multiple protective, mechanical, thermoregulatory, and cosmetic functions. Nails provide a rigid protective barrier for the distal digits [5]. The nail's free edge aids in grasping objects and scratching [5]. The nail also contributes to tactile perception by providing counter-pressure to the fingertips [5]. Glomus bodies help regulate the body's temperature by diverting blood flow from the capillaries [6].

If the nail matrix is damaged, onychodystrophy may ensue. The resulting onychodystrophy depends on the severity, duration, and location of the nail matrix injury [7]. A mild, transient, diffuse injury to the nail matrix can result in a transverse ridge across the nail plate, also known as Beau's line [7, 8]. Onychomadesis, which is the separation of the nail plate, can result if the injury to the matrix is more severe [7, 8]. Therefore, nail damage can cause cosmetic as well as functional challenges.

Cosmetic practices are often used to hide nail injuries and disorders, but they can have a profound impact on the structure and health of the nails. Excessive use of nail polish, especially those containing chemicals, including formaldehyde and toluene, can lead to nail brittleness and discoloration [1]. Moreover, frequent use of nail polish removers containing acetone can dry out and weaken the nail plate, causing discoloration and peeling [2]. Regular application of acrylic or gel nails may cause damage to the nail matrix and bed, potentially leading to onycholysis, or detachment of the nail from the nail bed [2].

Common Cosmetic Procedures and Products

Many people engage in nail cosmetic practices to make their nails more attractive and may also to camouflage nail disorders which they perceive are unsightly. While subjective, a nail is generally considered to be aesthetically pleasing if it has a smooth, glossy surface with the tip extending beyond the nail, an oval contour, and no overhanging cuticle [2].

Manicures and pedicures are at the center of the nail beautification industry. For a manicure and pedicure, the nails are cut to the desired length with clippers. The hands and feet are soaked in warm water with a mild detergent to soften the nail plate and cuticle. A foot scraper is often used to remove any rough skin or calluses. A cuticle softener comprising of alkaline substances like 0.4% sodium and potassium hydroxide is applied, which helps to dissolve the disulfide keratin bridges. The cuticle is then often pushed back with a metallic device and trimmed with a cuticle cutter. The surface of the nail is buffed to smoothen any ridges. Then, emollient cream is massaged into the skin. Following the preparation of the hands and feet, polish is applied to the nail with base coat, which has a high resin content to protect the nail from staining, followed by the polish and top coat, which instead of high resin contain more nitrocellulose to protect the polish from chipping [1, 2].

There are several types of nail polish and artificial nails that have gained popularity. Standard nail polish creates a colored film on the nail using components such as nitrocellulose and plasticizers. French manicures offer a natural look by applying pink nail polish with white tips. Nail extensions are used to alter the length of the nail, while press-on nails with adhesive backing change the nail appearance with a quick and convenient application. Acrylic nails are made from methacrylate monomers that harden through chemical or UV processes. Gel manicures are often used because of their durability and resistance to chipping, using UV-cured acrylic-based polish. Overall, these diverse nail polishes and manicures cater to varying needs and have different effects on the nail [1, 2]. Table 11.1 describes nail cosmetic types, ingredients, application methods, and technology [1, 2].

Despite the growing appeal of nail polish and professional manicures, there are inherent risks. Allergic contact dermatitis can occur from exposure to formaldehyde, toluene, or acrylates [6]. Prolonged exposure to phthalates and toluene, may pose respiratory risks and exacerbate asthma [2]. Additionally, the use of UV lamps during gel manicures raises concerns about solar lentigines, skin aging and increased skin cancer risk over time [6]. Moreover, inadequate hygiene practices in salons can lead to bacterial or fungal infections, and frequent use of acrylics or gel nails may weaken the natural nail, resulting in brittleness, thinning, and nail breakage [6].

Table 11.1 Nail cosmetic types, ingredients, application methods, and technology

Nail product	Main ingredients	Application method	Technology
UV gel	Acrylate oligomers, photoinitiators	Brush-on in layers, cured under UV/LED light	UV/LED polymerization
Nail lacquer (traditional polish)	Solvents (ethyl/butyl acetates), nitrocellulose, pigment suspender	Brush-on, air-dry	Solvent evaporation, polymer deposition
Dip powder	Cyanoacrylate resin, methacrylate powder, initiators	Brush resin, dip in powder, cure with activator	Cyanoacrylate polymerization
Liquid/powder sculptured nails (acrylics)	Methacrylate monomers, polymer powders, initiators	Liquid-powder mixture sculpted on nails	Polymerization reaction between powder and liquid
Nail polish remover	Acetone, moisturizers	Wipe or soak nails to remove polish/gel	Dissolves lacquer, softens UV gel/dip resin
Nail strengthener (solvent-based)	Alcohol, keratin crosslinkers	Brush-on, air-dry	Solvent evaporation, keratin crosslinking
Nail strengthener (lacquer-based)	Nail lacquer + reinforcing additives (starches, amino acids)	Brush-on, air-dry	Solvent evaporation, polymer deposition
Nail care (oils, creams, scrubs, masks)	Vegetable oils, botanical extracts, emulsifiers, sugar, clay	Applied by brush or hand	Various formulations (oil, emulsions, pastes)

Safety and Regulation of Nail Cosmetics

With the growing popularity of nail cosmetics products, United States and European countries have made efforts to ensure adequate quality and safety for consumers. The United States Food and Drug Administration (FDA) created the Federal Food, Drug, and Cosmetic Act for this purpose. These guidelines require that manufacturers and distributors provide the ingredient and safety information of all cosmetic products for consumers' knowledge. The FDA defines what can be considered a cosmetic product, provides regulation for adequate labeling of the products, and restricts ingredients and products with established adverse effects. It also requires clear warning statements on products with potential health hazards and statements if safety has not been tested or determined. The FDA also has implemented the Voluntary Cosmetics Regulation Program, which allows them to evaluate the safety of cosmetic products. The Cosmetic Ingredient Review Expert Panel is also part of the FDA and is an industry-funded panel of scientists with the goal of assessing the safety of different cosmetics products [9].

The European Union (EU) has similar requirements in the Cosmetic Regulation No. 1223/2009, which ensures that manufacturing information for each cosmetic product is readily available. It also ensures a "cosmetovigilance" system to report serious adverse effects of cosmetics. Under this act, the severity of adverse effects is analyzed and reported to the distributors and creators of the products as well as authorities nationwide. The EU implemented the European Community Cosmetics Directive in 2004, which mandates that all ingredients of cosmetic products be published on labels for consumers' review. Both the US and EU restricts the use of certain allergens if there is sufficient evidence from patch testing and literature [9]. These acts highlight the increasing emphasis on consumer safety, as the use of these cosmetic products become more widespread.

While these legislations are important for consumer safety, there are certain limitations. For example, there is often a delay in issuing warning or creating legislation for newly identified cosmetic allergens. For example, the EU had failed to appropriately regulate and prevent the use of methylisothiazolinone in cosmetic products in 2015, despite many reports of safety concerns [9]. Evidence-based literature on cosmetics also remains limited, resulting in increased reliance on animal studies by the FDA. However, the EU prohibits animal testing because of ethical concerns, which hinders ongoing research. Moreover, because of the increased use of online shopping, it becomes easy to import cosmetic products from other countries, where safety may be less regulated, resulting in increased exposure to harmful ingredients and potential adverse effects [9]. Therefore, increased knowledge about safety of nail cosmetic products is warranted.

Impact of Nail Cosmetics on Nail Health

Manicures and pedicures are generally safe, but there are several reported negative effects on nail and skin health. For example, cuticular cuts and "hang nails" are common with cuticle trimming, which can cause pain [2]. Irritant reactions following cuticle softeners are also observed [2]. Onychoschizia, which is peeling of the nail, can occur with aggressive nail clipping, which can cause the nails to become brittle and weak over time [1]. Buffing of the nail plate can also cause brittle and fragile nails [1]. Moreover, bacterial or fungal infections can spread from patient to patient with the use of pedicure tubs and inadequately sterilized equipment [8].

Cuticle damage is a common consequence of the nail cosmetic process, which can expose the nail to pathogens [2]. This can result in acute paronychia, an infection of the nail folds, which can then cause nail dystrophy [2]. Additionally, cuticle softeners also contain alkaline chemicals that can cause contact dermatitis [2].

Surface friability of the nail plate can occur due to use of nail products, particularly when nail polish is kept on for a while or reapplied without removing the first coat. This can result in pseudoleukonychia, or discoloration characterized by white longitudinal marks and patches, and can often mimic onychomycosis [2].

Bacterial and fungal infections may occur with nail manicures and pedicures due to inadequate sterilization of tools or disruption of the nail barrier [8]. A qualitative study of 72 establishments in Ontario reported that technicians reused almost all nail instruments without proper sterilization, and many did not wear gloves [9].

Prevention strategies include salon hygiene and appropriate sterilization of equipment as well as avoiding artificial nails, as they often trap moisture and contribute to the spread of infections [8]. Antifungal sprays or powders could be applied on their nails before applying polishes [8], but there is no evidence to suggest that they prevent fungal infections.

Nail polish, artificial nails, and nail polish removers are the most studied nail products. Dyes in nail polish, including Red no. 6, 7, and 34, and Yellow no. 5 Lake, may cause yellow-orange discoloration of the nail, which can often mimic onychomycosis, and longer use may lead to deeper penetration of the dye that only resolves if the nail is grown out [9]. Keratin degranulation can also occur with repeated use and removal of nail polish, which can result in pseudoleukonychia [2, 9].

Allergic contact dermatitis is common among people who engage in nail beautification processes. Toluene sulfonamide-formaldehyde resin (TSFR) in nail polish may cause allergic contact dermatitis of the hands, face, and eyes, often because of hand-to-face contact [9, 10]. One study of 119 people who were randomly patch tested found that 16 showed allergic reactions to TSFR [11]. Additionally, a 34-year-old woman developed a pruritic plaque involving the cheek due to allergic contact dermatitis from TSFR in nail polish [12]. Notably, one study investigating the allergic causes of periorbital eczema in 609 patients identified nail varnish as the contributing factor in 4% of cases [9]. One study of 18 patients with allergic contact dermatitis with TSFR found that 9 had to request sick leave, 4 were hospitalized due to severe dermatitis, and 2 had to change jobs entirely, thinking their work was the source of this issue [13]. Allergen metals such as nickel, chromium, and cobalt are in nail polish and can also cause allergic contact dermatitis [10]. For example, a study in Istanbul, Turkey found that 48 randomly tested cosmetic samples contained at least two allergen metals, with over 97% of products containing the metal at levels exceeding 1 μg/g, the target limit for sensitive populations [9]. Management of allergic contact dermatitis involves avoiding exposures to the allergen and using barrier creams [10].

Despite several reported reactions to TSFR, the FDA has not banned this compound, but has instead recommended caution if one has evidence of allergy. In 2015, Europe's Scientific Committee on Consumer Safety recommended the use of formaldehyde in nail products at a maximum level of 2.2%, which was decreased from the previous value of 5%. Phthalates have also been limited in Europe due to recent safety concerns such as allergic reactions, but the FDA has not restricted its use due to lack of concrete evidence of human toxicity. More studies are needed on the short- and long-term safety of nail products in humans [9]. It is also important to note the differences in regulation depending on the country where the cosmetic product is developed.

A study of 50 patients that evaluated pulse oximeter accuracy found that clear, red, and acrylic nails did not affect readings, while black and brown nail polish interfered significantly, preventing accurate readings in 12% and 64% of cases, respectively [9]. A study of 102 operating room nurses showed that there were greater number of bacterial colonies on fingernails with old, chipped nail polish that had been present for at least 4 days [14].

Artificial nails are associated with allergic contact dermatitis, particularly to methacrylate monomers [10] Reported findings have included paronychia, subungual swelling, severe pruritis, and nail dystrophy [9]. Methyl methacrylate (MMA) is associated neuropathy and permanent nail loss; therefore, its use has been largely decreased in nail products [9]. Other methacrylates, including 2-HEMA and HPMA have replaced its use, leading to other reports of allergic contact dermatitis, onycholysis, and eyelid dermatitis [9]. Additionally, cases of allergic contact dermatitis have been shown to hypoallergenic gel resins, highlighting the risk of allergic reactions even to products marketed towards sensitive skin [10].

UV-cured gel nails are associated with non-melanoma skin cancer [6]. While studies suggest that the UV dose per manicure session is relatively low, the cumulative effect of repeated exposure could lead to DNA damage over time [6]. Additional localized effects, such as nail plate thinning and degradation of the nail matrix caused by chemical and mechanical insults, further highlight the risks associated with gel nails [6].

Acetone, which is commonly used in nail polish removers, can cause dehydration of the nail plate and surrounding skin, resulting in brittleness [1]. Ingestion of acetone can cause lethargy and confusion [9]. These symptoms are often only temporary but require careful observation. Some nail polish removers contain N,N-dimethyl-p-toluidine and nitroethane, which can result in cyanosis and methemoglobinemia if ingested, requiring the use of IV fluids, oxygen, and methylene blue [9].

Impact of Nail Cosmetics on Nail Diseases

Many dermatological diseases can cause onychodystrophies, which are cosmetically cumbersome to the patient and reduce quality of life [7]. These patients may be therefore more likely to cover up the nails with nail polish, which can help conceal moderate nail dystrophy. For severe nail dystrophy, nail prosthesis may be an option for patients.

Nail psoriasis can cause pitting, ridges, thickening, and discoloration [7]. A study of 1728 nail psoriasis patients found that 93% of them were cosmetically unsatisfied with their nails [15]. Patients who conceal the nail with cosmetic nail products may have exacerbation of their nail disease, as polishes can introduce chemicals that increase nail fragility. Nail polish removers with acetone as well as nail hardeners can also dry out psoriatic nails, worsening brittleness [15]. Artificial nails, as well as manicures in general can cause acute paronychia or onycholysis, which can trigger more severe psoriatic symptoms [15]. For patients with nail psoriasis, dermatologists typically recommend nail polishes that are "hypoallergenic" and those free of formaldehyde, toluene, and other irritants [2]. Avoiding artificial nails as much as possible is also recommended [10]. Regular moisturizing of the nail and surrounding skin is also recommended to maintain nail health.

Nail lichen planus is another condition that can cause thinning and splitting of the nail [16]. Nail cosmetics can exacerbate fragility in nail lichen planus patients and cause worsening symptoms for patients. Gentle nail care, moisturizing, and avoiding harsh removers are recommended [2]. Artificial nails are not recommended, as they can exacerbate nail damage.

Alopecia areata is an inflammatory hair loss condition which can also affect the nails in some patients, causing ridging, leukonychia, and brittleness [17]. Nail cosmetics can also weaken the nails further. Dermatologists recommend regular moisturizing of the nail and surrounding skin, as well as opting for non-irritating nail products, which can help manage the cosmetic concerns without further damaging the nail integrity.

Special Populations and Considerations

Nail polishes and other cosmetic substances are generally not recommended for use in children. However, sometimes mothers use polishes on their children to avoid nail-biting habits [18]. Nail polish removers can rarely cause pneumothorax, pneumomediastinum, and respiratory obstruction in children. A 15-month-old who developed respiratory obstruction after consuming nail polish remover [18]. A similar event was observed in a 9-month-old, who ingested acetone-free nail polish remover. The child subsequently developed vomiting, hypotension, bradycardia, and a Glasgow Coma score of three. The child recovered fully in 8 h.

Tips for Consumers Visiting a Nail Salon

For people visiting nail salons, there are several things recommendations that physicians can make to their patients to optimize their health and safety. Firstly, the nail salon should be clean with sterilized equipment and clean pedicure tubs. Tools such as nail clippers, foot scrapers, and callus removers are best sterilized with autoclaving or soaking in 7.5% stabilized hydrogen peroxide for 6 h. Additionally, soaking nails in water for a few minutes before cutting prevents onychoschizia. Moreover, people should avoid cutting or excessive pushing back of the cuticle, as it can cause infection and pain. Lastly, any signs of infection, including pain, redness, swelling, or fever that is reported after going to a nail salon should be mentioned to a dermatologist for further evaluation [6].

Conclusions

Nail cosmetics, while widely used for aesthetic enhancement, can have significant effects on nail and skin health. Common concerns include cuticle damage, nail brittleness, and irritation from chemical exposure, all of which can lead to infections such as paronychia and onychomycosis. Frequent use of nail products, including polish and removers, may contribute to conditions, including pseudoleukonychia, allergic contact dermatitis, and nail plate fragility. Artificial nails and UV-cured gel nails pose additional risks, such as methacrylate-induced allergic reactions, nail dystrophy, and potential long-term UV exposure effects. Additionally, individuals with underlying nail disorders, such as psoriasis, lichen planus, or alopecia areata, may experience exacerbation of symptoms with the use of nail products. Despite these risks, preventive strategies—such as using breathable, water-based polishes, maintaining proper salon hygiene, and choosing hypoallergenic formulations—can help mitigate adverse effects. Further research is needed to better understand the long-term safety of nail cosmetics and improve regulatory guidelines for their use.

Contribution Statement Authors have all contributed substantially to the production of this manuscript.

Financial Disclosures Dr. Lipner has received research funding from Moberg Pharmaceuticals and BelleTorus Corporation.

Conflicts of Interest The authors have no conflicts of interest.

Ethical Considerations This retrospective study is exempt from informed consent. The data reviewed is a secondary analysis of existing data, does not involve intervention or interaction with human subjects, and is de-identified per the de-identification standard defined in Section §164.514(a) of the HIPAA Privacy Rule. The process by which the data is de-identified is attested to through a formal determination by a qualified expert as defined in Section §164.514(b)(1) of the HIPAA Privacy Rule. This formal determination by a qualified expert refreshed on December 2020.

References

1. Draelos ZD. Nail cosmetics and adornment. Dermatol Clin. 2021;39(2):351–9. https://doi.org/10.1016/j.det.2021.01.001. PMID: 33745645.
2. Madnani NA, Khan KJ. Nail cosmetics. Indian J Dermatol Venereol Leprol. 2012;78(3):309–17. https://doi.org/10.4103/0378-6323.95445. PMID: 22565430.
3. de Berker D. Nail anatomy. Clin Dermatol. 2013;31(5):509–15. https://doi.org/10.1016/j.clindermatol.2013.06.006. PMID: 24079579.
4. Yaemsiri S, Hou N, Slining MM, He K. Growth rate of human fingernails and toenails in healthy American young adults. J Eur Acad Dermatol Venereol. 2010;24(4):420–3. https://doi.org/10.1111/j.1468-3083.2009.03426.x. Epub 2009 Sept 8. PMID: 19744178.

5. Baswan S, Kasting GB, Li SK, Wickett R, Adams B, Eurich S, Schamper R. Understanding the formidable nail barrier: a review of the nail microstructure, composition and diseases. Mycoses. 2017;60(5):284–95. https://doi.org/10.1111/myc.12592. Epub 2017 Jan 18. PMID: 28098391; PMCID: PMC5383514.
6. Iorizzo M, Piraccini BM, Tosti A. Nail cosmetics in nail disorders. J Cosmet Dermatol. 2007;6(1):53–8. https://doi.org/10.1111/j.1473-2165.2007.00290.x. PMID: 17348997.
7. Lee DK, Lipner SR. Optimal diagnosis and management of common nail disorders. Ann Med. 2022;54(1):694–712. https://doi.org/10.1080/07853890.2022.2044511. PMID: 35238267; PMCID: PMC8896184.
8. Winthrop KL, Albridge K, South D, Albrecht P, Abrams M, Samuel MC, et al. The clinical management and outcome of nail salon acquired *Mycobacterium fortuitum* skin infections. Clin Infect Dis. 2004;38:38–44.
9. Arora H, Tosti A. Safety and efficacy of nail products. Cosmetics. 2017;4:24.
10. Lazzarini R, Duarte I, de Farias DC, Santos CA, Tsai AI. Frequency and main sites of allergic contact dermatitis caused by nail varnish. Dermatitis. 2008;19:319–22.
11. Groot AC, Bruynzeel DP, Bos JD, Meeren H, Joost TV, Jagtman BA, Weyland JW. The allergens in cosmetics. Arch Dermatol. 1988;124(10):1525–9.
12. Boehncke WH, Schmitt M, Zollner TM, Hensel O, Nail polish allergy. An important differential diagnosis in contact dermatitis. Dtsch Med Wochenschr. 1997;122:849–85.
13. Liden C, Berg M, Farm G, Wrangsjö K. Nail varnish allergy with far-reaching consequences. Br J Dermatol. 1993;128:57–62.
14. Wynd CA, Samstag DE, Lapp AM. Bacterial carriage on the fingernails of OR nurses. AORN J. 1994;60:99–805.
15. Dogra A, Arora AK. Nail psoriasis: the journey so far. Indian J Dermatol. 2014;59(4):319–33. https://doi.org/10.4103/0019-5154.135470. PMID: 25071247; PMCID: PMC4103264.
16. Gupta MK, Lipner SR. Review of nail lichen planus: epidemiology, pathogenesis, diagnosis, and treatment. Dermatol Clin. 2021;39(2):221–30. https://doi.org/10.1016/j.det.2020.12.002. Epub 2021 Feb 10. PMID: 33745635.
17. Pelzer C, Iorizzo M. Alopecia areata of the nails: diagnosis and management. J Clin Med. 2024;13(11):3292. https://doi.org/10.3390/jcm13113292. PMID: 38893003; PMCID: PMC11172645.
18. Brown JJ, Nanayakkara CS. Acetone-free nail polish removers: are they safe? Clin Toxicol (Phila). 2005;43:297–9.

Chapter 12
Hyperpigmentation Agents

Tamara Rogers and Ludger Kolbe

Abbreviations

AMPK	AMP-activated protein kinase
cAMP	Cyclic adenosine monophosphate
mTOR	Mammalian target of rapamycin
PIH	Post-inflammatory hyperpigmentation
TRP-1	Tyrosinase-related protein 1

Abstract

Hyperpigmentation disorders encompass a diverse range of skin conditions marked by increased melanin production or uneven melanin distribution, leading to significant psychological and emotional distress for affected individuals. The regulation of melanogenesis, primarily mediated by the enzyme tyrosinase, is discussed in detail in this chapter, highlighting its pivotal role in melanin synthesis and the challenges associated with targeting this pathway for therapeutic intervention.

Special emphasis is placed on the development of topical agents, particularly tyrosinase inhibitors, which have emerged as the primary focus in the search for effective treatments. While traditional agents like hydroquinone have been widely used, their associated side effects and regulatory restrictions have spurred interest in alternative compounds. The chapter critically evaluates the efficacy and safety profiles of emerging agents, including Thiamidol, which has shown to be the most effective inhibitor of human tyrosinase.

T. Rogers · L. Kolbe (✉)
R&D, Beiersdorf AG, Hamburg, Germany
e-mail: Tamara.Rogers@Beiersdorf.com; Ludger.Kolbe@Beiersdorf.com

P. Elsner et al. (eds.), *Cosmetics*, https://doi.org/10.1007/978-3-032-14644-1_12

In addition to tyrosinase inhibition, the chapter discusses alternative strategies, such as targeting the expression of tyrosinase and its regulatory factors. However, these approaches may carry a higher risk of side effects due to their broader impact on cellular functions.

As our understanding of melanogenesis deepens, the development of safe and effective depigmenting agents that target new mechanisms continues to evolve. Future treatments may involve multi-targeted approaches to enhance therapeutic efficacy while minimizing side effects, ultimately leading to improved outcomes for individuals affected by hyperpigmentation.

Introduction

Hyperpigmentation disorders represent a wide spectrum of skin conditions characterized by an increase in melanin production or uneven distribution of melanin. While these conditions are generally harmless, they can produce significant psychological and emotional distress [9, 84]. These dark, hyperpigmented lesions, especially on the face, neck, and hands, can lead to reduced self-esteem in affected individuals and impact their quality of life.

Hyperpigmentation affects all age groups and skin types, but primarily occurs in those with Fitzpatrick skin types III to VI [23]. The most common conditions of hyperpigmentation are solar lentigines, melasma and post-inflammatory hyperpigmentation (PIH). These skin conditions can be caused by both intrinsic factors like genetics and hormonal fluctuations, and extrinsic factors including sun exposure, medications, injuries or burns [31, 128]. Their etiology is complex, involving multiple biological pathways, making it a challenge for patients and dermatologists, as treatment often requires a multifaceted approach and long-term commitment.

Topical agents are the standard treatment for hyperpigmentation due to their accessibility and non-invasive nature. Hydroquinone has long been considered the gold standard for topical depigmentation [34]; however, it is associated with various side effects, including skin irritation, contact dermatitis, and exogenous ochronosis [86, 99, 137]. These safety concerns triggered regulatory restrictions in many countries. In 2020, the FDA banned the use of 2% hydroquinone in OTC products, therefore, hydroquinone is only available in prescription drugs and not in cosmetic skin care products. These restrictions and concerns on hydroquinone have driven the search for alternative agents with comparable efficacy and improved safety [64].

Regulation of Melanogenesis

Melanogenesis is a tightly regulated and complex biological process, responsible for the production of melanin within melanocytes. In these specialized cells, melanin is synthesized and stored in organelles knowns as melanosomes, which subsequently transfer the pigment to surrounding keratinocytes. This process is governed by the activation of various enzymes, the coordination of intracellular signaling pathways and the regulation of transcriptional mechanisms.

The synthesis of melanin starts with the amino acid L-tyrosine, which is converted into dopaquinone, resulting in the formation of melanin pigments. Tyrosinase, a melanocyte-specific enzyme, plays a crucial role in this process by catalyzing several reactions. Besides tyrosinase, there are currently over 125 genes identified as being directly or indirectly associated with melanogenesis, indicating a significant risk for dysregulation and the onset of pigmentary disorders [7, 13].

Various strategies to reduce hyperpigmentation have been described and used during the last decades. Since excessive melanin synthesis is the central event in hyperpigmentary disorders, these strategies can be separated into three groups [22] based on their interference with the melanogenesis. Interventions before melanin synthesis aim to reduce the transcription of important genes for pigmentation enzymes (Fig. 12.1). Interventions during melanin synthesis mainly aim to inhibit enzymes, mainly tyrosinase, to reduce melanin production. Mechanisms after melanin production mainly comprise inhibition of melanin transfer to keratinocytes or acceleration of epidermal turnover. Each target mechanism encompasses numerous agents that have demonstrated some efficacy in the treatment of pigmentary disorders.

The following chapter provides a comprehensive overview of the most promising hyperpigmentation agents, focusing on their mechanisms of action, clinical efficacy and safety.

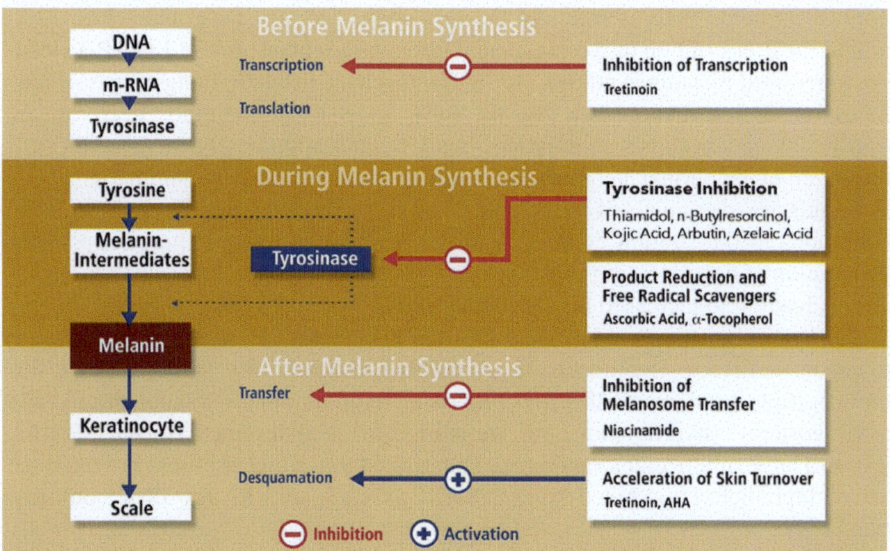

Fig. 12.1 Pigmentation targets and effective agents

Tyrosinase

The most prominent target for treating hyperpigmentation is tyrosinase, the key enzyme in melanin production. Tyrosinase, a copper-containing glycoprotein, is the rate-limiting, melanocyte-specific enzyme, catalyzing the conversion of tyrosine to melanin in the melanin biosynthesis pathway [109]. Tyrosinase has two enzyme activities. The monophenolase activity (hydroxylation of monophenols to diphenols) converts tyrosine to dopa, the diphenolase activity (oxidation of diphenols to quinones) catalyzes the oxidation of dopa to dopaquinone. These are complex reactions using molecular oxygen as co-substrate. The conversion rate (k_{cat}) of tyrosinase is about 140/s, which means that every tyrosinase produces 140 molecules dopaquinone/s [32]. This adds up to more than 12 million dopaquinone molecules per day per enzyme. Thus, only very efficient inhibitors would have an impact on skin hyperpigmentation.

Nevertheless, given its central role in melanogenesis, reduction of tyrosinase activity has emerged as a primary target in the treatment of hyperpigmentation disorders. For decades, downregulation of tyrosinase protein expression or inhibition of tyrosinase enzyme activity has been the main target for the development of depigmenting agents.

Downregulation of Melanocyte Activity

Retinoids

Topical retinoids such as tretinoin, retinol, adapalene, and tazarotene (Fig. 12.2) inhibit the transcription of tyrosinase and tyrosinase-related protein 1 (TRP-1) leading to reduced melanin synthesis [107]. The mechanisms underlying effects of retinoids on depigmentation are not yet fully understood. Retinoids decrease the transfer of melanosomes to keratinocytes [94] and additionally increase the cell turn-over of epidermal keratinocytes leading to accelerated melanin loss [141]. Retinoids are also involved in the control of cell differentiation. Retinoid-induced alterations in the stratum corneum and the permeability barrier may support the penetration of depigmenting substances in the epidermis and enhance their bioavailability, leading to increased loss of melanin [94].

For hyperpigmentation, retinoids are used in combination with other substances to enhance efficacy. The most common combination is known as the Kligman formula or triple combination therapy comprising hydroquinone, a topical retinoid and a corticosteroid (hydroquinone 5%, tretinoin 0.1%, and dexamethasone 0.1%) [62, 94]. In a large, multicenter, randomized controlled trial a higher efficacy of the three active ingredients combined was reported as compared to any dual combination [127].

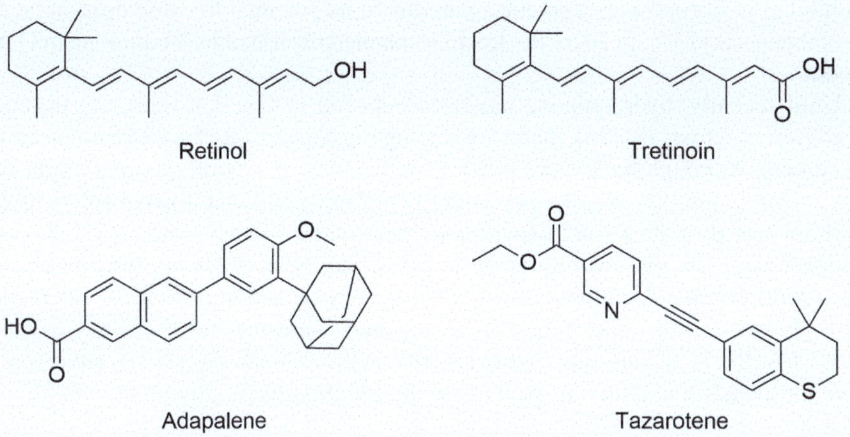

Fig. 12.2 Structures of retinol, tretinoin, adapalene and tazarotene

A study using a topical 0.1% tretinoin formulation in the treatment of melasma demonstrated a significant clinical improvement. However, this improvement took time and was first visible after 24 weeks of treatment [43]. Also, in melasma, the risk of secondary hyperpigmentation due to retinoid-induced irritation is high [100]. The most effective retinoids (tretinoin, tazarotene) are prescription drugs, adapalene and retinol are available in OTC products and/or cosmetic products.

Hydroquinone

Hydroquinone is a phenolic compound (Fig. 12.3) widely recognized as the gold standard for topical treatment of hyperpigmentation disorders such as melasma, lentigines, and post-inflammatory hyperpigmentation. Its clinical efficacy was first demonstrated in 1961, in a study where 45% of the patients treated with 1.5%–2% hydroquinone showed successful depigmentation [123]. In 1975, the triple combination cream by Kligman was introduced, combining 5% hydroquinone, 0.1% tretinoin and 0.1% dexamethasone acetate [62]. Since then, hydroquinone has become the most popular and one of the most efficient treatments of melasma. However, its topical use was associated with adverse effects including erythema, irritation and burning [127]. Long-term use of hydroquinone has been reported to increase the risk of developing exogenous ochronosis, a cutaneous disorder characterized by blue-black pigmentation [37, 53, 120, 126]. Currently, hydroquinone has been

Fig. 12.3 Structure of hydroquinone

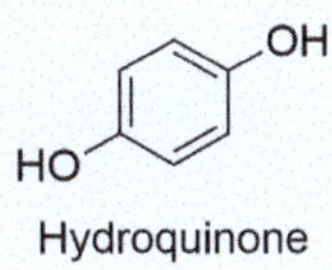

prohibited in Europe as a cosmetic agent due to its potential to cause drug-induced carcinogenesis [137]. In 2020, the US FDA banned the use of hydroquinone in OTC products.

Until recently, hydroquinone has been believed to function primarily through inhibition of tyrosinase [26], thereby reducing the conversion of tyrosine to melanin precursors. Although there were previous indications that hydroquinone might act as a substrate [45, 95, 96], the prevailing belief remained that it acted solely as an inhibitor based on data from experiments with *mushroom* tyrosinase [55]. Recent evidence suggests that hydroquinone is not an inhibitor of *human* tyrosinase, the IC_{50} (concentration for inhibition of 50% of enzyme activity) is above 4000 μM [78]. Hydroquinone rather functions as a pseudo-substrate for human tyrosinase [51]. Most likely, the ensuing highly reactive hydroquinone-derivatives are responsible for the adverse effects as well as for the efficacy [52].

Metformin

Metformin is widely known as a medication for managing diabetes, but recent research has revealed its potential effects on skin pigmentation (Fig. 12.4). This role is primarily due to its inhibitory effect on the AMP-activated protein kinase (AMPK)–mammalian target of rapamycin (mTOR) signaling pathway, which is essential for cellular metabolism and signaling processes [132]. It has been discovered that metformin not only decreases intracellular levels of cyclic adenosine monophosphate (cAMP), a well-known modulator of melanin synthesis [85], but also effectively modulates melanogenesis by reducing the basal levels of key melanogenic proteins, including tyrosinase, TRP-1, and TRP-2 [70]. Additionally, metformin was found to reduce forskolin and α-MSH-induced increases in these proteins, indicating its potential to inhibit melanin production at multiple points in the melanogenic pathway. In mice, the topical application of metformin on tail skin resulted in significant skin lightening. In human skin biopsies and reconstructed human epidermis, treatment with metformin also reduced melanin levels [70], although at very high concentrations (10,000 μM). Preliminary *in vivo* studies in melasma patients showed some efficacy but more studies with higher patient numbers are needed [88].

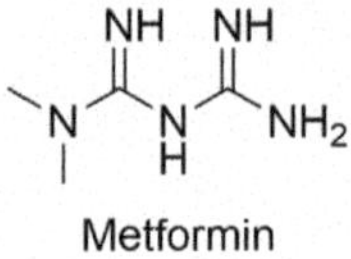

Fig. 12.4 Structure of metformin

Inhibition of Tyrosinase Enzyme Activity

As tyrosinase represents the most prominent and successful target for melanogenesis inhibitors, many commercially available topical skin lightening substances in cosmetic products belong to this group of inhibitors [101].

The three-dimensional structures of several tyrosinases were recently resolved, among them the structures of mushroom tyrosinase [49] and of two bacterial enzymes from Streptomyces castaneoglobisporus [83] and Bacillus megaterium [115]. However, very little kinetic or structural information is available for human tyrosinase, mainly because of substantial difficulties in obtaining sufficient amounts of human tyrosinase from natural sources or by heterologous expression. It has been transiently expressed in various animal cell lines [93, 113, 129, 136], but yields were always very low. More recently, several groups have developed more efficient expression systems [27, 40, 66], but data on the three-dimensional structure are still missing.

Therefore, a commercially available tyrosinase derived from the mushroom *Agaricus bisporus* is often utilized in *in vitro* models in search for new depigmenting agents targeting human tyrosinase. However, tyrosinase enzymes differ significantly across species and substances tested with a tyrosinase from one species may not significantly inhibit tyrosinase from another species. Therefore, most tyrosinase inhibitors screened to inhibit mushroom tyrosinase, display only limited efficacy against human tyrosinase [27, 69] and clinical efficacy often remains unsatisfactory.

The below paragraphs describe various tyrosinase inhibitors used in topical formulations. The selection is based on the significance of the available scientific data and the usage in topical cosmetic/dermatological products on the market. The substances are listed in alphabetical order. When available, data on inhibition of recombinant human tyrosinase [27] are given as $IC_{50,}$ the concentration needed to inhibit 50% of the enzyme activity.

Arbutin

Arbutin is the β-d-glucopyranoside of hydroquinone (Fig. 12.5) and is found in the leaves of bearberries (*Arctostaphylos uva-ursi*) and in smaller quantities in cranberry and blueberry leaves [140, 146].

In cultured human melanocytes, arbutin inhibited tyrosinase activity at noncytotoxic concentrations in the millimolar range [76]. It did not affect the expression of tyrosinase mRNA. For the inhibition of recombinant human tyrosinase, the IC_{50} was found to be above 4000 μM [78]. Arbutin also inhibited melanosome maturation and was in cell-based antioxidant assays utilizing erythrocytes and skin fibroblasts demonstrated to exerted strong antioxidant activity [19, 125]. However, it was also reported that arbutin-containing formulations might not be free of hydroquinone

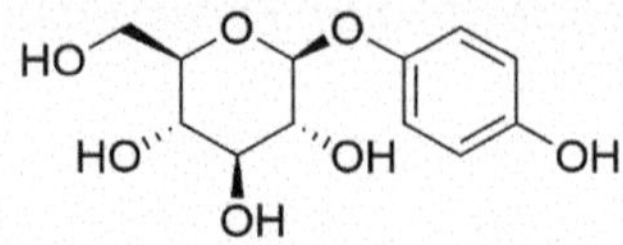

Fig. 12.5 Structure of arbutin

due to arbutin's decomposition to hydroquinone induced by either the skin's natural microbiota [11] or UV radiation [24].

In vivo, it was shown in women suffering from melasma and lentigines, that treatment with an arbutin cream twice daily for 8 weeks leads to skin lightening and evenness of skin tone [89].

Azelaic Acid

Azelaic acid is a dicarboxylic acid which is naturally produced by *Malassezia* spp. [111] (Fig. 12.6). Azelaic acid was initially developed as a topical anti-acne agent but due to its effect on tyrosinase, it has also been used to treat hyperpigmentation disorders like melasma [10]. Azelaic acid competitively inhibits tyrosinase activity effectively reducing melanogenesis [20]. Inhibition of recombinant human tyrosinase is weak with an IC_{50} above 2800 μM. By targeting the mitochondrion, azelaic acid damages human hyperactive and malignant melanocytes without affecting normal cells [104]. *In vitro*, azelaic acid can reduce DNA synthesis leading to decreased proliferation and differentiation of melanocytes [72]. Additionally, azelaic acid exerts a significant anti-inflammatory activity and was shown to be a scavenger of free radicals [97, 98].

In patients with melasma, treatment with a skin cream containing 20% azelaic acid for 6 months resulted in the same melasma-reducing efficacy as therapy with 4% hydroquinone [8].

Topical application of up to 20% azelaic acid is generally well tolerated, with the primary side effects being mild and temporary sensations of stinging, burning or itching [2, 38].

Butylresorcinol, Hexylresorcinol and Phenylethylresorcinol

The 4-substituted resorcinol motif has been known for a long time as a chemical moiety for the inhibition of human tyrosinase [59] (Fig. 12.7). Many natural compounds, mainly flavonoids, known as whitening ingredients, contain this resorcinol

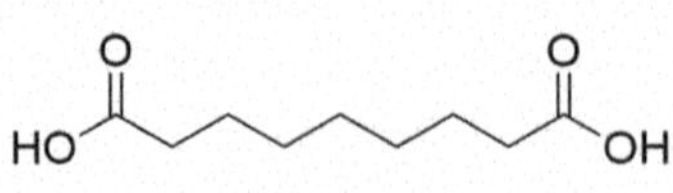

Fig. 12.6 Structure of azelaic acid

motif [6, 118]. Unfortunately, the bioavailability of flavonoids is generally very low, and therefore smaller resorcinols with high effectiveness and good bioavailability were developed.

Among these resorcinol-motif containing compounds, 4-butylresorcinol has been characterized as a strong mushroom tyrosinase and TRP-1 inhibitor [58, 60]. The IC_{50} for mushroom tyrosinase is 0.6 μM, however, for human tyrosinase the IC_{50} is 21 μM [78]. In artificial skin models, butylresorcinol inhibits melanin production with an IC_{50} of 13.5 μM. Butylresorcinol-containing formulations have been shown to be effective in treatment of melasma, age spot and post-inflammatory hyperpigmentation [18, 63, 75].

For hexyresorcinol the IC_{50} for mushroom tyrosinase is around 1 μM, inhibition of human tyrosinase is significantly less efficient with an IC_{50} of 94 μM. For the treatment of hyperpigmentation, hexylresorcinol is often combined with other active ingredients like niacinamide, resveratrol, silymarin and vitamin C [28, 33, 35, 116].

Phenylethylresorcinol is another resorcinol-motif containing compound used in many cosmetic products. Tyrosinase inhibition was determined with an IC_{50} of 0.2 μM for mushroom tyrosinase and 131 μM for the human enzyme [63, 112, 131]. Stable formulation and effective topical delivery are challenging, and several investigations on topical delivery and carrier systems were published [4, 65, 73, 144].

In a study directly comparing 0.3% butylresorcinol, 0.3% hexylresorcinol and 0.5% phenylethylresorcinol, it was found that butylresorcinol is more effective than hexylresorcinol which is more effective than phenylethylresorcinol [63].

Cysteamine

Cysteamine is a naturally occurring aminothiol, first recognized in the mid-twentieth century as a byproduct from the degradation pathway of Coenzyme A [16, 25] (Fig. 12.8). It has since been identified as a modulator of melanogenesis, primarily through its ability to suppress tyrosinase activity and reduce melanocyte overstimulation [50, 103]. Its precise mechanism of action remains only partially elucidated, however, cysteamine is known to increase intracellular glutathione levels, shifting from eumelanin to pheomelanin production [30, 121]. Its thiol structure may contribute to its depigmenting effects, as thiol-containing compounds are capable of

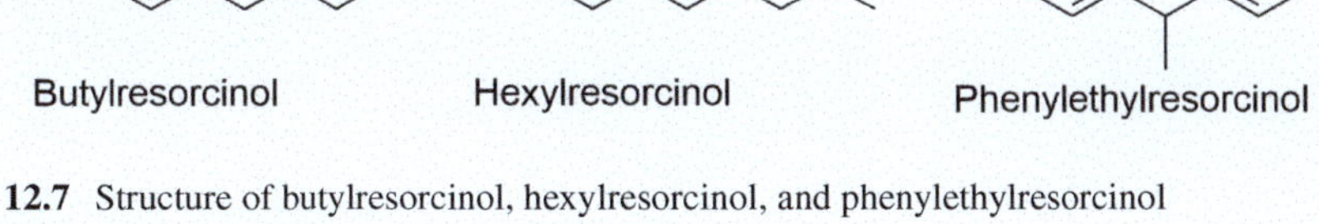

Fig. 12.7 Structure of butylresorcinol, hexylresorcinol, and phenylethylresorcinol

Fig. 12.8 Structure of cysteamine

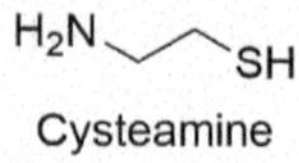

inhibiting both tyrosinase and peroxidase [57]. Additionally, these compounds can scavenge dopaquinone and chelate metal ions such as iron and copper, thereby disrupting oxidative reactions that facilitate pigment formation [12, 117]. However, cysteamine does not significantly inhibit purified recombinant human tyrosinase and IC_{50} could not be calculated.

In a double-blinded, randomized controlled study, its therapeutic efficacy has been demonstrated, leading to a 20% reduction in MASI after application of 5% cysteamine over 16 weeks [92].

Cysteamine is generally well tolerated but side effects include erythema, dryness, itching, burning, and irritation, with itching and burning being the most common [36, 56, 82].

Glabridin

Cosmetic products containing licorice extracts for skin whitening has a long history of use [74] and is available in many skin care products today. Glabridin is the main ingredient in licorice for treatment of hyperpigmentation (Fig. 12.9). Glabridin binds to tyrosinase with a reversible noncompetitive mode and inhibits with an IC_{50} value of 0.43 μM [26]. However, inhibition of recombinant human tyrosinase is low, only 19% at 30 μM, and no IC_{50} was achieved because higher concentrations were insoluble. Despite its popularity, data on clinical efficacy is scarce. In an uncontrolled open-label study to evaluate the appearance of epidermal melasma, a gel formulation containing glabridin, andrographolide, and apolactoferrin showed some efficacy. Commercial licorice extracts usually contain low concentrations of glabridin and its pure solubility make it difficult to formulate effective concentrations.

Fig. 12.9 Structure of glabridin

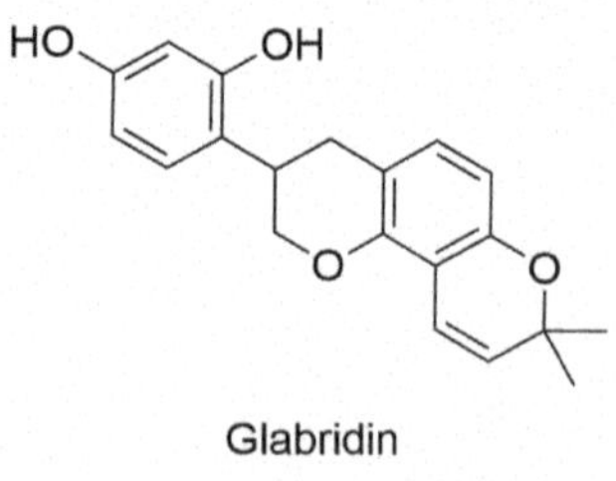

Glutathione

Glutathione (γ-glutamyl-cysteinylglycine) is a small, water-soluble thiol-tripeptide with important functions in the cellular redox cycle (Fig. 12.10). It has gained some popularity as oral and intravenous skin whitening ingredient but there is only limited evidence for efficacy [122]. Oral glutathione had only limited efficacy even at high concentrations. Intravenous application is contraindicated due to lack efficacy and high risk of severe side effects. The available research indicated that glutathione has moderate to low efficacy as a skin-lightening agent in topical formulations [110].

Kojic Acid

Kojic acid (5-hydroxy-2-hydroxymethyl-4-pyrone) is an organic acid produced by fungal species such as Acetobacter, Aspergillus, and Penicillium [108] (Fig. 12.11). Kojic acid acts as a tyrosinase inhibitor, but additionally exerts antioxidant, antimicrobial and antiaging effects [108, 114, 147]. However, the essential mechanism of the inhibition of tyrosinase is the chelation of the active copper site of the enzyme. Inhibition of purified recombinant human tyrosinase revealed an IC_{50} of >500 μM [78]. Also, the suppression of the tautomerization of dopachrome to 5,6-dihydroxyindole-2-carboxylic acid contributes to kojic acid's depigmenting activity [41, 147]. Kojic acid is not oil soluble, displays a sensitivity to light and heat resulting in a low stability [67] which makes the development of topical formulations challenging. Side effects of kojic acid include contact dermatitis, sensitization, redness and erythema [41, 147]. Considering concerns related to potential endocrine disrupting properties of kojic acid, the Scientific Committee for Consumer Safety (European Commission) has the opinion that kojic acid—as a skin lightening agent in cosmetic products—is safe for the consumer up to a maximum concentration of 0.7% kojic acid in the final product [14].

In vivo, in the treatment of photodamage, lentigines, and hyperpigmented scars, kojic acid was shown to be efficacious [108, 114].

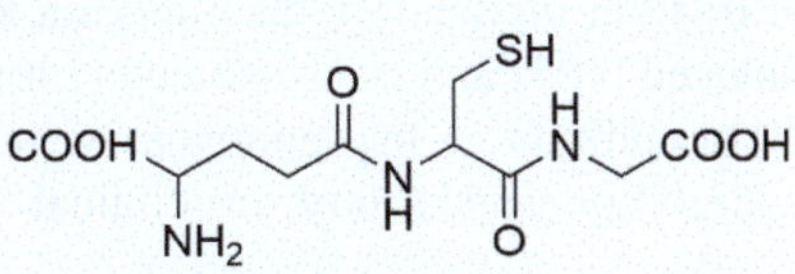

Glutathione

Fig. 12.10 Structure of glutathione

Fig. 12.11 Structure of kojic acid

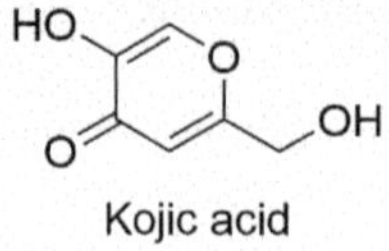

4-Methoxysalicylate (4-MSK)

Potassium 4-methoxysalicylate (4MSK) is a derivative of salicylic acid that was approved in 2003 in Japan as a skin lightening active ingredient (Fig. 12.12). 4-MSK suppresses melanin production by inhibiting tyrosinase. The IC_{50} for mushroom tyrosinase is with 4020 µM rather high. Inhibition of recombinant human tyrosinase was not detectable. Therefore, the mode of action is probably not tyrosinase inhibition. A recent publication [119] showed that 4-MSK slightly reduces melanin production in cultured melanocytes and also changes the expression of keratinocyte markers, like keratin 1, keratin 10, filaggrin and involucrin. 4-MSK might have a mild peeling effect. A clinical study with 3% 4-MSK showed an increase in skin lightness.

Thiamidol

Thiamidol (isobutylamido thiazolyl resorcinol) is a synthetic compound specifically developed to target hyperpigmentation by inhibiting human tyrosinase (Fig. 12.13). Unlike previous compounds that were screened using mushroom tyrosinase—often resulting in limited clinical relevance—Thiamidol was identified in a screening of over 50,000 molecules as the most effective candidate against the human form of the enzyme [78, 79]. The IC_{50} of Thiamidol is 1.1 µM, which makes it the most effective inhibitor of human tyrosinase. Thiamidol acts by reversibly binding to the active site of the enzyme, thereby blocking the conversion of L-DOPA to melanin. Interestingly, Thiamidol is a relatively weak inhibitor of mushroom tyrosinase with an IC_{50} of 108 µM, showing how misleading screening of inhibitors with mushroom tyrosinase can be. The targeted mechanism of Thiamidol makes it highly effective in treating pigmentary disorders such as melasma [5], solar lentigines [78], acne-induced [105] and laser-induced [130] post-inflammatory hyperpigmentation.

In addition to its depigmenting action, Thiamidol has demonstrated excellent tolerability and safety in clinical trials. Patients using topical formulations

Fig. 12.12 Structure of 4-MSK

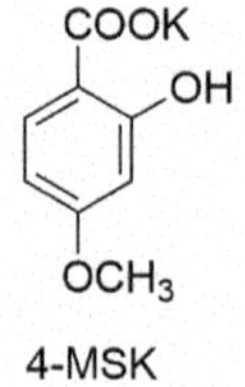

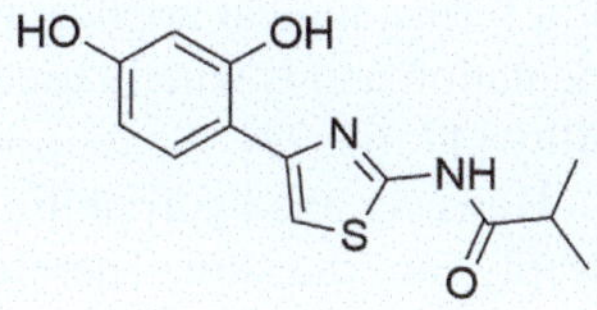
Thiamidol

Fig. 12.13 Structure of thiamidol

containing Thiamidol showed significant reductions in melanin levels and visible improvements in skin tone within as little as 4 weeks. In a 24-week treatment study, Thiamidol continuously improved melasma over the entire period in comparison to the sunscreen group. After cessation, the MASI scores of the Thiamidol group increased to the level of the sunscreen group, showing the reversibility of Thiamidol's mode of action [106]. When compared to hydroquinone (2%) in a double-blind randomized study, 0.2% thiamidol was found to be significantly more efficacious than hydroquinone [5]. In another study the original Kligman's trio (5% hydroquinone, 0.1% retinoic acid, and 0.1% dexamethasone acetate) was compared to a new trio, where they combined 0.1% Thiamidol, 0.1% retinoic acid, and 0.1% dexamethasone acetate [15]. The authors found that the new trio improved melasma at least as good as the original Kligman's trio, but with much better skin tolerability. The quality of life (MelasQoL score) was significantly improved only by the new trio with Thiamidol.

The mild and reversible efficacy of Thiamidol makes it a safe treatment for long-term use against hyperpigmentation.

Tranexamic Acid

Tranexamic acid (TXA) is well-known anti-fibrinolytic oral drug, the efficacy on skin hyperpigmentation was identified as a side effect (Fig. 12.14). Its mechanism of action is not fully understood; however, it has been shown that TXA not only reduces inflammation by inhibiting plasmin [1, 46, 68, 138], but also reduces melanogenesis by interfering with tyrosinase activity [143]. However, recombinant human tyrosinase was not inhibited significantly, no IC_{50} could be determined [80]. Additionally, TXA suppresses the release of inflammatory mediators such as prostaglandins and leukotrienes—substances known to stimulate melanocyte activity and pigment formation [48, 134, 139].

Clinical studies have shown that both oral and topical formulations of TXA can significantly improve conditions like melasma over time. Although slower than its

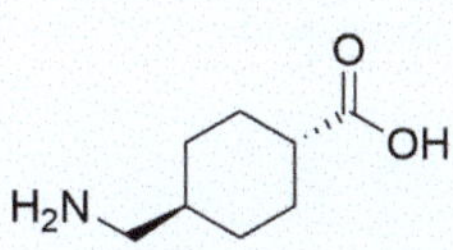
Tranexamic acid

Fig. 12.14 Structure of tranexamic acid

oral forms, topical application of 2%–5% TXA can effectively suppress hyperpigmentation and is widely used despite reported skin irritation and formulation instability [47, 61, 77].

However, the hydrophilic nature of tranexamic acid limits its ability to penetrate deeply into the skin. Therefore, liposomal formulations and ester derivatives have been developed. Both strategies have shown to improve the skin penetration and reduce the risk for skin irritation [81, 142].

Antioxidants for the Treatment of Hyperpigmentation

Oxidative stress, often triggered by UV radiation, pollution, or inflammation, can activate melanocytes and upregulate tyrosinase activity, leading to increased melanin synthesis. Antioxidants, therefore, can be used to treat skin hyperpigmentation by scavenging free radicals and reducing the oxidative conversion of melanin precursors [91]. However, antioxidants can only reduce the excessive stimulation of melanin production. Therefore, they can be used to reduce UV-induced darkening of hyperpigmented spots but not to lighten established spots to background skin color [29].

Many antioxidants are used in topical products, mainly in combination with other ingredients because their efficacy as single compound is too low for significant effects on human skin.

Many tyrosinase inhibitors also have antioxidative properties but the only antioxidant discussed in this section is vitamin C (ascorbic acid). While ascorbic acid is also a tyrosinase inhibitor, its main function in treatment of hyperpigmentation is prevention of melanin oxidation.

Ascorbic Acid and Derivatives

Ascorbic acid or vitamin C is a natural antioxidant isolated from citrus fruits and certain green vegetables (Fig. 12.15). Vitamin C acts as an antioxidant to help neutralize reactive oxygen species which can stimulate melanocyte activity and increase pigmentation [135]. Additionally, it interacts with copper ions at the active site of tyrosinase, thereby blocking the conversion of tyrosine to melanin [90]. The IC_{50} for inhibition of recombinant human tyrosinase is around 65 μM [80]. Interestingly, in

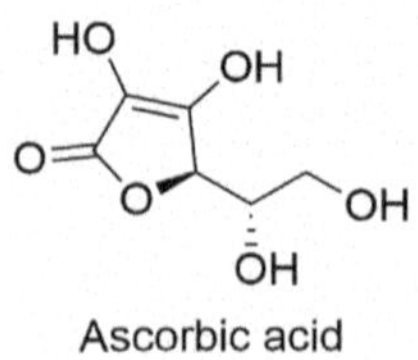

Fig. 12.15 Structure of ascorbic acid

melanoDerm skin models no significant inhibition was found, probably because the skin models use ascorbic acid completely for their redox homeostasis.

Vitamin C is an unstable compound, which oxidizes quickly and decomposes in aqueous solutions. The penetration of vitamin C into the skin is limited. As acidity improves stability as well as penetration, the pH of ascorbic acid in formulation must be below 4 [3, 124]. Further, several lipid-soluble analogues and derivatives have been developed, to overcome the repulsion of vitamin C by epidermal cells and to improve its penetration [102, 124]. The inhibition of recombinant human tyrosinase by the vitamin C derivatives ascorbic acid 2-glucoside, 3-o-cetyl ascorbic acid, Mg ascorbyl palmitate and ascorbyl tetraisopalmitate is rather low, not achieving an IC_{50}. These derivatives probably have to be metabolized in skin to the free ascorbic acid to be effective.

Ascorbic acid and its more stable derivatives are widely used as antioxidant in cosmetics products. Although its efficacy against hyperpigmentation as single active ingredient is rather low, it is often used in combination with other anti-pigment ingredients to boost efficacy.

Inhibition of Melanosome Transfer

Reducing the transfer of melanosomes from melanocytes to keratinocytes is another method to inhibit skin pigmentation. Melanosome transfer is a biological process, in which the melanin-containing melanosomes are transferred from melanocytes to surrounding keratinocytes [21]. In hyperpigmentation disorders, this transfer process becomes dysregulated or overactive, leading to excessive pigment deposition in the upper layers of the skin.

Niacinamide

Niacinamide, the physiologically active amide of vitamin B3, has variable effects on melanogenesis, with reports showing increased, decreased, or no effect on tyrosinase activity and melanin synthesis [71, 133] (Fig. 12.16). Despite controversial results, niacinamide is a known topical agent in the treatment of hyperpigmentation, primarily due to its capability to inhibit melanosome transfer from melanocytes to keratinocytes [42, 44]. *In vitro* studies have shown that niacinamide at very high concentration (1000 μM) can inhibit melanosome transfer by 35%–68%, and that

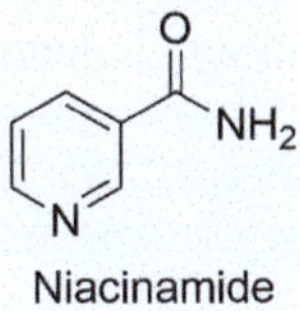

Fig. 12.16 Structure of niacinamide

disrupting the interaction between melanocytes and keratinocytes, can lead to the downregulation of melanogenesis.

In vivo studies have demonstrated that niacinamide significantly reduces hyperpigmentation and increased skin lightness, with visible improvements observed after 4 weeks of use [44].

Besides, niacinamide exhibits antioxidant properties by preventing oxidation of lipids and proteins, and by inhibiting the generation of reactive oxygen species [54, 145]. It has also been shown that niacinamide reduces UV-induced erythema by suppressing the production of pro-inflammatory cytokines, e.g. IL-6, IL-8 and TNF-α [17, 87].

Discussion

Hyperpigmentation disorders, including melasma, lentigines, and post-inflammatory hyperpigmentation, are complex biological processes, regulated many different genes. However, with tyrosinase playing a crucial role in its etiology it has become the primary target for treatment against hyperpigmentation, and a wide spectrum of agents has been developed to inhibit its activity or modulate related pathways.

Inhibition of tyrosinase enzyme activity has gained high interest because it leads to a very specific downregulation of melanogenesis if only this single key enzyme is blocked. Thus, adverse side effects can be avoided if an inhibitor only targets tyrosinase and, therefore, tyrosinase inhibition is not only the most effective but also the safest mode of action for the treatment of hyperpigmentation. Among the 20 most commonly used ingredients against hyperpigmentation in cosmetic/dermatological products, 17 are claimed to tyrosinase inhibitors (Beiersdorf AG, data on file).

Other approaches, like downregulation of tyrosinase expression/ maturation e.g. by targeting MITF expression or activation are much more prone to side effects because nuclear factors like MITF control the expression of many proteins not only involved in melanogenesis but also in melanocyte proliferation and differentiation. Scavenging of the tyrosinase-produced melanin precursor dopaquinone with thiol-containing compounds like cysteamine and 2-mercaptanicotinoyl glycine is also a challenging approach since 12 million scavenger molecules would be needed per day (tyrosinase turnover rate: 140/s) to capture all precursors while only 1 inhibitor molecule is enough to completely block enzyme activity.

Therefore, screening for tyrosinase inhibitors has been the most attractive approach to identify ingredients to treat hyperpigmentation ever since Fitzpatrick published his Science paper 75 years ago [39] where he showed that tyrosinase is present in human skin and important for the production of melanin.

Hundreds of tyrosinase inhibitors are discovered and published every year (Fig. 12.17). This not only shows the high demand for effective treatment of skin hyperpigmentation but also that most of these molecules do not fulfill the promise and never make it to the market. While in principle tyrosinase inhibition is safe,

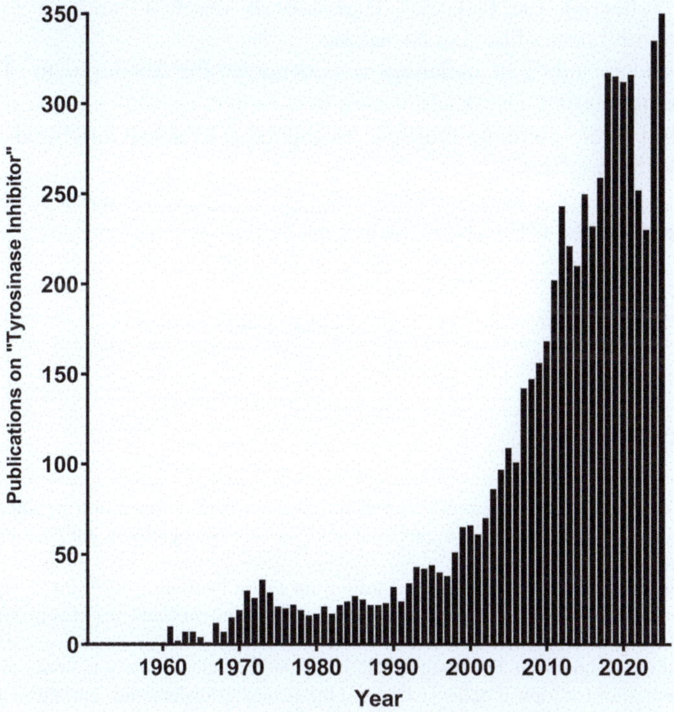

Fig. 12.17 Pubmed search for 'tyrosinase inhibitors', publications per year from 1950 to 2024

some of these molecules cause side effects because they interfere with other cellular functions. Hydroquinone is described as tyrosinase inhibitor in dozens of publications but actually is a pseudo-substrate and is converted to a toxic hydroquinone-derivative by tyrosinase (Ito). Rhododendrol introduced as tyrosinase inhibitor had to be removed from the market in 2013 after causing leukoderma in almost 20,000 of around 800,000 consumers using products containing rhododendrol [51]. It turned out that rhododendrol is not a competitive inhibitor of tyrosinase as originally thought but a substrate which is converted to rhododendrol-quinone and is toxic to melanocytes.

How was it possible that tyrosinase substrates were originally determined as tyrosinase inhibitors? Almost all tyrosinase inhibitors were tested on mushroom tyrosinase since this enzyme is commercially available and, until recently, it was not possible to purify a recombinant human tyrosinase in high enough amounts to screen for inhibitors. The advent of a soluble human tyrosinase [27] allowed to compare the efficacy of well-known inhibitors on mushroom versus human tyrosinase. It turned out that hydroquinone as well as rhododendrol are not effective inhibitors of the human enzyme with IC_{50} of >4000 μM and >1200 μM, respectively [78]. In contrast, the most effective inhibitor of human tyrosinase, Thiamidol, shows an IC_{50} of 1 μM with human tyrosinase but only an IC_{50} of 108 μM with mushroom tyrosinase, reflecting the fact that Thiamidol is the first inhibitor exclusively designed for inhibition of human tyrosinase.

As our understanding of melanogenesis deepens, the development of safe and effective depigmenting agents addressing new targets continues to evolve. Future therapies will likely combine multiple mechanisms to achieve optimal outcomes with minimal side effects.

Acknowledgments The authors would like to thank Dr. Silke Gallinat for expert scientific writing support.

List of contributions Tamara Rogers: writing; Ludger Kolbe: writing.

References

1. Abiko Y, Iwamoto M. Plasminogen-plasmin system: VII. Potentiation of antifibrinolytic action of a synthetic inhibitor, tranexamic acid, by α2-macroglobulin antiplasmin. Biochim Biophys Acta. 1970;214:411–8.
2. Akhavan A, Bershad SV. Topical acne drugs. Am J Clin Dermatol. 2003;4:473–92.
3. Al-Niaimi F, Chiang NYZ. Topical vitamin C and the skin: mechanisms of action and clinical applications. J Clin Aesthet Dermatol. 2017;10(7):14–7.
4. Amnuaikit T, Limsuwan T, Khongkow P, Boonme P. Vesicular carriers containing phenylethyl resorcinol for topical delivery system; liposomes, transfersomes and invasomes. Asian J Pharm Sci. 2018;13(5):472–84.
5. Arrowitz C, Schoelermann AM, Mann T, Jiang LI, Weber T, Kolbe L. Effective tyrosinase inhibition by thiamidol results in significant improvement of mild to moderate melasma. J Invest Dermatol. 2019;139(8):1691–1698.e6.
6. Arung ET, Shimizu K, Kondo R. Artocarpus plants as a potential source of skin whitening agents. Nat Prod Commun. 2011;6:1397–402.
7. Bajpai VK, Swigut T, Mohammed J, Naqvi S, Arreola M, Tycko J, Kim TC, Pritchard JK, Bassik MC, Wysocka J. A genome-wide genetic screen uncovers determinants of human pigmentation. Science. 2023;381(6658):eade6289.
8. Baliña LM, Graupe K. The treatment of melasma. 20% azelaic acid versus 4% hydroquinone cream. Int J Dermatol. 1991;30(12):893–5.
9. Balkrishnan R, McMichael AJ, Camacho FT, Saltzberg F, Housman TS, Grummer S, et al. Development and validation of a health-related quality of life instrument for women with melasma. Br J Dermatol. 2003;149(3):572–7.
10. Bandyopadhyay D. Topical treatment of melasma. Indian J Dermatol. 2009;54(4):303–9.
11. Bang SH, Han SJ, Kim DH. Hydrolysis of arbutin to hydroquinone by human skin bacteria and its effect on antioxidant activity. J Cosmet Dermatol. 2008;7(3):189–93. https://doi.org/10.1111/j.1473-2165.2008.00387.x. PMID: 18789053.
12. Benathan M, Labidi F. Cysteine-dependent 5-S-cysteinyldopa formation and its regulation by glutathione in normal epidermal melanocytes. Arch Dermatol Res. 1996;288:697–702.
13. Bennett DC, Lamoreux ML. The color loci of mice—a genetic century. Pigment Cell Res. 2003;16(4):333–44.
14. Bernauer U, Bodin L, Chaudhry Q, Coenraad PJ, Dusinska M, et al. SCCS Opinion on Kojic Acid—SCCS/1637/21—final version. ND-AQ-12-014-EN-N, Scientific Committee for Consumer Safety (European Commission); 2022. hal-03612741.

15. Bertold C, et al. Efficacy and safety of a novel triple combination cream compared to Kligman's trio for melasma: a 24-week double-blind prospective randomized controlled trial. J Eur Acad Dermatol Venereol. 2023;37(12):2601–7.
16. Besouw M, Masereeuw R, van den Heuvel L, Levtchenko E. Cysteamine: an old drug with new potential. Drug Discov Today. 2013;18:785–92.
17. Bierman JC, Laughlin T, Tamura M, Hulette B, Mack CE, Sherrill JD, Tan CYR, Morenc M, Bellanger S, Oblong JE. Niacinamide mitigates SASP-related inflammation induced by environmental stressors in human epidermal keratinocytes and skin. Int J Cosmet Sci. 2020;42:501–11.
18. Bohnsack K, Koop U, Hiddemann S, Kolbe L, Rippke F. Pigmentation reducing efficacy and tolerability of six new face care formulations containing 4-n-butylresorcinol, poster no. P864. In: 21st EADV congress. 2012.
19. Boo YC. Arbutin as a skin depigmenting agent with antimelanogenic and antioxidant properties. Antioxidants (Basel). 2021;10(7):1129.
20. Breathnach AS. Pharmacological properties of azelaic acid. Clin Drug Investig. 1995;10(Suppl 2):27–33.
21. Brenner M, Hearing VJ. Modifying skin pigmentation—approaches through intrinsic biochemistry and exogenous agents. Drug Discov Today Dis Mech. 2008;5(2):e189–99.
22. Briganti S, Camera E, Picardo M. Chemical and instrumental approaches to treat hyperpigmentation. Pigment Cell Res. 2003;16:101–10.
23. Cestari TF, Dantas LP, Boza JC. Acquired hyperpigmentations. An Bras Dermatol. 2014;89(1):11–25.
24. Chang NF, Chen YS, Lin YJ, Tai TH, Chen AN, Huang CH, et al. Study of hydroquinone mediated cytotoxicity and hypopigmentation effects from UVB-irradiated arbutin and deoxyarbutin. Int J Mol Sci. 2017;18(5):969.
25. Chavin W, Schlesinger W. Some potent melanin depigmentary agents in the black goldfish. Naturwissenschaften. 1966;53:413–4.
26. Chen J, Yu X, Huang Y. Inhibitory mechanisms of glabridin on tyrosinase. Spectrochim Acta A Mol Biomol Spectrosc. 2016;5(168):111–7.
27. Cordes P, Sun W, Wolber R, Kolbe L, Klebe G, Röhm KH. Expression in non-melanogenic systems and purification of soluble variants of human tyrosinase. Biol Chem. 2013;394(5):685–93.
28. Davis A, Furtak A, Paterson S, Velthuizen R, Shen J, Nip J, Bappal A, Lathrop W, Villa A, Lee JM, Guelakis M. Topical application of retinyl propionate, 4 hexyl resorcinol, and niacinamide reverses molecular and clinical features of ageing. Int J Cosmet Sci. 2024;46(5):761–74.
29. De Dormael R, Bastien P, Sextius P, Gueniche A, Ye D, Tran C, Chevalier V, Gomes C, Souverain L, Tricaud C. Vitamin C prevents ultraviolet-induced pigmentation in healthy volunteers: Bayesian meta-analysis results from 31 randomized controlled versus vehicle clinical studies. J Clin Aesthet Dermatol. 2019;12(2):E53–9.
30. de Matos DG, Furnus CC. The importance of having high glutathione (GSH) level after bovine *in vitro* maturation on embryo development effect of beta-mercaptoethanol, cysteine and cystine. Theriogenology. 2000;53:761–71.
31. Del Bino S, Duval C, Bernerd F. Clinical and biological characterization of skin pigmentation diversity and its consequences on UV impact. Int J Mol Sci. 2018;19(9):2668.
32. Dolinska MB, Kus NJ, Farney SK, Wingfield PT, Brooks BP, Sergeev YV. Oculocutaneous albinism type 1: link between mutations, tyrosinase conformational stability, and enzymatic activity. Pigment Cell Melanoma Res. 2017;30(1):41–52.
33. Draelos ZD, Diaz I, Cohen A, Mao J, Boyd T. A novel skin brightening topical technology. J Cosmet Dermatol. 2020;19(12):3280–5.
34. Ennes SBP, Paschoalick RC, Alchorne MMDA. A double-blind, comparative, placebo-controlled study of the efficacy and tolerability of 4% hydroquinone as a depigmenting agent in melasma. J Dermatol Treat. 2000;11(3):173–9.

35. Farris P, Zeichner J, Berson D. Efficacy and tolerability of a skin brightening/ anti-aging cosmeceutical containing retinol 0.5%, niacinamide, hexylresorcinol, and resveratrol. J Drugs Dermatol. 2016;15(7):863–8.
36. Farshi S, Mansouri P, Kasraee B. Efficacy of cysteamine cream in the treatment of epidermal melasma, evaluating by Dermacatch as a new measurement method: a randomized double blind placebo controlled study. J Dermatol Treat. 2018;29:182–9.
37. Findlay GH, Morrison JG, Simson IW. Exogenous ochronosis and pigmented colloid milium from hydroquinone bleaching creams. Br J Dermatol. 1975;93:613–22.
38. Fitton A, Goa KL. Azelaic acid: a review of its pharmacological properties and therapeutic efficacy in acne and hyperpigmentary skin disorders. Drugs. 1991;41:780–98.
39. Fitzpatrick TB, Becker SW Jr, Lerner AB, Montgomery. Tyrosinase in human skin: demonstration of its presence and of its role in human melanin formation. Science. 1950;112(2904):223–5.
40. Fogal S, Carotti M, Giaretta L, Lanciai F, Nogara L, Bubacco L, Bergantino E. Human tyrosinase produced in insect cells: a landmark for the screening of new drugs addressing its activity. Mol Biotechnol. 2015;57:45–57.
41. Gillbro JM, Olsson MJ. The melanogenesis and mechanisms of skin-lightening agents—existing and new approaches. Int J Cosmet Sci. 2011;33(3):210–21.
42. Greatens A, Hakozaki T, Koshoffer A, Epstein H, Schwemberger S, Babcock G, Bissett D, Takiwaki H, Arase S, Wickett RR, et al. Effective inhibition of melanosome transfer to keratinocytes by lectins and niacinamide is reversible. Exp Dermatol. 2005;14:498–508.
43. Griffiths CE, Finkel LJ, Ditre CM, Hamilton TA, Ellis CN, Voorhees JJ. Topical tretinoin (retinoic acid) improves melasma. A vehicle-controlled, clinical trial. Br J Dermatol. 1993;129(4):415–21.
44. Hakozaki T, Minwalla L, Zhuang J, Chhoa M, Matsubara A, Miyamoto K, et al. The effect of niacinamide on reducing cutaneous pigmentation and suppression of melanosome transfer. Br J Dermatol. 2002;147(1):20–31.
45. Havens MB, Tramposch KM. Hydroquinone inhibits tyrosinase activity by acting as an alternate substrate. J Invest Dermatol. 1986;87:409.
46. Hseu JH, Chan CI, Vadivalagan C, Chen SJ, Yen HR, Hseu YC, Yang HL, Wu PY. Tranexamic acid improves psoriasis-like skin inflammation: evidence from *in vivo* and *in vitro* studies. Biomed Pharm. 2023;166:115307.
47. Igarashi M, Tomita Y, Seiji M. Hydroquinone therapy for chloasma. Rinsho Derma. 1977;19:761–5.
48. Ishihara Y, Kitamura S, Kosaka K, Harasawa M. Tranexamic acid no prostaglandin gouseisogai ni kansuru kenkyu. Jpn Pharmacol Ther. 1978;6:398–402.
49. Ismaya WT, Rozeboom HJ, Weijn A, Mes JJ, Fusetti F, Wichers HJ, Dijkstra BW. Crystal structure of Agaricus bisporus mushroom tyrosinase: identity of the tetramer subunits and interaction with tropolone. Biochemistry. 2011;50:5477–86.
50. Ito Y, Jimbow K, Ito S. Depigmentation of black guinea pig skin by topical application of cysteaminylphenol, cysteinylphenol, and related compounds. J Invest Dermatol. 1987;88:77–82.
51. Ito S, Kolbe L, Weets G, Rogers T, Bushdid C, Nishimaki-Mogami T, Tanaka H, Passeron T, Ojika M, Wakamatsu K. Exogenous ochronosis by hydroquinone is not caused by inhibition of homogentisate dioxygenase but potentially by tyrosinase-catalyzed metabolism of hydroquinone. Br J Dermatol. 2025;193(5):959–67.
52. Jimbow K, Obata H, Pathak MA, Fitzpatrick TB. Mechanism of depigmentation by hydroquinone. J Invest Dermatol. 1974;62(4):436–49.
53. Jow T, Hantash BM. Hydroquinone-induced depigmentation: case report and review of the literature. Dermatitis. 2014;25:e1–5.
54. Kamat JP, Devasagayam TPA. Nicotinamide (vitamin B-3) as an effective antioxidant against oxidative damage in rat brain mitochondria. Redox Rep. 1999;4:179–84.

55. Kang HH, Rho HS, Hwang JS, Oh SG. Depigmenting activity and low cytotoxicity of alkoxy benzoates or alkoxy cinnamte in cultured melanocytes. Chem Pharm Bull (Tokyo). 2003;51(9):1085–8.
56. Karrabi M, David J, Sahebkar M. Clinical evaluation of efficacy, safety and tolerability of cysteamine 5% cream in comparison with modified Kligman's formula in subjects with epidermal melasma: a randomized, double-blind clinical trial study. Skin Res Technol. 2020;27:24–31.
57. Kasraee B. Peroxidase-mediated mechanisms are involved in the melanocytotoxic and melanogenesis-inhibiting effects of chemical agents. Dermatology. 2002;205:329–39.
58. Katagiri T, Okubo T, Oyobikawa M, et al. Inhibitory action of 4-n-butylresorcinol on Melanogenesis and its skin whitening effect. J Soc Cosmet Chem Jpn. 2001;35:42–9.
59. Khatib S, Nerya O, Musa R, Shmuel M, Tamir S, Vaya J. Chalcones as potent tyrosinase inhibitors: the importance of a 2,4-substituted resorcinol moiety. Bioorg Med Chem. 2005;13:433–41.
60. Kim DS, Kim SY, Park SH, et al. Inhibitory effects of 4-n-butylresorcinol on tyrosinase activity and melanin synthesis. Biol Pharm Bull. 2005;28:2216–9.
61. Kita Y, Sugai T. Effect of bleach agents on chloasma. Skin Res. 1992;34:142–6.
62. Kligman AM, Willis I. A new formula for depigmenting human skin. Arch Dermatol. 1975;111(1):40–8. PMID: 1119822.
63. Kolbe L, Mann T, Gerwat W, Batzer J, Ahlheit S, Scherner C, Wenck H, Stäb F. 4-n-Butylresorcinol, a highly effective tyrosinase inhibitor for the topical treatment of hyperpigmentation. J Eur Acad Dermatol Venereol. 2013;27(s1):19–23. https://doi.org/10.1111/jdv.12051.
64. Kooyers TJ, Westerhof W. Toxicology and health risks of hydroquinone in skin lightening formulations. J Eur Acad Venereol. 2006;20:777–80.
65. Köpke D, Müller RH, Pyo SM. Phenylethyl resorcinol smartLipids for skin brightening—increased loading & chemical stability. Eur J Pharm Sci. 2019;137:104992.
66. Lai X, Soler-Lopez M, Wichers HJ, Dijkstra BW. Large-scale recombinant expression and purification of human tyrosinase suitable for structural studies. PLoS ONE. 2016;11:e0161697.
67. Lajis AF, Hamid M, Ariff AB. Depigmenting effect of Kojic acid esters in hyperpigmented B16F1 melanoma cells. J Biomed Biotechnol. 2012;2012:952452.
68. Law RHP, Wu G, Leung EWW, Hidaka K, Quek AJ, Caradoc-Davies TT, et al. X-ray crystal structure of plasmin with tranexamic acid-derived active site inhibitors. Blood Adv. 2017;1:766–71.
69. Lee SY, Baek N, Nam TG. Natural, semisynthetic and synthetic tyrosinase inhibitors. J Enzyme Inhib Med Chem. 2016;31:1–13.
70. Lehraiki A, Abbe P, Cerezo M, et al. Inhibition of melanogenesis by the antidiabetic metformin. J Invest Dermatol. 2014;134:2589–97.
71. Lei TC, Virador VM, Vieira WD, Hearing VJ. A melanocyte-keratinocyte coculture model to assess regulators of pigmentation *in vitro*. Anal Biochem. 2002;305:260–8.
72. Leibl H, Stingl G, Pehamberger H, Korschan H, Konrad K, Wolff K. Inhibition of DNA synthesis of melanoma cells by azelaic acid. J Invest Dermatol. 1985;85(5):417–22.
73. Limsuwan T, Boonme P, Khongkow P, Amnuaikit T. Ethosomes of phenylethyl resorcinol as vesicular delivery system for skin lightening applications. Biomed Res Int. 2017;2017:8310979.
74. Liu J, Xu X, Jian M, Guo Y, Zhai L, Sun G, Sun L, Jiang R. Glycyrrhiza glabra extract as a skin-whitening agent: identification of active components and CRTC1/MITF pathway-inhibition mechanism. J Ethnopharmacol. 2025;349:119948.
75. Madan Mohan NT, Gowda A, Jaiswal AK, Sharath Kumar BC, Shilpashree P, Gangaboraiah B, Shamanna M. Assessment of efficacy, safety, and tolerability of 4-n-butylresorcinol 03% cream: an Indian multicentric study on melasma. Clin Cosmet Investig Dermatol. 2016;9:21–7.
76. Maeda K, Fukuda M. Arbutin: mechanism of its depigmenting action in human melanocyte culture. J Pharmacol Exp Ther. 1996;276(2):765–9.

77. Maeda K, Naganuma M. Topical trans-4-aminomethylcyclohexanecarboxylic acid prevents ultraviolet radiation-induced pigmentation. J Photochem Photobiol B Biol. 1998;47:136–41.
78. Mann T, Gerwat W, Batzer J, Eggers K, Scherner C, Wenck H, et al. Inhibition of human tyrosinase requires molecular motifs distinctively different from mushroom tyrosinase. J Invest Dermatol. 2018;138(7):1601–8.
79. Mann T, Scherner C, Röhm KH, Kolbe L. Structure-activity relationships of thiazolyl resorcinols, potent and selective inhibitors of human tyrosinase. Int J Mol Sci. 2018;19(3):690.
80. Mann T, Welge V, Weise J, Roggenkamp D, Kolbe L. 29th EADV Congress 2020. Poster no P1240. Medicom Medical Publishers; 2020.
81. Manosroi A, Podjanasoonthon K, Manosroi J. Development of novel topical tranexamic acid liposome formulations. Int J Pharm. 2002;235(1-2):61–70.
82. Mansouri P, Farshi S, Hashemi Z, Kasraee B. Evaluation of the efficacy of cysteamine 5% cream in the treatment of epidermal melasma: a randomized double-blind placebo-controlled trial. Br J Dermatol. 2015;173:209–17.
83. Matoba Y, Kumagai T, Yamamoto A, Yoshitsu H, Sugiyama M. Crystallographic evidence that the dinuclear copper center of tyrosinase is flexible during catalysis. J Biol Chem. 2006;281:8981–90.
84. Maymone MBC, Neamah HH, Wirya SA, Patzelt NM, Secemsky EA, Zancanaro PQ, et al. The impact of skin hyperpigmentation and hyperchromia on quality of life: a cross-sectional study. J Am Acad Dermatol. 2017;77:775–8.
85. Miller RA, Chu Q, Xie J, et al. Biguanides suppress hepatic glucagon signalling by decreasing production of cyclic AMP. Nature. 2013;494:256–60.
86. Mishra SN, Dhurat RS, Deshpande DJ, Nayak CS. Diagnostic utility of dermatoscopy in hydroquinone-induced exogenous ochronosis. Int J Dermatol. 2013;52(4):413–417.
87. Monfrecola G, Gaudiello F, Cirillo T, Fabbrocini G, Balato A, Lembo S. Nicotinamide downregulates gene expression of interleukin-6, interleukin-10, monocyte chemoattractant protein-1, and tumour necrosis factor-alpha gene expression in HaCaT keratinocytes after ultraviolet B irradiation. Clin Exp Dermatol. 2013;38:185–8.
88. Mongkhon P, Ruengorn C, Awiphan R, Phosuya C, Ruanta Y, Thavorn K, Jamjanya S, Chuamanochan M, Nochaiwong S. Efficacy and safety of metformin for melasma treatment: a systematic review and meta-analysis. Front Pharmacol. 2023;14:1281050.
89. Morag M, Nawrot J, Siatkowski I, Adamski Z, Fedorowicz T, Dawid-Pac R, et al. A double-blind, placebo-controlled randomized trial of Serratulae quinquefoliae folium, a new source of β-arbutin, in selected skin hyperpigmentations. J Cosmet Dermatol. 2015;14(3):185–90.
90. Munoz-Munoz JL, Garcia-Molina F, García-Ruiz PA, Varon R, Tudela J, García-Canovas F, Rodriguez-Lopez JN. Stereospecific inactivation of tyrosinase by L-and D-ascorbic acid. Biochim Biophys Acta Proteins Proteomics. 2009;1794(2):244–53.
91. Nahhas AF, Abdel-Malek ZA, Kohli I, Braunberger TL, Lim HW, Hamzavi IH. The potential role of antioxidants in mitigating skin hyperpigmentation resulting from ultraviolet and visible light-induced oxidative stress. Photodermatol Photoimmunol Photomed. 2019;35:420–8.
92. Nguyen J, Remyn L, Chung IY, Honigman A, Gourani-Tehrani S, Wutami I, Wong C, Paul E, Rodrigues M. Evaluation of the efficacy of cysteamine cream compared to hydroquinone in the treatment of melasma: a randomised, double-blinded trial. Australas J Dermatol. 2021;62(1):e41–6.
93. Olivares C, Garcia-Borron JC, Solano F. Identification of active site residues involved in metal cofactor binding and stereospecific substrate recognition in mammalian tyrosinase. Implications to the catalytic cycle. Biochemistry. 2002;41:679–86.
94. Ortonne JP. Retinoid therapy of pigmentary disorders. Dermatol Ther. 2006;19(5):280–8.
95. Palumbo A, d'Ischia M, Misuraca G, Prota G. Mechanism of inhibition of melanogenesis by hydroquinone. Biochim Biophys Acta. 1991;1073(1):85–90.
96. Passi S, Nazzaro-Porro M. Molecular basis of substrate and inhibitory specificity of tyrosinase: phenolic compounds. Br J Dermatol. 1981;104:659–65.

97. Passi S, Picardo M, De Luca C, Breathnach AS, Nazzaro-Porro M. Scavenging activity of azelaic acid on hydroxyl radicals "*in vitro*". Free Radic Res Commun. 1991;11(6):329–38.
98. Passi S, Picardo M, Zompetta C, De Luca C, Breathnach AS, Nazzaro-Porro M. The oxyradical-scavenging activity of azelaic acid in biological systems. Free Radic Res Commun. 1991;15(1):17–28.
99. Penneys NS. Ochronosislike pigmentation from hydroquinone bleaching creams. Arch Dermatol. 1985;121(10):1239–40.
100. Philipp-Dormston WG. Melasma: a step-by-step approach towards a multimodal combination therapy. Clin Cosmet Investig Dermatol. 2024;17:1203–16.
101. Pillaiyar T, Manickam M, Namasivayam V. Skin whitening agents: medicinal chemistry perspective of tyrosinase inhibitors. J Enzyme Inhib Med Chem. 2017;32(1):403–25.
102. Pullar JM, Carr AC, Vissers MCM. The roles of vitamin C in skin health. Nutrients. 2017;9(8):866.
103. Qiu L, Zhang M, Sturm RA, Gardiner B, Tonks I, Kay G, Parsons PG. Inhibition of melanin synthesis by cystamine in human melanoma cells. J Invest Dermatol. 2000;114:21–7.
104. Robins EJ, Breathnach AS, Bashin YP, Ethridge L, Nazzaro-Porro M, Passi S, et al. Effectiveness of azelaic acid as a depigmenting and chemotherapeutic agent. J Invest Dermatol. 1986;87(2):293–4.
105. Roggenkamp D, Dlova N, Mann T, Batzer J, Riedel J, Kausch M, Zoric I, Kolbe L. Effective reduction of post-inflammatory hyperpigmentation with the tyrosinase inhibitor isobutylamido-thiazolyl-resorcinol (Thiamidol). Int J Cosmet Sci. 2021;43:292–301.
106. Roggenkamp D, Sammain A, Fürstenau M, Kausch M, Passeron T, Kolbe L. Thiamidol® in moderate-to-severe melasma: 24-week, randomized, double-blind, vehicle-controlled clinical study with subsequent regression phase. J Dermatol. 2021;48(12):1871–6.
107. Roméro C, Aberdam E, Larnier C, Ortonne JP. Retinoic acid as modulator of UVB-induced melanocyte differentiation. Involvement of the melanogenic enzymes expression. J Cell Sci. 1994;107(Pt 4):1095–103.
108. Saeedi M, Eslamifar M, Khezri K. Kojic acid applications in cosmetic and pharmaceutical preparations. Biomed Pharmacother. 2019;110:582–93.
109. Sánchez-Ferrer A, Rodríguez-López JN, García-Cánovas F, García-Carmona F. Tyrosinase: a comprehensive review of its mechanism. Biochim Biophys Acta. 1995;1247(1):1–11.
110. Sarkar R, Yadav V, Yadav T, Janaani P, Mandal I. Glutathione as a skin-lightening agent and in melasma: a systematic review. Int J Dermatol. 2025;64(6):992–1004.
111. Sauer N, Oślizło M, Brzostek M, Wolska J, Lubaszka K, Karłowicz-Bodalska K. The multiple uses of azelaic acid in dermatology: mechanism of action, preparations, and potential therapeutic applications. Postepy Dermatol Alergol. 2023;40(6):716–24.
112. Schmaus G, Vielhabe G, Jacobs K, Franke H. 4-(1-Phenylethyl)1,3-benzenediol: a new highly potent lightening agent. J Cosmet Sci. 2006;57:197–8.
113. Schweikardt T, Olivares C, Solano F, Jaenicke E, Garcia-Borron JC, Decker H. A three-dimensional model of mammalian tyrosinase active site accounting for loss of function mutations. Pigment Cell Res. 2007;20:394–401.
114. Searle T, Al-Niaimi F, Ali FR. The top 10 cosmeceuticals for facial hyperpigmentation. Dermatol Ther. 2020;33(6):e14095.
115. Sendovski M, Kanteev M, Ben-Yosef VS, Adir N, Fishman A. First structures of an active bacterial tyrosinase reveal copper plasticity. J Mol Biol. 2011;405:227–37.
116. Shariff R, Du Y, Dutta M, Kumar S 5th, Thimmaiah S, Doraiswamy C, Kumari A, Kale V, Nair N, Zhang S, Joshi M, Santhanam U, Qiang Q, Damodaran A. Superior even skin tone and anti-ageing benefit of a combination of 4-hexylresorcinol and niacinamide. Int J Cosmet Sci. 2022;44(1):103–17.
117. Shibata T, Prota G, Mishima Y. Non-melanosomal regulatory factors in melanogenesis. J Invest Dermatol. 1993;100:274s–80s.
118. Shimizu K, Kondo R, Sakai K. Inhibition of tyrosinase by flavonoids, stilbenes and related 4-substituted resorcinols: structure-activity investigations. Planta Med. 2000;66:11–5.

119. Shirasugi Y, Shibata T, Koike S, Hara M, Hasegawa K, Iino M, Sonoki A, Funasaka Y. Potassium 4-methoxysalicylate (4MSK) exerts a skin lightening effect by acting on melanocytes and keratinocytes. J Cosmet Dermatol. 2025;24(3):e70112.
120. Simmons BJ, Griffith RD, Bray FN, Falto-Aizpurua LA, Nouri K. Exogenous ochronosis: a comprehensive review of the diagnosis, epidemiology, causes, and treatments. Am J Clin Dermatol. 2015;16:205–12.
121. Smit NP, Van der Meulen H, Koerten HK, Kolb RM, Mommaas AM, Lentjes EG, Pavel S. Melanogenesis in cultured melanocytes can be substantially influenced by L-tyrosine and L-cysteine. J Invest Dermatol. 1997;109:796–800.
122. Sonthalia S, Daulatabad D, Sarkar R. Glutathione as a skin whitening agent: facts, myths, evidence and controversies. Indian J Dermatol Venereol Leprol. 2016;82(3):262–72.
123. Spencer MC. Hydroquinone bleaching: submitted for publication March 6, 1961. This study was approved by the Veterans Administration Hospital, Danville, Ill. From the Department of Dermatology, Northwestern University Medical School, Chicago. JAMA Dermatol. 1961;84:131–4.
124. Stamford NP. Stability, transdermal penetration, and cutaneous effects of ascorbic acid and its derivatives. J Cosmet Dermatol. 2012;11(4):310–7.
125. Takebayashi J, Ishii R, Chen J, Matsumoto T, Ishimi Y, Tai A. Reassessment of antioxidant activity of arbutin: multifaceted evaluation using five antioxidant assay systems. Free Radic Res. 2010;44(4):473–8.
126. Tan SK. Exogenous ochronosis in ethnic Chinese Asians: a clinicopathological study, diagnosis and treatment. J Eur Acad Dermatol Venereol. 2011;25:842–50.
127. Taylor SC, Torok H, Jones T, Lowe N, Rich P, Tschen E, Menter A, Baumann L, Wieder JJ, Jarratt MM, Pariser D, Martin D, Weiss J, Shavin J, Ramirez N. Efficacy and safety of a new triple-combination agent for the treatment of facial melasma. Cutis. 2003;72(1):67–72.
128. Taylor S, Grimes P, Lim J, Im S, Lui H. Postinflammatory hyperpigmentation. J Cutan Med Surg. 2009;13(4):183–91. https://doi.org/10.2310/7750.2009.08077.
129. Tripathi RK, Hearing VJ, Urabe K, Aroca P, Spritz RA. Mutational mapping of the catalytic activities of human tyrosinase. J Biol Chem. 1992;267:23707–12.
130. Vachiramon V, Sakpuwadol N, Yongpisarn T, Anuntrangsee T, Palakornkitti P. Efficacy of isobutylamido thiazolyl resorcinol for prevention of laser-induced post-inflammatory hyperpigmentation: a randomized, controlled trial. J Cosmet Dermatol. 2024;23(7):2450–7.
131. Vielhaber G, Schmaus G, Jacobs K, Franke H, Lange S, Herrmann M, et al. 4-(1-phenylethyl)1,3-benzenediol: a new, highly efficient lightening agent. Int J Cosmet Sci. 2007;29:65–6.
132. Viollet B, Guigas B, Sanz Garcia N, et al. Cellular and molecular mechanisms of metformin: an overview. Clin Sci (Lond). 2012;122:253–70.
133. Virador VM, Kobayashi N, Matsunaga J, Hearing VJ. A standardized protocol for assessing regulators of pigmentation. Anal Biochem. 1999;270:207–19.
134. Weide I, Tippler B, Syrovets T, Simmet T. Plasmin is a specific stimulus of the 5-lipoxygenase pathway of human peripheral monocytes. Thromb Haemost. 1996;76:561–8.
135. Wen YT, Liang YQ, Chai WM, Wei QM, Yu ZY, Wang LJ. Effect of ascorbic acid on tyrosinase and its anti-browning activity in fresh-cut Fuji apple. J Food Biochem. 2021;45(12):e13995.
136. Wendt M. Rationales design neuer tyrosinase-inhibitoren. PhD thesis, University of Marburg Medical School; 2006.
137. Westerhof W, Kooyers TJ. Hydroquinone and its analogues in dermatology—a potential health risk. J Cosmet Dermatol. 2005;4(2):55–9.
138. Wu G, Mazzitelli BA, Quek AJ, Veldman MJ, Conroy PJ, CaradocDavies TT, et al. Tranexamic acid is an active site inhibitor of urokinase plasminogen activator. Blood Adv. 2019;3:729–33.
139. Xing X, Xu Z, Chen L, Jin S, Zhang C, Xiang L. Tranexamic acid inhibits melanogenesis partially via stimulation of TGF-β1 expression in human epidermal keratinocytes. Exp Dermatol. 2022;31:633–40.

140. Xu WH, Liang Q, Zhang YJ, Zhao P. Naturally occurring arbutin derivatives and their bioactivities. Chem Biodivers. 2015;12(1):54–81.
141. Yoshimura K, Tsukamoto K, Okazaki M, Virador VM, Lei TC, Suzuki Y, et al. Effects of all-trans retinoic acid on melanogenesis in pigmented skin equivalents and monolayer culture of melanocytes. J Dermatol Sci. 2001;27(Suppl 1):S68–75.
142. Zeng Y, Ma M, Chen Y, Xie H, Ding P, Zhang K. Enhancing skin delivery of tranexamic acid via esterification: synthesis and evaluation of alkyl ester derivatives. RSC Adv. 2024;14(47):34996–5004.
143. Zhang XY, Yang XH, Yang H, Yang YP. Study of inhibitory effect of acidum tranexamicum on melanin synthesis. Chin J Dermatovenerol Int Tradit West Med. 2003;2:227–9.
144. Zhang Y, Sil BC, Kung CP, Hadgraft J, Heinrich M, Sinko B, Lane ME. Characterization and topical delivery of phenylethyl resorcinol. Int J Cosmet Sci. 2019;41(5):479–88.
145. Zhen AX, Piao MJ, Kang KA, Fernando PDSM, Kang HK, Koh YS, Yi JM, Hyun JW. Niacinamide protects skin cells from oxidative stress induced by particulate matter. Biomol Ther. 2019;27:562–9.
146. Zhou H, Zhao J, Li A, Reetz MT. Chemical and biocatalytic routes to arbutin[†]. Molecules. 2019;24(18):3303.
147. Zilles JC, Dos Santos FL, Kulkamp-Guerreiro IC, Contri RV. Biological activities and safety data of kojic acid and its derivatives: a review. Exp Dermatol. 2022;31(10):1500–21.

Chapter 13
Reversers for Neuromodulators

Jean Carruthers Cosmetic and Apul Parikh

Introduction

Background

After antibiotics, the newest class of generational drug to reach world-wide acceptance is that of the Botulinum neuromodulators. This drug class was first recognized as a terrible poison, and only after nearly a century and a half of scientific investigation was it found to be a potent pluripotential drug extremely helpful in treating a variety of medical conditions [1].

The poisoning effects of Botulinum toxin were first recognized in southern Germany in the 1820s when Dr Justinus Kerner, the young Medical Superintendent of Weinsberg, Germany, studied the deaths that followed social gatherings in his region in the aftermath of the Napoleonic Wars. In these mysterious poisoning outbreaks, groups of local people who had eaten contaminated blood sausages became paralysed, stopped breathing, and died. Dr Kerner tried some of the "fatty acid" in the sausages on his own tongue and observed that his oral cavity became dry. He hypothesised "The fatty acid from the blood sausages could be useful in many diseases [1]". He was absolutely correct.

Between 1895 and 1897, the Belgian Immunologist, Emile-Pierre van Ermengem isolated, identified and characterized the bacterium known as *Clostridium botulinum* and confirmed it produced a deadly exotoxin that caused the sausage poisoning, now called *botulism* (The name relates to the Latin for "sausage" being "botulus") [2].

J. Carruthers Cosmetic (✉)
Clinical Professor, Department of Ophthalmology, University of British Columbia, Vancouver, BC, Canada
e-mail: drjean@carruthers.net

A. Parikh
Dr. Apul Parikh Clinic, London, UK

P. Elsner et al. (eds.), *Cosmetics*, https://doi.org/10.1007/978-3-032-14644-1_13

In 1977, nearly 120 years after Kerner's superbly detailed 1822 manuscript, the first clinical usage of Botulinum toxin A (BoNT-A) was described by the California Ophthalmologist, Dr. Alan Scott [3]. His initial research was to compare the effects of the injection of different chemicals into the extraocular muscles of macaque monkeys; the most successful molecule injected was Botulinum toxin A as there was a change in the monkeys' ocular alignment. In addition, no BoNT-A treated experimental macaque monkey died, unlike those treated with abungaroneurotoxin and Diisofluorophosphate [4].

Scott followed the animal experiments with larger human studies—a National Institutes of Health (NIH) multicenter international study, where BoNT-A was injected into human extra-ocular muscles to treat misaligned eyes (strabismus). It was also injected into the orbicularis oculi to treat blepharospasm, hemifacial spasm and spastic lower eyelid entropion [5]. This study showed that BoNT-A in the miniscule doses used clinically in human extraocular muscles was effective and safe. This was an extremely important change of reputation for this amazing molecule—to go from "Most poisonous poison" to world class therapeutic and cosmetic drug [6].

At present there are 6 FDA approved botulinum toxin type A neuromodulators; onabotulinumtoxin, abobotulinumtoxin, incobotulinumtoxin, prabotulinumtoxin, letbotulinumtoxin, daxxify, and one type B rimabotulinumtoxin. The first type E toxin (trenibotulinumtoxinE (BoNT/E)) is currently under FDA analysis for clinical safety and efficacy [7].

The first approved BoNT-A, onabotulinumtoxin A, has over 30 approved indications in 100 countries [8] and an exemplary safety profile. There is however a small risk of severe adverse events relating to the dosage given. This was recognised by the U.S Food and Drug Administration (FDA) who in 2009 made changes to BoNT product labelling, including a 'black box' warning. This outlined the potential local and distant spread, as well as the resultant signs and symptoms of systemic botulism [9].

Systemic toxicity is very rare. It is generally felt that recommended doses in cosmetic treatments are too low to cause systemic botulism. Diffusion of the injected material into adjacent muscle groups can lead to iatrogenic local overcorrections. The commonest example of this being iatrogenic ptosis of the eyelids or brows with treatments for glabellar and forehead lines. Due to this potential systemic toxicity, BoNT was one of the first agents to be considered for use as a biological weapon, and initially much research was dedicated during the Second World War to weaponize this toxin [10].

Signs and Symptoms of Systemic Botulism

The onset, severity and specific symptoms of botulism vary significantly. They may vary depending on the patient, any pre-existing health issues, the route by which the BoNT was introduced into the body, as well as the quantity of the toxin introduced into the body [11].

As food-borne botulism is the most common variety, gastrointestinal signs and symptoms may be present, and these include nausea, vomiting, diarrhoea, as well as abdominal pain. These symptoms aften precede or accompany a descending flaccid paralysis, as well as the other neurological manifestations of botulism [12].

Autonomic symptoms are often the earliest signs of botulism. These include a dry mouth or throat and is often misdiagnosed as pharyngitis [13]. The main neurological symptoms include dysarthria, dysphonia, dysphagia, which may be accompanied by visual disturbances in the form of diplopia, blurred vision, fixed mydriasis, and bilateral ptosis [14]. In severe cases there can be serious clinical deterioration, culminating in inspiratory stridor, progressing to respiratory failure [15].

What is especially interesting is the onset of the botulism toxicity. This may vary from 1 day to 2–3 weeks post exposure [10]. The mechanism of the delayed and distant effects is also poorly understood. It is generally accepted that BoNT is a locally acting agent, and animal studies have shown that botulinum toxin can spread to 30–45 mm from the injection site [16]. However, the timing and distant sites of adverse events, may suggest that haematogenous spread, as well as retrograde axonal transport of BoNT may occur [17]. Another theory is that the BoNT injections may uncover an underlying neuromuscular disorder in patients [18].

Aetiology of Systemic Botulism

There are several causes of botulism that have been established:

1. **Foodborne botulism**

   This is caused by oral ingestion of foods contaminated with BoNT. This has historically been the most common form of botulism. Improperly canned foods and fermented foods that are consumed without cooking, have often been implicated as a source of contamination. Clostridium botulinum multiplies and grows toxin in food that have a pH of <4.5, a low salt and sugar content, as well as a temperature of 4° to 121 °C [7]. Most food related cases are sporadic and are usually small in terms of numbers of people involved. This often makes it difficult for clinicians to pinpoint BoNT as a causative factor. It is thus essential in these cases to obtain a detailed food history from the patient, as well as from close contacts who may have ingested the food too [19].
2. **Infantile botulism**

   This is caused by ingestion of the BoNT, followed by colonisation of the intestines. There is a higher incidence in children below the age of 1, where normal florae that could compete with C. botulinum have not been fully established. Other predisposing factors could include previous bowel or gastric surgery, congenital bowel abnormalities, inflammatory bowel disease, antimicrobial therapy, and immunosuppressive medications [18]. This is the most common type of botulism in the United States, and studies have also implicated honey consumption as a risk factor in 20% of all cases [11].

3. **Adult intestinal toxaemia botulism**

   This is similar to infantile botulism, in that the botulism results from colonisation of the intestines by botulinum-toxin producing Clostridia. Patients often have an underlying bowel disorder or altered bowel flora after usage of antimicrobials [13].

4. **Wound Botulism**

   As the name implies, this occurs as a result of wound contamination with C. botulinum spores from the surrounding environment, and subsequent germination of these spores and production of the toxin in an anaerobic environment of an abscess [19]. This condition was extremely rare, however has recently experienced a dramatic increase. Almost all the cases relate to injections of illicit drugs, the so-called "Black tar heroin", where the drug is injected into soft tissues [13].

5. **Iatrogenic botulism**

   In 2004 in Florida an unfrocked osteopathic physician bought Research grade BoNT-A from a California company, without fully appreciating the vial contents. He injected about 20 million units of BoNT-A into 4 people, one of whom was himself. The fact that all four people developed systemic botulism but survived is due to the marvellous skills of the intensivist physicians in the hospital Intensive Care Unit [20].

   Iatrogenic botulism typically occurs due to accidental overdose or potentially the usage of non-approved product [15]. A very recent (April 2024) outbreak of clinical botulism was seen in 9 US states [21] in which 19 people were affected of whom 4 were hospitalized. This situation was extremely worrying with regards to the health outcomes of the injected victims, as well as the motivations of the injectors of these products. The usage of illegal non approved generic botulinum toxins with non-standardised dosages, are potentially most likely to cause botulism [20].

6. **Inhalational botulism**

   Inhalation botulism is rare and does not occur naturally. Purified botulinum toxin, produced and weaponized by military biological warfare programs, could be dispersed as an aerosol and cause inhalational botulism [10]. The median lethal dose for humans has been estimated at 2 nanograms of botulinum toxin per kilogram of bodyweight, which is approximately 3 times greater than in foodborne cases.

Treatment and Reversal of Systemic Botulism

The main aspects in the treatment of botulism mainly focus on:

(i) Support of the respiratory system
(ii) Gastrointestinal decontamination in cases of food-borne botulism
(iii) Antitoxin or antidote treatments [22].

In this chapter, the focus will be principally on antitoxin, or antidote treatments.

1. Botulinum Antitoxin (BAT)

   Botulinum antitoxin (equine derived Botulism Antitoxin Heptavalent (BAT), produced by Emergent BioSolutions inc.) [22] is comprised of antibodies or antibody antigen-binding fragments, that block the neurotoxin produced by Clostridium botulinum. The main goal of this antitoxin treatment is to neutralise the unbound BoNT at the presynaptic level at the neuromuscular junction [22] and attempt to reduce thc involvement of new nerve endings. It is thus ineffective once the BoNT has been internalised into the presynaptic neurons.

   However, the antitoxin efficacy has only been established in experimental animal studies, and no human-based studies have been performed to evaluate the safety and efficacy profile of BAT [17]. The usage of BAT in humans is thus based on case reports and clinical experience. There is also limited data linking the dosage, and the toxin neutralising effect of BAT [23]. BAT was approved by the US Food and Drug Administration (FDA) in 2013, to treat all serotypes of botulism [24]. There are various formulations available, containing different amounts of the antitoxin. However, the recommended dosage is one vial 20 mL (1 vial) IV infusion. This is diluted further with 0.9% NaCl to 1:10 ratio before administering at an initial rate of 0.5 mL per minute [25].

   The main challenges surrounding BAT administration are that it is an equine-derived medication, and that patients need to be closely monitored for any immediate hypersensitivity reaction. This can be an anaphylaxis type reaction, or a delayed Type III serum sickness reaction that can occur weeks after the infusion [25]. Early botulism symptoms may be nonspecific, and often the BAT administration is often delayed whilst other differential diagnoses are being excluded. This delay can be clinically significant and may result in generalised muscle paralysis, requiring intubation and ventilation [26].

2. Monoclonal Antibodies

   There has recently been extensive research into creating new drugs such as monoclonal antibodies, to prevent and block the catalytic activity of the BoNT [27]. Considering that it is the ability of the BoNT light chain, as well as the intraneuronal cleaved SNARE proteins to prevent neurotransmission of acetylcholine at the neuromuscular junction, much of the research has focused on interfering with the light chain activity. Recently there has been development of an antidote to BoNT serotype A1 intoxication named B8C1ad or Cyto-111 (atoxic derivative). B8c1ad has been shown to be able to enter the neuronal cytosol and protect the SNARE proteins by inhibiting the light chain activity in situ.

   Animal studies in mice, guinea pigs and Chinese-origin rhesus macaques demonstrated that toxic signs of botulism were successfully treated after administration of B8C1ad [28]. It was also felt that given the mechanism of action of B8C1ad is intracellular, it would have a broader therapeutic window over BAT. Although animal studies have been largely positive, there will be a need for costly and time-consuming human studies, to establish the safety parameters, the dosage as well as the number of treatments required.

3. Pyridostigmine (Mestinon)

   Pyridostigmine is a drug that is used in the treatment of myasthenia gravis. It is a reversible acetylcholinesterase inhibitor that works by preventing the breakdown of acetylcholine in the cholinergic neuromuscular junction. It has also been used off label in emergencies to reverse neuromuscular junction blockers in anaesthesia [29]. Based on this it is used in BoNT toxicity by potentiating the neuromuscular junction transmission. It can be used in the oral or intravenous form. There is currently research underway to produce a local subcutaneous injectable formulation of pyridostigmine to treat small areas of BoNT overexpression such as iatrogenic eyelid ptosis [30].

4. Experimental

   There are also several experimental medications that are being trialled, based on their interference with the different stages of BoNT pathways. The first group aims to block the binding of BoNT to receptors at the presynaptic membrane. These include ganglioside receptors such as quinic and thearubigin. The next group of medications aim to interfere with the internalisation process. These include methylamine hydrocholoride, bafilomycin A and quinolol [31]. There is one other group of medicines that can be used in the recovery of affected nerve terminals. These include 3,4 diaminopyridine (3,4 DAP) which is a potassium channel blocker. These act by increasing the duration of the presynaptic action potential, and thus increasing acetylcholine release [31]. There have also been a plethora of medications used to try and improve the outcomes in botulism, with little or no success. These included steroids, guanidine, immunoglobulins as well as chloroquine [17].

Aesthetic Use of Neuromodulators

The worldwide demand for aesthetic procedures continues to grow [32]. There was a 73% increase from 2018 (5,043,057 cosmetic neuromodulator procedures) to 2022 (8,736,591 procedures), a 73% increase [32]. Cosmetic neuromodulators have a pristine safety record. Serious adverse events such as suspected toxin-related anaphylaxis are extremely rare [33]. Reports of iatrogenic botulism have largely associated with therapeutic rather than cosmetic uses [34]. In 2004 and 2024 USA based cosmetic health care providers have used nonapproved neuromodulators in unsafe doses [20, 21]. Unwanted effects are rarely seen when approved neurotoxins are used for facial rejuvenation, such as neutralizing antibodies [35], facial flaccidity [36] and eyelid ptosis [37]. We can presume that they will continue to be produced as more injectors who are less well trained on both facial and neck anatomy and injection technique enter the worldwide aesthetic provider arena.

Neutralizing Antibodies

Aesthetic BoNT-A injections are on occasion hindered by immunity caused by neutralizing antibodies that have formed against the active toxin (150 KD) or associated complexing proteins [38]. While not planned "reversers" primary or secondary immunogenicity does prevent the expected neuromodulator effects.

Primary Nonresponsivsemess

Primary nonresponsiveness can also be a cause of neuromodulator treatment failure. Reasons for this include neuromuscular disorders, such as myasthenia gravis, poor injection technique, or reduced BoNT-A potency due to inadequate storage and improper reconstitution [39].

Individual genetic variability is another possibility [39]. The Major Histocompatibility Complex (MHC) plays a crucial role in immunity. Human Leukocyte antigens (HLA) are located on chromosome 6 at position 21.31. The region comprises over 200 genes. Of which a small subset of the HLA region's genes are implicated in the immune response to neuromodulators, namely those that code for the classical class I (A, B, and C) and class II (DR, DQ, and DP) antigens. The carrier of DQB1*06:04 (associated with primary biliary cholangitis and narcolepsy) and DQA1*01:02 (associated with Type I diabetes, multiple sclerosis, thyroiditis, and autoimmune hepatitis) has a significant association with immunogenicity to BoNT-A. These alleles are distributied in the Mediterranean, north and central Africa; central Europe; North, Central Australia and Queensland; Western Asia and the Indochina belt. In the United States, non-Hispanic whites having the highest incidence and Native North Americans having the lowest frequency [39].

Secondary Nonresponsiveness

Case Report

A 40 year old white female patient presented to JC Clinic with secondary clinical resistance to three Health Canada-approved types of botulinum toxin A (BoNT-A), namely onabotulinumtoxinA, abobotulinumtoxinA, and incobotulinumtoxinA given to treat glabellar frown lines.

Her excellent initial treatment response became diminished with subsequent treatments. Her last onabotulinumtoxinA injection of the glabella (30 U) and horizontal forehead lines (10 U) gave no clinical response after 3 weeks. The test used for suspected secondary nonresponsiveness used was the Extensor digitorum brevis

(EDB) test which uses electromyography to measure the compound muscle action potential [40]. 20 units of onabotulinumtoxinA were injected into the extensor digitorum brevis muscle on the lateral dorsum of her right foot. Using electromyography, her mean baseline compound muscle action potential (CMAP) following peroneal nerve stimulation was 8.2 mV (normal ≥2 mV). After 30 days, the CMAP was essentially unchanged (7.9 mV). As the expected decrease in CMAP of a responsive individual would be at least a 50% reduction, the <20% reduction suggests blockade by neutralizing antibodies.

Additional research immunologic testing includes direct measurement of neutralizing antibodies [41]. The mouse bioassay and immunoprecipitation assay are other research tools which are relatively unavailable to most clinicians.

Subsequently she was treated with botulinum toxin B (rimabotulinumtoxinB) on the glabella (3000 U), lateral canthal lines (375 U), and frontalis (1125 U) with excellent results. She achieved as a good response with rimabotulinumtoxin A (BoNT-B) as onabototulinumtoxin A despite 30% heavy chain homology in their molecular structure [39].

Secondary nonresponsiveness is characterized by intentional immunization [38], or treatment failure following initial successes with antibody formation against the 150 kD neuromodulator core protein, the binding domain, or the accessory proteins. A large meta-analysis in 2010 showed only 11 of 2240 subjects (0.5%) treated with onabotulinumtoxinA for five different indications developed neutralizing antibodies against BoNT-A [42]. When subjects only treated on the glabella were assessed, only 2 of 718 subjects (0.3%) developed neutralizing antibodies.

A more recent meta-analysis of neutralizing antibody formation against onabotulinumtoxinA [43] was performed across multiple indications including cervical dystonia, post-stroke spasticity, axillary hyperhidrosis, neurogenic overactive bladder, and glabellar lines. The study found that among evaluable subjects, 27 of 5876 (0.5%) developed neutralizing antibodies after onabotulinumtoxinA treatment. Due to their low incidence, no evidence of a relationship was apparent between the presence of neutralizing antibodies and gender, treatment indication, dose, dosing interval, treatment cycle, or the injection site. Subjects who developed neutralizing antibodies had no immunological disorders.

Risk factors for developing neutralizing antibodies include high doses of neuromodulator per treatment (e.g., 400 to 500 U for cervical dystonia), booster injections 2 weeks after primary treatment which is analogous to immunization, and the use of products with containing accessory proteins (e.g., onabotulinumtoxinA, abobotulinumtoxinA, nivoboltulinumtoxinA) versus those containing the core 150 kD molecule (e.g., daxibotulinumtoxinA, incobotulinumtoxinA) [44].

Patients who are nonresponsive to BoNT-A may respond to a type-B toxin. Among 36 patients with cervical dystonia and a secondary non-response to type-A toxin, 13 (36%) had an acceptable clinical response to rimabotulinumtoxinB and were able to continue therapy. Among 20 patients with spasticity and were nonresponsive to type-A resistant, seven responded to rimabotulinumtoxinB [44]. For subjects becoming nonresponsive, response may return after waiting 30 months.

Treating Eyelid Ptosis Following Cosmetic Facial BoNT-A Injection

Eyelid ptosis or drooping (blepharoptosis) occurs when a misplaced BoNT-A injection causes the upper eyelid to droop. Fortunately, there is a second muscle deep in the upper eyelid called Muller's muscle which is adrenergically innervated. It originates from the under surface of the levator aponeurosis at the level of Whitnall's ligament and inserts into the superior border of the tarsus. It contributes ~2 mm of eyelid elevation.

Stimulating Müller's muscle can be done with one of several available topical alpha-adrenergic agonists. Apraclonidine 0.5% is a prescription eyedrop indicated to control or prevent post-surgical elevations in intraocular pressure. The eyelid will elevate 1–2 mm for approximately 4 h. Other eyedrops are available over-the-counter, such as oxymetazoline and naphazoline, with and without an antihistamine. As they do not provide long-lasting relief, patients should choose when they wish to use them.

Another means for treating ptosis is to inject BoNT-A into the pretarsal portion of the orbicularis oculi, the purse-string muscle that protects the eye. Contraction of the pretarsal portion of orbicularis oculi is responsible for blinking of the eyelid. Injection of 1 unit of BoNT-A at the far medial and far lateral pretarsal orbicularis oculi is helpful [45] in reversing the ptosis.

Pyridostigmine (Mestinon)

Pyridostigmine is a drug that is used in the clinical treatment of myasthenia gravis and also in anesthesia in the operating room to reverse neuromuscular blockade by nondepolarizing muscle relaxants. It is a reversible acetylcholinesterase inhibitor that works by preventing the breakdown of acetylcholine by the enzyme acetylcholinesterase at the neuromuscular junction [29]. In BoNT-A toxicity it potentiates the neuromuscular junction transmission of acetyl choline. It is at present used in the oral form or intravenously [29]. There is currently research underway to produce an injectable formulation of pyridostigmine [30] that could be injected locally in the aesthetic clinic if a patient presented with iatrogenic eyelid or eyebrow ptosis.

There are also several experimental medications that are being trialled, based on their interference with the different stages of BoNT pathways. The first group aims to block the binding of BoNT to receptors at the presynaptic membrane. These include ganglioside receptors such as quinic and thearubigin. The next group of medications aim to interfere with the internalisation process. These include methylamine hydrocholoride, bafilomycin A and quinolol [17]. There is one other group of medicines that can be used in the recovery of affected nerve terminals. These include 3,4 diaminopyridine (3,4 DAP) which is a potassium channel blocker. These act by increasing the duration of the presynaptic action potential, and thus increasing acetylcholine release [46]. There have also been a plethora of medications used in desperation to try and improve the outcome in systemic botulism, with little or no success. So far, the scientific approach has been much more successful.

Summary

Clinical use of the botulinum neurotoxins has exploded worldwide due to their efficacy and safety when used with detailed knowledge of human anatomy and the careful use of approved neuromodulators in recommended doses. We cannot overemphasise the positive effect of the health regulatory agencies such as the FDA, Health Canada and the European and Asian agencies in maintaining the high level of safety which has permitted this therapeutic and cosmetic expansion.

Reversal of neuromodulator effect is accomplished in the eyelid by using eyedrops such as apraclonidine and oxymetazoline to stimulate Muller's muscle, an adrenergically innervated muscle which also lifts the lid. Recent research into a new indication for an approved anticholinesterase, Pyridostigmine, as a local injectable reverser for all neuromodulators looks very promising [30].

Clinical botulism is a rare, but potentially severe, life-threatening condition. It is important to report every case to national agencies, as every case is potentially a public health emergency. To date there have been 2 recent clinical botulism outbreaks in the USA- one in 2004 and one 20 years later in 2024 which is still being investigated. In the first outbreak, all 4 subjects were saved by the skill and dedication of the hospital intensivists. The outcomes of the victims in the 2024 outbreak are still unknown as their hospital stays have just begun. To date, apart from supportive treatments, BAT is the only antitoxin available. Systemic treatment is also currently available using oral or intravenous Pyridostigmine (Mestinon). However, there are many side effects such as nausea, vomiting, diarrhoea, and blurred vision which make it less attractive. There are several studies underway to produce new medications which affect the neuromuscular junction to attempt to treat systemic botulism which at present would be fatal without the dedicated supportive care of our hospital Intensive Care Units [20].

References

1. Erbguth FJ. From poison to remedy: the chequered history of botulinum toxin. J Neural Transm (Vienna). 2008;115(4):559–65. https://doi.org/10.1007/s00702-007-0728-2. Epub 2007 Apr 26.
2. Münchau A, Bhatia KP. Uses of botulinum toxin injection in medicine today. BMJ. 2000;320(7228):161–5. https://doi.org/10.1136/bmj.320.7228.161.
3. Scott AB. Botulinum toxin injection into extraocular muscles as an alternative to strabismus surgery. J Pediatr Ophthalmol Strabismus. 1980;17(1):21–5. https://doi.org/10.3928/0191-3913-19800101-06.

4. Scott AB, Rosenbaum A, Collins CC. Pharmacologic weakening of extraocular muscles. Investig Ophthalmol. 1973;12(12):924–7.
5. Carruthers J, Carruthers A. Botox: beyond wrinkles. Clin Dermatol. 2004;22(1):89–93. https://doi.org/10.1016/j.clindermatol.2003.11.013.
6. Carruthers A, Carruthers J. History of the cosmetic use of Botulinum A exotoxin. Dermatologic Surg. 1998;24(11):1168–70. https://doi.org/10.1111/j.1524-4725.1998.tb04092.x.
7. Yoelin SG, Dhawan SS, Vitarella D, Ahmad W, Hasan F, Abushakra S. Safety and efficacy of EB-001, a novel type e botulinum toxin, in subjects with glabellar frown lines: results of a phase 2, randomized, placebo-controlled, ascending-dose study. Plast Reconstr Surg. 2018;142(6):847e–55e. https://doi.org/10.1097/PRS.0000000000005029.
8. "Botox® (onabotulinumtoxinA) for injection". Prescribing Information. North Chicago: AbbVie Inc. Available from: [insert website].
9. International Commission on Microbiological Specifications for Foods. Clostridium botulinum. In: Microorganisms in foods 5: characteristics of microbial pathogens is the only book that examines the characteristics of foodborne pathogens in relation to HACCP. London: Blackie Academic & Professional; 1996. ISBN: 041247350X.
10. Arnon SS, Schechter R, Inglesby TV, Henderson DA, Bartlett JG, Ascher MS, Eitzen E, Fine AD, Hauer J, Layton M, Lillibridge S, Osterholm MT, O'Toole T, Parker G, Perl TM, Russell PK, Swerdlow DL, Tonat K, Working Group on Civilian Biodefense. Botulinum toxin as a biological weapon: medical and public health management. JAMA. 2001;285(8):1059–70. https://doi.org/10.1001/jama.285.8.1059. Erratum in: JAMA 2001 Apr 25;285(16):2081.
11. Spika JS, Shaffer N, Hargrett-Bean N, Collin S, MacDonald KL, Blake PA. Risk factors for infant botulism in the United States. Am J Dis Child. 1989;143(7):828–32. https://doi.org/10.1001/archpedi.1989.02150190078026.
12. Chia JK, Clark JB, Ryan CA, Pollack M. Botulism in an adult associated with food-borne intestinal infection with Clostridium botulinum. N Engl J Med. 1986;315(4):239–41. https://doi.org/10.1056/NEJM198607243150407.
13. Passaro DJ, Werner SB, McGee J, Mac Kenzie WR, Vugia DJ. Wound botulism associated with black tar heroin among injecting drug users. JAMA. 1998;279(11):859–63. https://doi.org/10.1001/jama.279.11.859.
14. Thirunavukkarasu N, Johnson E, Pillai S, Hodge D, Stanker L, Wentz T, Singh B, Venkateswaran K, McNutt P, Adler M, Brown E, Hammack T, Burr D, Sharma S. Botulinum neurotoxin detection methods for public health response and surveillance. Front Bioeng Biotechnol. 2018;6:80. https://doi.org/10.3389/fbioe.2018.00080.
15. Bakheit AM, Ward CD, McLellan DL. Generalised botulism-like syndrome after intramuscular injections of botulinum toxin type A: a report of two cases. J Neurol Neurosurg Psychiatry. 1997;62(2):198. https://doi.org/10.1136/jnnp.62.2.198.
16. Hughes JM, Blumenthal JR, Merson MH, Lombard GL, Dowell VR Jr, Gangarosa EJ. Clinical features of types A and B food-borne botulism. Ann Intern Med. 1981;95(4):442–5. https://doi.org/10.7326/0003-4819-95-4-442.
17. Lonati D, Schicchi A, Crevani M, Buscaglia E, Scaravaggi G, Maida F, Cirronis M, Petrolini VM, Locatelli CA. Foodborne botulism: clinical diagnosis and medical treatment. Toxins (Basel). 2020;12(8):509. https://doi.org/10.3390/toxins12080509.
18. Geyer HL. Botulism. In: Nelson LS, et al., editors. Goldfrank's toxicologic emergencies. 11th ed. McGraw-Hill Education; 2019. Available from: https://accessemergencymedicine.mhmedical.com/content.aspx?bookid=2569&sectionid=210271082.
19. Sobel J. Botulism. Clin Infect Dis. 2005;41(8):1167–73. https://doi.org/10.1086/444507. Epub 2005 Aug 29.
20. Chertow DS, Tan ET, Maslanka SE, Schulte J, Bresnitz EA, Weisman RS, Bernstein J, Marcus SM, Kumar S, Malecki J, Sobel J, Braden CR. Botulism in 4 adults following cosmetic injections with an unlicensed, highly concentrated botulinum preparation. JAMA. 2006;296(20):2476–9. https://doi.org/10.1001/jama.296.20.2476.

21. Tilley C. CDC investigating botched Botox shots in 9 states hospitalizing women. Daily Mail. 16 Apr 2024. Available from: https://www.msn.com/en-us/health/medical/cdc-investigating-botched-botox-shots-in-9-states-hospitalizing-women/ar-BB1lICXs?ocid=socialshare&cvid=daf27a574841465a831423795486483e&ei=7&sc=shoreline.
22. Emergent Biosolutions [website]. Available from: https://www.emergentbiosolutions.com/products-services/our-products/. Accessed 13 Apr 2024.
23. Hatheway CH, Snyder JD, Seals JE, Edell TA, Lewis GE Jr. Antitoxin levels in botulism patients treated with trivalent equine botulism antitoxin to toxin types A, B, and E. J Infect Dis. 1984;150(3):407–12. https://doi.org/10.1093/infdis/150.3.407.
24. Ni SA, Brady MF. Botulism antitoxin. [Updated 2023 Sep 4]. In: StatPearls [Internet]. Treasure Island (FL): StatPearls Publishing; 2024. Available from: https://www.ncbi.nlm.nih.gov/books/NBK534807/.
25. Lawley TJ, Bielory L, Gascon P, Yancey KB, Young NS, Frank MM. A prospective clinical and immunologic analysis of patients with serum sickness. N Engl J Med. 1984;311(22):1407–13. https://doi.org/10.1056/NEJM198411293112204.
26. Chaudhry R. Botulism: a diagnostic challenge. Indian J Med Res. 2011;134(1):10–2.
27. Anniballi F, Lonati D, Fiore A, Auricchio B, De Medici D, Locatelli CA. New targets in the search for preventive and therapeutic agents for botulism. Expert Rev Anti-Infect Ther. 2014;12(9):1075–86. https://doi.org/10.1586/14787210.2014.945917. Epub 2014 Aug 4.
28. McNutt PM, Vazquez-Cintron EJ, Tenezaca L, Ondeck CA, Kelly KE, Mangkhalakhili M, Machamer JB, Angeles CA, Glotfelty EJ, Cika J, Benjumea CH, Whitfield JT, Band PA, Shoemaker CB, Ichtchenko K. Neuronal delivery of antibodies has therapeutic effects in animal models of botulism. Sci Transl Med. 2021;13(575):eabd7789. https://doi.org/10.1126/scitranslmed.abd7789.
29. Katz RL. Pyridostigmin (mestinon) as an antagonist of d-tubocurarine. Anesthesiology. 1967;28(3):528–34. PMID: 6023525.
30. Delnova [website]. Available from: https://delnova.net/aesthetic-solution/#:~:text=ReViVox%C2%AE%20is%20a%20safe,botulinum%2DType%20A%20toxin%20injections. Accessed 13 Apr 2024.
31. Qiao J, Hayes KC, Hsieh JTC, Potter PJ, Delaney GA. Effects of 4-aminopyridine on motor evoked potentials in patients with spinal cord injury. J Neurotrauma. 1997;14:135–49.
32. American Society of Plastic Surgeons. Plastic surgery statistics 2022. Available: https://www.plasticsurgery.org/plastic-surgery-statistics. Accessed 13 Apr 2024.
33. Li M, Goldberger BA, Hopkins C. Fatal case of BOTOX-related anaphylaxis? J Forensic Sci. 2005;50(1):169–72.
34. Coban A, Matur Z, Hanagasi HA, Parman Y. Iatrogenic botulism after botulinum toxin type a injections. Clin Neuropharmacol. 2010;33(3):158–60. https://doi.org/10.1097/WNF.0b013e3181d479e0. Effects of 4-aminopyridine on motor evoked potentials in patients with spinal cord injury. J Neurotrauma. 1997.
35. Albrecht P, Jansen A, Lee JI, Moll M, Ringelstein M, Rosenthal D, Bigalke H, Aktas O, Hartung HP, Hefter H. High prevalence of neutralizing antibodies after long-term botulinum neurotoxin therapy. Neurology. 2019;92(1):e48–54. https://doi.org/10.1212/WNL.0000000000006688. Epub 2018 Nov 21. Erratum in: Neurology. 2022 Feb 22;98(8):341.
36. Yin Y, Li T, Wang C, Ma Q, Fan X. Treatment of facial flaccidity and sagging after botulinum toxin A injection into the masseter. Plast Reconstr Surg. 2023;151(3):521–5. https://doi.org/10.1097/PRS.0000000000009909. Epub 2022 Nov 19.
37. Omoigui S, Irene S. Treatment of ptosis as a complication of botulinum toxin injection. Pain Med. 2005;6(2):149–51. https://doi.org/10.1111/j.1526-4637.2005.05029.x.
38. Bellows S, Jankovic J. Reply to comment on re-visiting immunogenicity associated with botulinum toxin treatment. Toxins 2019, 11, 491. Toxins (Basel). 2020;12(2):72. https://doi.org/10.3390/toxins12020072.
39. Rahman E. Neuromodulator immunogemicity. In: Carruthers J, Carruthers A, Dover J, Alam M, editors. Botulinum toxin. Procedures in cosmetic dermatology. Elsevier; Netherlands. 2023. p. 264–70.

40. Gordon PH, Gooch CL, Greene PE. Extensor digitorum brevis test and resistance to botulinum toxin type A. Muscle Nerve. 2002;26(6):828–31. https://doi.org/10.1002/mus.10231.
41. Dressler D, Wohlfahrt K, Meyer-Rogge E, Wiest L, Bigalke H. Antibody-induced failure of botulinum toxin a therapy in cosmetic indications. Dermatologic Surg. 2010;36(Suppl 4):2182–7. https://doi.org/10.1111/j.1524-4725.2010.01710.x. PMID: 21134050.
42. Naumann M, Carruthers A, Carruthers J, Aurora SK, Zafonte R, Abu-Shakra S, Boodhoo T, Miller-Messana MA, Demos G, James L, Beddingfield F, VanDenburgh A, Chapman MA, Brin MF. Meta-analysis of neutralizing antibody conversion with onabotulinumtoxinA (BOTOX®) across multiple indications. Mov Disord. 2010;25(13):2211–8. https://doi.org/10.1002/mds.23254.
43. Jankovic J, Carruthers J, Naumann M, Ogilvie P, Boodhoo T, Attar M, Gupta S, Singh R, Soliman J, Yushmanova I, Brin MF, Shen J. Neutralizing antibody formation with onabotulinumtoxinA (BOTOX®) treatment from global registration studies across multiple indications: a meta-analysis. Toxins (Basel). 2023;15(5):342. https://doi.org/10.3390/toxins15050342. PMID: 37235376; PMCID: PMC10224273.
44. Barnes MP, Best D, Kidd L, Roberts B, Stark S, Weeks P, Whitaker J. The use of botulinum toxin type-B in the treatment of patients who have become unresponsive to botulinum toxin type-A—initial experiences. Eur J Neurol. 2005;12(12):947–55. https://doi.org/10.1111/j.1468-1331.2005.01095.x.
45. Fagien S. Temporary management of upper lid ptosis, lid malposition, and eyelid fissure asymmetry with botulinum toxin type A. Plast Reconstr Surg. 2004;114(7):1892–902. https://doi.org/10.1097/01.prs.0000142744.55379.8d.
46. Qiao J, Hayes KC, Hsieh JT, Potter PJ, Delaney GA. Effects of 4-aminopyridine on motor evoked potentials in patients with spinal cord injury. J Neurotrauma. 1997;14(3):135–49. https://doi.org/10.1089/neu.1997.14.135.

Chapter 14
Hypoallergenic Cosmetics

Stanley B. Levy and Howard I. Maibach

Strictly speaking hypoallergenic refers to a cosmetic or skin care formulation less likely to cause an allergic (Type IV hypersensitivity) reaction than a similar product type in the marketplace. This claim implies to both consumers and professionals a reduced risk of adverse effects from all forms of irritation, as these are more common than true allergy. A responsible manufacturer making this claim formulates products and performs pre-market testing considering all forms of adverse skin reactions including the various possible forms of irritation.

History

In the early 1930's Alfred Woititz, a chemist in New Yok City, began developing cosmetic formulations for his wife, Fannie May, who was having difficulties tolerating available products. He consulted with Dr. Marion Sulzberger, a noted dermatologist expert in skin allergies, for assistance in developing safer formulations. He soon began getting requests dermatologists for these formulations. Dr. Sulzberger also proposed adding complete ingredient disclosures and that patch test materials be supplied by manufacturers to physicians. Utilizing both his and his wife's names Woititz formed a company, Almay Pharmaceutical Corporation. Other companies with similar product lines soon followed including Marcelle and A-Rex in Chicago.

Professional distribution and ingredient labeling initially distinguished hypoallergenic cosmetics from other cosmetic products. In the early1970's another cosmetic brand, Clinique, began suggesting improved safety of its products with the

S. B. Levy (✉)
Department of Dermatology, Duke University, Durham, NC, USA

H. I. Maibach
Department of Dermatology, University of California, San Francisco, CA, USA

P. Elsner et al. (eds.), *Cosmetics*, https://doi.org/10.1007/978-3-032-14644-1_14

claim "allergy-tested". Ingredient labeling became mandatory in the US in 1973. In 1975 the U.S. Food and Drug Administration (FDA) proposed a definition for the term hypoallergenic and the regulating of this claim ([5]). Almay and Clinique both contested the validity and practicality of such regulation. The U.S. Court of Appeals in 1977 declared the FDA regulation invalid. The hypoallergenic claim remains unregulated in the USA. Mandatory ingredient labeling for cosmetics in Europe did not come into effect until 1997. In the European Union (EU) the term hypoallergenic can be used, as recommended by a sub-working committee on cosmetic claims (https://ec.europa.eu/docsroom/documents/24847), if a cosmetic product has been designed to minimize allergic potential by avoidance of known sensitizers and appropriate risk assessment of skin sensitization (https://ec.europa.eu/docsroom/documents/24847). No final regulation has been approved.

Perception

Consumers interpret hypoallergenic to mean a reduced risk or elimination of all types of reactions indicating physiologic intolerance to the extent that a product cannot be used safely or comfortably. Arguably, dermatologists also have this same expectation. A mailed questionnaire study to members of the American Academy of Dermatology assessing their perception of hypoallergenicity indicated that most respondents also had a broader interpretation of the term to include all forms or irritation [3]. Although Type IV cell mediated reactions are the most studied and best understood, most adverse reactions associated with cosmetics are not allergic (Table 14.1). They include visible irritant dermatitis, acneiform eruptions or contact folliculitis, contact urticaria and subjective irritation.

Between 50% and 70% of the general population self identifies as having some form of sensitive skin [4] often solely based on having experienced purely subjective symptoms including stinging, burning or itching, wherein a product cannot be used comfortably. A disproportionate number of atopic individuals are prone to subjective irritation [10] as well as visible irritant dermatitis. A weakened or defective skin barrier, vasomotor instability (flushing or blushing easily), and heightened

Table 14.1 Cosmetic intolerance

Subjective or sensory irritation	Contact urticaria
Stinging	Immunologic
Burning	Non-immunologic
Itching	Acneiform/folliculits
Contact dermatitis	Conjunctivitis
Irritant	Cheilitis
Allergic (type IV)	Pigmentary change
Photosensitivity	Hair and nail changes
	Respiratory/inhalant

neurosensory awareness all contribute to a wider notion of sensitive skin. As consumers have difficulty differentiating various types of skin reactions, cosmetic manufacturers can assume that products claiming to be hypoallergenic are more likely to be self-selected by atopic individuals and consumers prone to both irritant contact dermatitis and sensory irritation expecting a reduced risk for the full range of sensitivity. Likewise, professional recommendations for specific brands and products are based on the expectation that the responsible manufacturer has considered all these possibilities.

Formulation

Ingredient selection is fundamental to formulating hypoallergenic cosmetics as many known sensitizers and irritants can simply be avoided at this earliest stage of product development (Table 14.2) [9]. Irritation, not allergy accounts for most adverse cosmetic reactions. Ideally fewer and the most necessary ingredients are used in a single formulation. There should be clear justification for all selected Ingredients. Ingredients with possible allergic or irritation potential are used at the lowest effective concentration to ensure product safety. Ingredient rating systems have been developed attempting to validate ingredient selection [16]. A responsible manufacturer continually reviews and monitors the dermatologic and toxicologic literature as part of this process.

Fragrances are complex mixtures of ingredients and a leading cause of allergic contact sensitivity in skin care and cosmetic products [13]. Ideally fragrance ingredients are completely avoided in hypoallergenic formulations, i.e., 100% fragrance free. However, some manufacturers claiming that a product is fragrance-free may include masking agents or botanical ingredients in their formulations that have

Table 14.2 Guidelines for formulating hypoallergenic products

Eliminate known sensitizers
Utilize safe alternatives
Minimize and use safest available ingredients
Avoid fragrance
Utilize mild surfactants
Reduce concentration of certain ingredients
Use pure materials
Avoid cross-sensitizers
Consider using quenchers or anti-irritants
Label product ingredients accurately
Always test final formulations thoroughly

fragrance properties to improve product aesthetics and still claim the product is free of fragrance or unscented. These ingredients are also best avoided.

Preservatives are a common cause of allergic contact dermatitis in cosmetics [1]. Adequate preservation of products is necessary for prolonging shelf life and preventing bacterial contamination with repeat usage of a product by consumers. Most cosmetic products need proper preservation due to their water-based formulations. Ingredients with antimicrobial properties present a higher risk of true allergic reactions as a function of their chemical structure. These can include methylchloroisothiazolinone, the most sensitizing isothiazolinone, formaldehyde and formaldehyde releasers (imidazolidinyl urea, diazonidyl urea, and quaternium 15). Formaldehyde releasers should be utilized at the lowest concentration necessary for adequate preservation to minimize free formaldehyde release. Parabens are associated with a lower incidence of sensitization than the previously mentioned preservatives; but their weak estrogenic properties have been cited limiting the concentration used [6]. Preservatives and fragrances are responsible for most contact urticaria associated with cosmetics, the majority of which is nonimmunologic and underdiagnosed [7].

Other commonly used ingredients in cosmetic formulations have allergic potential. Substitutes for propylene glycol, lanolin alcohol, organic chemical sunscreens and some surfactants are available. Nail enamels can be formulated without the use of tosylamide formaldehyde resin. Acrylates employed in nail enamels are polymerized and unlikely to sensitize. Artificial nails or nail extenders contain acrylates in monomeric form and are potentially more sensitizing. More challenging is formulating cosmetically acceptable permanent hair dyes without p-phenylendiamine and its derivatives. Semi-permanent hair color products are less reactive but still contains some unreacted components at lower concentrations. Plant based colors including henna and other vegetable dyes can be utilized as alternatives for hair coloring but are less long lasting and less likely to result in a natural appearance.

Consumers select hypoallergenic cosmetics with the expectation that the potential for all forms of irritation are reduced. Potential irritants need to be avoided. This includes ingredients deliberately selected for inclusion in a formulation to induce sensory responses such as menthol. Surfactants and emulsifiers should be chosen carefully and employed at the lowest possible effective concentration in formulations as they can be disruptive to intercellular skin lipids affecting barrier function [14]. Exfoliants and hydroxy acids can potentially damage the skin barrier and are best avoided. Volatile ingredients such as light weight alcohols evaporating rapidly from the skin may be perceived negatively. Conversely, occlusive hydrophobic agents may improve barrier function by reducing transepidermal water loss. Formulations that are slightly acidic (pH 5.2–5.6) more closely simulate the skin's "acid mantle" normally present and are better tolerated. Strict raw material guidelines ensuring ingredient purity are a necessity.

Testing

The cornerstone predictive pre-market test for delayed Type IV hypersensitivity is the Human Repeat Insult Patch Test (HRIPT) [15]. Mounting pressure from both consumers and animal rights groups has resulted in testing methods with laboratory animals being utilized much less frequently in the cosmetic and skin care industry. The European Union no longer allows cosmetic product testing using animal models. The most rigorous protocols employ 48-h patches in place continuously for 3 weeks followed by a 10 day to 2 week rest period and a subsequent challenge patch. Protocols utilizing 48-h patches as opposed to 24-h (with a rest day between the patch applications) are more rigorous comparable to a Cumulative Irritation Study. The latter can be useful in developing and claiming a particular formulation to be less irritating than an alternative by comparative testing. Additional phototesting may be added when formulation assessment suggests the risk of phototoxic and photoallergic reactions.

Supervised or Controlled Product Use Testing is fundamental to screening for the wider range of objective and subjective irritation potential. Test subjects can be identified by their dermatologic and product use history to identify irritation prone individuals. Special panels can be recruited for specific concerns such as aggravation of acne, eye area and lip irritation.

Carefully developed questionnaires can be employed to recruit individuals prone to sensory forms of irritation [11]. Product use diaries kept by the test subjects themselves during use studies are important. The lactic acid stinging test [12] can be utilized to select test panelists prone to this form of sensory irritation. "Stingers" are selected who consistently experience this sensation when 5%–10% lactic acid is applied to the nasolabial fold or malar area. Methods are being refined to precisely identify these individuals through questionnaires and lipid profiling, though significant challenges remain [8, 17].

Conclusion

There is no universally agreed upon standard or regulatory definition for the claim of hypoallergenicity as applied to cosmetic and skin care products. Complete consensus may not be realistic or achievable considering the wide range of opinions among physicians, cosmetic scientists and regulatory agencies regarding this claim. Ideally a hypoallergenic formulation is fragrance free and formulated with the least sensitizing preservatives and other ingredients. All potential forms of sensitivity are considered in product development. The full range of available premarket safety testing is employed appropriate to the product type and its intended use. Professional recommendations for specific brands claiming hypoallergenicity are very much dependent on the standards and integrity of the specific manufacturer making this claim.

References

1. Deza G, Giménez-Arnau A. Allergic contact dermatitis in preservatives: current standing and future options. Curr Opin Allergy Clin Immunol. 2017;17(4):263–8. https://doi.org/10.1097/ACI.0000000000000373.
2. Do LHD, Azizi N, Maibach H. Sensitive skin syndrome: an update. Am J Clin Dermatol. 2020;21(3):401–9. https://doi.org/10.1007/s40257-019-00499-7. PMID: 31834575.
3. Draelos ZD, Rietschel RL. Hypoallergenicity and the dermatologist's perception. J Am Acad Dermatol. 1996;35(2 Pt 1):248–51. https://doi.org/10.1016/s0190-9622(96)90342-4.
4. Farage MA. The prevalence of sensitive skin. Front Med. 2019;6:98. https://doi.org/10.3389/fmed.2019.00098. PMID: 31157225; PMCID: PMC6533878.
5. Federal Register, Hypoallergenic and other claims of relative safety. 1975;40(110):24450.
6. Fransway AF, Fransway PJ, Belsito DV, Yiannias JA. Paraben Toxicology. Dermatitis. 2019;30(1):32–45. https://doi.org/10.1097/DER.0000000000000428. PMID: 30570577.
7. Giménez-Arnau AM, Pesqué D, Maibach HI. Contact urticaria syndrome: a comprehensive review. Curr Dermatol Rep. 2022;11(4):194–201. https://doi.org/10.1007/s13671-022-00379-0.
8. Kim S, Joo KM, Oh M, An S, Han J, Park S, Kwak I, Lee DH, Cho JY. Improving sensitive skin diagnosis by integrating diagnostic questionnaires, lactic acid sting test, and lipid profiling. J Cosmet Dermatol. 2025;24(3):e70099. https://doi.org/10.1111/jocd.70099. PMID: 40029145; PMCID: PMC118750.
9. Levy SB. Hypoallergenic cosmetics. In: Schlossman ML, editor. The chemistry and manufacture of cosmetics, vol. III. 3rd ed. Carol Stream: Allured; 2002. p. 503–26.
10. Maarouf M, Kromenacker B, Capozza KL, Kempton D, Hendricks A, Tran K, Shi VY. Pain and itch are dual burdens in atopic. Dermatitis. 2018;29(5):278–81. https://doi.org/10.1097/DER.0000000000000406. PMID: 30179978.
11. Misery L, Loser K, Ständer S. Sensitive skin. J Eur Acad Dermatol Venereol. 2016;30(Suppl 1):2–8. https://doi.org/10.1111/jdv.13532. PMID: 26805416.
12. Pan Y, Ma X, Song Y, Zhao J, Yan S. Questionnaire and lactic acid sting test play different role on the assessment of sensitive skin: a cross-sectional study. Clin Cosmet Investig Dermatol. 2021;14:1215–25. https://doi.org/10.2147/CCID.S325166. PMID: 34548802; PMCID: PMC8449876.
13. Reeder MJ. Allergic contact dermatitis to fragrances. Dermatol Clin. 2020;38(3):371–7. https://doi.org/10.1016/j.det.2020.02.009. Epub 2020 May 4. PMID: 32475515.
14. Salomon G, Giordano-Labadie F. Surfactant irritations and allergies. Eur J Dermatol. 2022;32(6):677–81. https://doi.org/10.1684/ejd.2022.4290. PMID: 36856374; PMCID: PMC10195118.
15. Strickland J, Daniel AB, Allen D, et al. Skin sensitization testing needs and data uses by US regulatory and research agencies. Arch Toxicol. 2019;93(2):273–91. https://doi.org/10.1007/s00204-018-2341-6. Epub 2018 Oct 30. PMID: 30377734; PMCID: PMC6363849.
16. Verallo-Rowell VM. The validated hypoallergenic cosmetic rating system: its 30-year evolution and effect on the prevalence of cosmetic reactions. Dermatitis. 2011;22(2):80–97. https://doi.org/10.2310/6620.2011.1004.
17. Yan S, Zhao J, Han Y, Wang R, Bai K, Ge J, Pan Y, Zhao H. The challenges in investigating the pathogenesis of sensitive skin by noninvasive measurements: a systematic review. Clin Cosmet Investig Dermatol. 2023;16:237–51. https://doi.org/10.2147/CCID.S392925. PMID: 36726811; PMCID: PMC9885880.

Chapter 15
The Use of Sensitive Skin Panels to Substantiate Cosmetic Claims

L. Misery

Sensitive skin is consensually recognized as "a syndrome defined by the occurrence of unpleasant sensations (stinging, burning, pain, pruritus, and tingling sensations) in response to stimuli that normally should not provoke such sensations. These unpleasant sensations cannot be explained by lesions attributable to any skin disease. The skin can appear normal or be accompanied by erythema. Sensitive skin can affect all body locations, especially the face" [1]. Hence, sensitive skin is a primary disorder (with many etiologies), and there is no "secondary sensitive skin." The occurrence of sensory symptoms in patients with atopic dermatitis or any other skin disease is a manifestation of this skin disease itself, but this is not sensitive skin.

The same expert group published a second position paper on the pathophysiology and management of sensitive skin [2]. A multifactorial origin was suggested after discussion of many putative mechanisms. However, it was concluded that sensitive skin is not an immunological disorder but is related to alterations of the skin nervous system and that skin barrier abnormalities are frequently associated, but without any direct relationship. Growing evidence suggest that sensitive skin is a neuropathic disorder [3].

Consequently, co-cultures of skin/epidermis/keratinocytes and sensory neurons could be adequate models for in vitro studies of sensitive skin [4], while other models are rather interesting for the evaluation of skin irritation [5, 6]. The main concern is that sensitive is strongly associated with individuals and that a clinical evaluation is needed.

A meta-analysis including 13 studies has shown that cosmetics and physical (variations in temperature, cold, heat, wind, sun, air conditioning, wet air, and dry

L. Misery (✉)
Laboratory Interactions Epitheliums-Neurons (LINK), University of Western Brittany, Brest, France

Department of Dermatology and Allergology, University Hospital of Brest, Brest, France
e-mail: laurent.misery@chu-brest.fr

P. Elsner et al. (eds.), *Cosmetics*, https://doi.org/10.1007/978-3-032-14644-1_15

air), chemical (water and pollution), or psychological (emotional) factors could be associated with sensitive skin. The most important factors are cosmetics, far ahead of the other factors [7].

In order to substantiate cosmetic claims about sensitive skin, panels of subjects with sensitive skin are frequently used, with the aim to demonstrate that cosmetic products do not aggravate sensitive skin and sometimes ameliorate sensitive skin. Unfortunately, a number of evaluations have no value because sensitive skin panels are not adequately defined.

A sensitive skin panel must be defined by two criteria:

- No skin disease is associated, because an evaluation of sensitive skin is not possible if we do not know if we are evaluating sensitive skin, a skin disease, or both
- Positive criteria for the assessment of sensitive skin are clearly defined.

These criteria can be assessed with different methods, which will be cited in the following paragraphs.

Chemical Tests

Stinging test remains the most commonly technique used to define sensitive skin panels [8]. Many other objectification techniques have been proposed: chromametry, laser Doppler, thermal sensitivity test, capsaicin test, sodium lauryl sulfate, dimethyl sulfoxide, ethanol or other chemical compounds, etc. [9–11]. These tests try to evaluate the sensory and/or the erythemal response of the skin to some factors.

Stinging Test

The famous lactic acid stinging test (LAST) of Frosch and Kligman is the first standardized test [8]. It consists of the application of 0.5 mL of 10% (or 5%) lactic acid to the nasolabial fold with subsequent assessment of the severity of the subjective symptoms. Erythema is sometimes evaluated. Control is provided by the application of a saline solution to the other fold.

Stinging test is very commonly used and is very useful for the follow-up of sensitive skin. However, it is a poor instrument to assess sensitive skin [12]. Hence, Marriott et al. tested four chemicals commonly used to induce different sensory effects (lactic acid, stinging; capsaicin, burning; menthol, cooling; and ethanol, a mixture of burning and stinging), then noted a high number of variations in reactivity to the tested substances and a lack of predictive value of increased reactivity among the different materials [13]. An important intra-individual variability was also observed comparing the responses to only two chemicals [14]. Nonetheless, other authors found lactic acid stinging test was predictive of sensitive skin [15].

Another controversy is the quantification of the intensity of unpleasant sensory responses [16, 17]. The semiquantitative assessment is frequently used [18]. Measuring cerebral responses to the LAST with functional magnetic resonance imaging (fMRI) may allow a more objective assessment [19] but is certainly not possible in routine practice. In any case, there is a discrepancy between lactic acid response and self-perception of sensitive skin [20]. Consequently, it is recommended to associate LAST with a concomitant questionnaire [16].

Capsaicin Test

Capsaicin test was more recently described, to assess the hyperactivation of TRPV1 in subjects with sensitive skin [21]. A 0.075% emulsion of capsaicin is applied. Similar to the LAST, it is based on a subjective individual pain scale.

Interestingly, the capsaicin detection threshold (CDT) test combines the specific reactivity of sensitive skin to capsaicin, the application simplicity of the LAST, and a method of detection threshold. It does not rely anymore on the quantification of the intensity of the response but on the determination of detection thresholds of topically applied capsaicin. Five capsaicin concentrations are used in 10% ethanol aqueous solution (3.16×10^{-5}%, 1×10^{-4}%, 3.16×10^{-4}%, 1×10^{-3}%, 3.16×10^{-3}%) [21]. The method used to attain the detection threshold consists of applying increasing concentrations of capsaicin onto the nasolabial folds (3-min interval between each application). The vehicle is simultaneously applied following a split-face, single-blind plan. The test is stopped as soon as the subject reports a specific sensation on the capsaicin side.

Neurophysiological Techniques

These methods are used for studying the impairment of somatosensory function in neurologic diseases. They are based on different stimuli: thermal (cold, warm), electrical, or mechanical. Their use is more restricted to specialized centers, and they are rarely used to assess sensitive skin.

Current Perception Threshold (CPT)

Sensitivity evaluations using the CPT method are based on the distinction of the types of involved nerve fibers thanks their activation by three different current frequencies produced by the Neurometer® CPT® device (Neurotron Inc., Aurora, CO, USA). Transcutaneous electrical stimuli are applied through two electrodes. The frequencies produced by the Neurometer® CPT® provide selective stimulation of three subsets of nerve fibers: the 2000-Hz current stimulates large myelinated Aβ fibers (touch and pressure sensation), the 250-Hz current stimulates small myelinated Aδ fibers (temperature, pressure, fast pain, and prickling itch sensation), and the 5-Hz current stimulates unmyelinated C-fibers (temperature, slow pain, and burning itch sensation). Ham et al. analyzed the relationship between the frequency of response at each sensation (stinging, burning, and itching) during a lactic acid sting test and the CPT value of each frequency [22]. To reconfirm this relationship, they analyzed differences of the CPT value (5 Hz) between the itch responder and non-itch responder groups. There was a significant correlation between itch sensation and CPT values of 5 Hz. The itch responder group showed significantly lower sensory perception value of 5 Hz than the non-itch responder group.

Quantitative Sensory Testing (QST)

QST is a psychophysical validated method that uses different stimuli of increasing intensity to measure somatosensory perception [23]. This method allows evaluation of the participation of small and large nerve fibers. Currently, QST is used mainly in neuropathic pain or neuropathic pruritus to look for small-fiber neuropathies [24]. The detection thresholds of heat pain (HPT), vibration pain (VDT), and cold pain (CDT) can be tested using the Computer-Assisted Sensory Examination (CASE) system IV (WR Medical Electronics Co., Maplewood, MN, USA) [25, 26]. A thermal electrode of 10 cm^2 is placed on the dorsum of the dominant hand of the subject or elsewhere. The CASE IV software program automatically calculates the pain ratings of HP 0.5, HP 5.0, and HP 5–0.5 with a quadratic regression equation. HP 0.5 is defined as the midpoint between the smallest stimulus that created pain and the largest no-painful stimulus. HP 5.0 corresponded to the stimulus that created a rating of 5 from the subject. HP 5–0.5 was the difference between these two values. In subjects with sensitive skin, the HPT is significantly lower (14.5 ± 2.8) than in the controls (17.8 ± 2.5) ($p < 0.001$) [25]. Intermediate pain (HPT 5.0) is also significantly decreased.

Cutaneous Thermal Sensation

This psychophysical test is only based on the assessment of peripheral sensitivity to thermal stimuli. This test involved the use of a thermal testing instrument—for example, the Thermal Sensory Analyser (TSA 2001) manufactured by Medoc, Ramat Yishai, Israel—to assess the thermal functional components of cutaneous nerve endings [16, 27]. The thermode delivers thermal stimuli capable of heating or cooling the skin.

Skin Biopsies

Histological analysis of skin biopsies in sensitive skin areas shows a decrease of intraepidermal nerve density, like in small-fiber neuropathies [28]. However, it is difficult to use this invasive technique routinely.

Parallel Tests

The aim of many other tests is to evaluate skin properties which can be modified in subjects with sensitive skin but are not directly related to sensitive skin: transepidermal water loss (TEWL), cutaneous pH, epidermal thickness (measured by ultrasonography, optical microscopy, or confocal microscopy), skin penetrability (assessed with UV light), molecular composition of stratum corneum (using confocal Raman microspectroscopy), or others [12, 29–32]. All these tests are commonly used in studies on sensitive skin, but they never measure skin hypersensitivity.

Questionnaires

It is obviously not possible to objectively discriminate the presence or absence of sensitive skin [33] because sensitive skin is first and foremost a sensory disorder. Nonetheless, the concept of diagnosis of sensitive skin using questionnaires came a long time after the reactivity tests. Many scales were proposed, but they were frequently used only by a company or an author and even only for an only study.

Some have been more widely used because they were created, validated, and translated in many languages using the currently recommended methodology: the Sensitive Scalp Severity (3S) questionnaire for the sensitive scalp [34] and the Sensitive Scale for sensitive skin in general [35]. More recently, a scale called BoSS has been proposed to measure the burden of sensitive skin [36].

Sensitive Scale

Sensitive Scale (SS-10) is a 10-item scale (Fig. 15.1) that was initially tested in 11 countries in different languages on 2966 participants [35]. The internal consistency was high. Correlations with the dry skin type, higher age, female gender, fair phototypes, and the Dermatology Quality of Life Index (DLQI) were found. DLQI is a tool to evaluate the quality of life in patients with skin disorders [37]. Using the 10-item version appeared to be preferable to the 14-item because it was quicker and easier to complete, with the same internal consistency and the supplementary 4

DEGREE OF OVERALL SKIN IRRITATION DURING THE PAST 3 DAYS

Using a vertical line, indicate the symptoms felt during the past 3 days on the horizontal line (0 = absence of irritation, 10 = intolerable irritation).

Important: To be completed by the patient

Skin irritation 0 Min. ——— 10 Max

SEVERITY OF SKIN CONDITION DURING THE PAST 3 DAYS

Please indicate the intensity of each of the following symptoms during the past 3 days. (0 = zero intensity, 10 = intolerable intensity): darken one number between 0 and 10.

Important : To be completed by the patient

Skin condition felt:

Tingling	⓪	①	②	③	④	⑤	⑥	⑦	⑧	⑨	⑩
Burning	⓪	①	②	③	④	⑤	⑥	⑦	⑧	⑨	⑩
Sensations of heat	⓪	①	②	③	④	⑤	⑥	⑦	⑧	⑨	⑩
Tautness	⓪	①	②	③	④	⑤	⑥	⑦	⑧	⑨	⑩
Itching	⓪	①	②	③	④	⑤	⑥	⑦	⑧	⑨	⑩
Pain	⓪	①	②	③	④	⑤	⑥	⑦	⑧	⑨	⑩
General discomfort	⓪	①	②	③	④	⑤	⑥	⑦	⑧	⑨	⑩
Hot flashes	⓪	①	②	③	④	⑤	⑥	⑦	⑧	⑨	⑩

Visible skin conditions:

Redness	⓪	①	②	③	④	⑤	⑥	⑦	⑧	⑨	⑩

Fig. 15.1 Sensitive scale

items that were excluded were very rarely observed in patients. The mean initial score was around 37/100 (and 44/140 in the initial 14-item version). More recently, a SS-10 cut-off value of 12.7 to detect sensitive skin was identified (with a sensitivity of 72.4% and specificity of 90.3%) [38]. For practical reasons, we propose that a score greater than 13 on the SS-10 can be used as the cut-off to diagnose sensitive skin, and a score greater than 5 can be used as the cut-off to diagnose slightly sensitive skin.

For each of the 5 following symptoms (do you feel itching, prickling, tightness, pain or burning on your scalp?), which of the statements below best describes how it affects you.
No, I do not feel it
Yes, but it is not troublesome
Yes, and it is slightly troublesome
Yes, and it is sufficiently troublesome to alter my lifestyle
Yes, and it is unbearable

Fig. 15.2 The 3S questionnaire

3S Questionnaire

The 3S Questionnaire was created to assess sensitive scalp [34] (Fig. 15.2). The total score is obtained by multiplying score severity of abnormal sensations by the number of these sensations. The 3S questionnaire allowed discrimination between subjects with slightly sensitive, sensitive, and very sensitive scalps. Itching and prickling were the most frequent symptoms. The 3S questionnaire is a convenient and effective tool for investigating the severity and symptomatology of the sensitive scalp.

BoSS Questionnaire

The burden of a disease is made of the physical, psychological, sociological, and economic consequences. The BoSS Questionnaire was designed to evaluate all these aspects in patients with sensitive skin [36]. This questionnaire was developed using standardized methods for creating and validating quality of life questionnaires, consisting in three phases: a design phase, a development phase, and a validation phase. The BoSS Questionnaire was found psychometrically robust, with excellent internal consistency and good item-scale, convergent, and construct validity. This questionnaire was also significantly correlated with both components of the SF-12 and with the DLQI, confirming its concurrent validity, with a higher correlation with DLQI. Internal and external validities are high, and we showed clear reliability with the severity of sensitive skin and other factors.

The BoSS Questionnaire could be also used a diagnostic tool for sensitive skin. A positive and statistically significant correlation was observed between the SS-10 score and the BoSS score [38], and the mean BoSS score is very different according the severity of sensitive skin [39]. A cut-off definition is currently in progress.

Conclusion

Although there are a large number of techniques for sensitive skin testing, there is and there will be no objective technique for the diagnosis of sensitive skin and the diagnosis, as well as the building of sensitive skin panels, is mainly based on questionnaires.

Another limitation is the fact that it is not possible to separate normal skin from sensitive skin. Some cut-offs were proposed and are very useful. However, all authors have to keep in mind that there is a continuum between a completely normal skin and all graduations of sensitive skin.

References

1. Misery L, Ständer S, Szepietowski JC, Reich A, Wallengren J, Evers AW, et al. Definition of sensitive skin: an expert position paper from the special interest group on sensitive skin of the International Forum for the Study of Itch. Acta Derm Venereol. 2017;97:4–6.
2. Misery L, Weisshaar E, Brenaut E, Evers AWM, Huet F, Ständer S, et al. Pathophysiology and management of sensitive skin: position paper from the special interest group on sensitive skin of the International Forum for the Study of Itch (IFSI). J Eur Acad Dermatol Venereol. 2020;34:222–9.
3. Misery L. Sensitive skins may be neuropathic disorders: lessons from studies on skin and other organs. Cosmetics. 2021;8:14.
4. Sakka M, Leschiera R, Le Gall-Ianotto C, Gouin O, L'herondelle K, Buscaglia P, et al. A new tool to test active ingredient using lactic acid in vitro, a help to understand cellular mechanism involved in stinging test: an example using a bacterial polysaccharide (Fucogel®). Exp Dermatol. 2018;27:238–44.
5. Harding AL, Murdoch C, Danby S, Hasan MZ, Nakanishi H, Furuno T, et al. Determination of chemical irritation potential using a defined gene signature set on tissue-engineered human skin equivalents. JID Innov. 2021;1(2):100011.
6. Misery L. Irritated skin is not sensitive skin. JID Innov. 2021;1:10031.
7. Brenaut E, Barnetche T, Le-Gall Ianotto C, Roudot AC, Misery L, Ficheux AS. Role of the environment in sensitive skin from the worldwide patient's point of view: a literature review and meta-analysis. J Eur Acad Dermatol Venereol. 2020;34:230–8.
8. Frosch PJ, Kligman AM. A method of appraising the stinging capacity of topically applied substances. J Soc Cosmet Chem. 1977;28:197–209.
9. Honari G, Andersen RM, Maibach HI. Sensitive skin syndrome. 2nd ed. Boca Raton: CRC Press; 2017. 222 p.
10. Berardesca E, Fluhr JW, Maibach HI. What is sensitive skin ? In: Berardesca E, Fluhr JW, Maibach HI, editors. Sensitive skin syndrome. New York: Taylor & Francis; 2006. p. 1–6.
11. Farage MA, Katsarou A, Maibach HI. Sensory, clinical and physiological factors in sensitive skin: a review. Contact Derm. 2006;55(1):1–14.
12. Maroñas-Jiménez L, González-Guerra E, Guerra-Tapia A. Challenges of investigation. In: Honari G, Andersen RM, Maibach HI, editors. Sensitive skin syndrome. 2nd ed. Boca Raton: CRC Press; 2017.
13. Marriott M, Holmes J, Peters L, Cooper K, Rowson M, Basketter DA. The complex problem of sensitive skin. Contact Derm. 2005;53:93–9.
14. Green BG, Shaffer GS. Psychophysical assessment of the chemical irritability of human skin. J Soc Cosmet Chem. 1992;43:131–47.

15. Darlenski R, Kazandjieva J, Fluhr JW, Maurer M, Tsankov N. Lactic acid sting test does not differentiate between facial and generalized skin functional impairment in sensitive skin in atopic dermatitis and rosacea. J Dermatol Sci. 2014;76:151–3.
16. Jourdain R. Neurosensory assessment. In: Honari G, Andersen RM, Maibach HI, editors. Sensitive skin syndrome. 2nd ed. Boca Raton: CRC Press; 2017.
17. Slodownik D, Williams J, Lee A, Tate B, Nixon R. Controversies regarding the sensitive skin syndrome. Expert Rev Dermatol. 2007;2:579–84.
18. Fauger A, Lhoste A, Chavagnac-Bonneville M, Sayag M, Jourdan E, Ardiet N, et al. Effects of a new topical combination on sensitive skin. J Cosmet Sci. 2015;66:79–86.
19. Querleux B, Dauchot K, Jourdain R, Bastien P, Bittoun J, Anton JL, et al. Neural basis of sensitive skin: an fMRI study. Skin Res Technol. 2008;14(4):454–61.
20. Seidenari S, Francomano M, Mantavoni L. Baseline biophysical parameters in subjects with sensitive skin. Contact Dermat. 1998;38:311–5.
21. Jourdain R, Bastien P, de Lacharriere O, Rubinstenn G. Detection thresholds of capsaicin: a new test to assess facial skin neurosensitivity. J Cosmet Sci. 2005;56:153–66.
22. Ham H, An SM, Lee EJ, Lee E, Kim HO, Koh JS. Itching sensation and neuronal sensitivity of the skin. Skin Res Technol. 2016;22(1):104–7.
23. Dyck PJ, Zimmerman I, Gillen DA, et al. Cool, warm, and heat-pain detection thresholds: testing methods and inferences about anatomic distribution of receptors. Neurology. 1993;43:1500–8.
24. Misery L, Brenaut E, Le Garrec R, Abasq C, Genestet S, Marcorelles P, et al. Neuropathic pruritus. Nat Rev Neurol. 2014;10(7):408–16.
25. Dyck PJ, Zimmerman IR, Johnson DM, et al. A standard test of heat-pain responses using CASE IV. J Neurol Sci. 1996;136:54–63.
26. Huet F, Dion A, Batardière A, Nedelec AS, Le Caër F, Bourgeois P, et al. Sensitive skin can be small fibre neuropathy: results from a case-control quantitative sensory testing study. Br J Dermatol. 2018;179:1157–62.
27. Yosipovitch G, Maibach HI. Thermal sensory analyzer, boon to the study of C and Aδ fibers. In: Curr Probl Dermatol, vol. 26; 1998. p. 84–9.
28. Buhé V, Vié K, Guéré C, Natalizio A, Lhéritier C, Le Gall-Ianotto C, et al. Pathophysiological study of sensitive skin. Acta Derm Venereol. 2016;96:314–8.
29. Primavera G, Berardesca E. Sensitive skin: mechanisms and diagnosis. Int J Cosmet Sci. 2005;27:1–10.
30. Inamadar AC, Palit A. Sensitive skin: an overview. Indian J Dermatol Venereol Leprol. 2013;79:9–16.
31. Bornkessel A, Flach M, Arens-Corell M, Elsner P, Fluhr JW. Functional assessment of a washing emulsion for sensitive skin: mild impairment of stratum corneum hydration, pH, barrier function, lipid content, integrity and cohesion in a controlled washing test. Skin Res Technol. 2005;11:53–60.
32. Falcone D, Uzunbajakava NE, van Erp PEJ, van de Kerkhof PCM. Confocal Raman microspectroscopy: a new paradigm in the diagnosis of sensitive skin? In: Honari G, Andersen RM, Maibach HI, editors. Sensitive skin syndrome. 2nd ed. Boca Raton: CRC Press; 2017.
33. Diogo L, Papoila L. Is it possible to characterize objectively sensitive skin ? Skin Res Technol. 2010;16:30–7.
34. Misery L, Rahhali N, Ambonati M, Black D, Saint-Martory C, Schmitt AM, et al. Evaluation of sensitive scalp severity and symptomatology by using a new score. J Eur Acad Dermatol Venereol. 2011;25:1295–8.
35. Misery L, Jean-Decoster C, Mery S, Georgescu V, Sibaud V. A new ten-item questionnaire for assessing sensitive skin: the sensitive scale-10. Acta Derm Venereol. 2014;94:635–9.
36. Misery L, Jourdan E, Abadie S, Ezzedine K, Brenaut E, Huet F, et al. Development and validation of a new tool to assess the burden of sensitive skin (BoSS). J Eur Acad Dermatol Venereol. 2018;32:2217–23.

37. Finlay AY, Khan GK. Dermatology Life Quality Index (DLQI) – a simple practical measure for routine clinical use. Clin Exp Dermatol. 1994;19:210–6.
38. Legeas C, Misery L, Fluhr JW, Roudot AC, Ficheux AS, Brenaut E. Proposal for cut-off scores for sensitive skin on sensitive scale-10 in a group of adult women. Acta Derm Venereol. 2021;101:adv00373.
39. Polena H, Chavagnac-Bonneville M, Misery L, Sayag M. Burden of sensitive skin (BoSS) questionnaire and current perception threshold: use as diagnostic tools for sensitive skin syndrome. Acta Derm Venereol. 2021;101:adv00606.

Chapter 16
Fragrances and Contact Sensitization: Prevalence and Mechanisms Involved

B. Blömeke and H. F. Merk

Introduction

Products with Fragrances

Approximately 3000 synthetic and 300–400 natural fragrances are known to be used by different industries [1]. Fragrance materials (natural fragrances, synthetic fragrances, natural essential oils, and fragrances mixtures representing combinations of different materials) are ubiquitously used, and fragrances are a primary factor in consumer choice. Fragrance materials are used to create perfumes, refine cosmetic, hygiene and present in products such as soaps, shampoos, lotions, facial and toilet tissues, air fresheners, disinfectants, vaporizers, household cleansers and detergents. Moreover, fragrances also play a considerable role in masking undesirable smells arising from fatty acids, oils and surfactants that are commonly used in cosmetic formulations, medicaments, food, plastics, paper, or paints. Fragrance materials are also utilized in other contexts, including but not limited to drinks, food flavoring, medicine, and aromatherapy. Furthermore, fragrances are components of smokeless tobacco pouches [2].

Given the potential critical conception associated with synthetic fragrances, natural fragrances and minimally processed natural constituents of plants (botanical extracts or essential oils) are increasingly been produced. Thus, essential oils are an important asset to the cosmetics industry as they are emitting pleasant scents and

B. Blömeke (✉)
Department of Environmental Toxicology, Trier University, Trier, Germany
e-mail: bloemeke@uni-trier.de

H. F. Merk
Department of Dermatology and Allergology, Medical Faculty, RWTH Aachen University, Talbothof, Aachen, Germany
e-mail: Hans.Merk@post.rwth-aachen.de

P. Elsner et al. (eds.), *Cosmetics*, https://doi.org/10.1007/978-3-032-14644-1_16

may be active agents and preservatives (anti-aging, antimicrobial, sun protection, and whitening). Table 16.1 provides examples of fragrances found in household products tested worldwide (adapted from [3]). For their usage in cosmetics see Guzmán et al. 2021 [4].

Sources of Fragrances

Extracts from animal secretions and plants are natural sources of raw materials for fragrances. Most natural fragrances are extracted from essential plant oils. Essential oils are volatile, complex mixtures of compounds characterized by a strong scent and are formed by aromatic plants as secondary metabolites. In nature, they play an important role in protection of plants, for example as antibacterials, antivirals, antifungals, insecticides and against herbivores by reducing their appetite for such plants. They also may attract some insects to favor the dispersion of pollen and seeds or repel undesirable others.

Two different types of essential oil cells are known, superficial cells, for example, glandular hairs located on the surface of the plant (e.g., oregano, mint, lavender), and cells embedded in plant tissue. Examples for the latter are the secretions of citrus fruits and eucalyptus leaves, or layers of cells surrounding intercellular space (canals or secretory cavities), for example, resin canals of pine.

Table 16.1 Frequencies (%) of fragrances in 450 household products tested worldwide. Adapted from [3]

Fragrances	Percentage
Limonene	72
α-Pinene	40
β-Pinene	43
Camphene	29
α-Terpinene	30
γ-Terpinene	20
β-Terpinene	23
α-Terpinolene	18
Linalool	45
β-Phellandrene	26
Citronellol	44
Eucalyptol	35
Geraniol	34
4-Terpineol	28
ρ-Cymene	28
Eugenol	31
Myrcene	32
Lilial	33
Citral	27

About 300 essential oils are commercially relevant. Volatile components account for 85–99%, mainly consisting of terpenoids (monoterpenes) and derivates thereof i.e. oxygenated monoterpenes and sesquiterpenes (see Sect. 1.3). Essential oils obtained from various fruits (oranges, mandarins, lime, lemons and grapefruits) of the *Citrus* genus are very popular, accounting for the largest commercial share of natural fragrances and flavors. Their essential oil is present in the fruit's peel in great quantities consisting of limonene, linalool, linalyl acetate, β-pinene, and α-terpineol among others. Another important essential oil is Lavender oil derived from lavender (*Lavendula angustifolia*). The primary components of lavender oil are linalool, linalyl acetate, and caryophyllene. Peppermint oil is also widely utilized in several industries, including food, perfumes, pharmaceuticals, and flavoring. It is derived from *Mentha piperita L.*, a sterile hybrid of the species *M. aquatica L. and M. spicata*. Mint oils include menthol, menthone, and menthyl acetate as their primary components.

Essential oils have been widely used all over the world, and their use is growing due to the strong demand for pure natural ingredients in various fields. Thus, the large quantities of essential oils are generated by the industrial culture of essential oil donors and adulteration of essential oils. Separately, the greater insight and understanding of olfaction, synthesis of classical fragrances and new molecules with diverse structures and odor characters is increasingly accomplished in recent years. The group of synthetic fragrances includes derivates of several chemical structures and organic functions: acids, alcohols, esters, aldehydes, acetals, nitrogen heterocycles, oximes, amides, amines, nitriles, Schiff base, oxygen heterocyclics, lactones, coumarins, ethers, sulfur heterocycles, thiols, sulfides, thiocyanates, dithiazides, and hydrocarbons. For example, the transformation of alkenes, alkynes, dienes, and enynes results in carbo- and heterocyclic fragrances with natural and tunable scents. Hence, many industries use synthetic fragrances that are developed to mimic the aromatic and chemical constituents of natural, plant-based oils that are more expensive to manufacture. For a comprehensive review see Lin and colleagues [5].

Chemistry of Fragrances

Essential plant oils are very complex mixtures which can contain 20–60 substances at different concentrations. Typically, they are characterized by two or three major components at high concentrations (20–70%) compared to other components present in smaller amounts. The components are heterogeneous regarding their chemical structures; they can be assigned as lipophilic terpenoids, phenylpropanoids, or short-chain aliphatic hydrocarbon derivatives, all characterized by low molecular weight (<500–1000 Da). Different chemical groups make up a major part of essential oils, such as hydrocarbons, alcohols, phenols, aldehydes, ketones, esters, ethers, and phenylpropanoids (Fig. 16.1). Quantitatively, the main components are frequently belonging to the terpene family. Their classification is mainly based on the number of

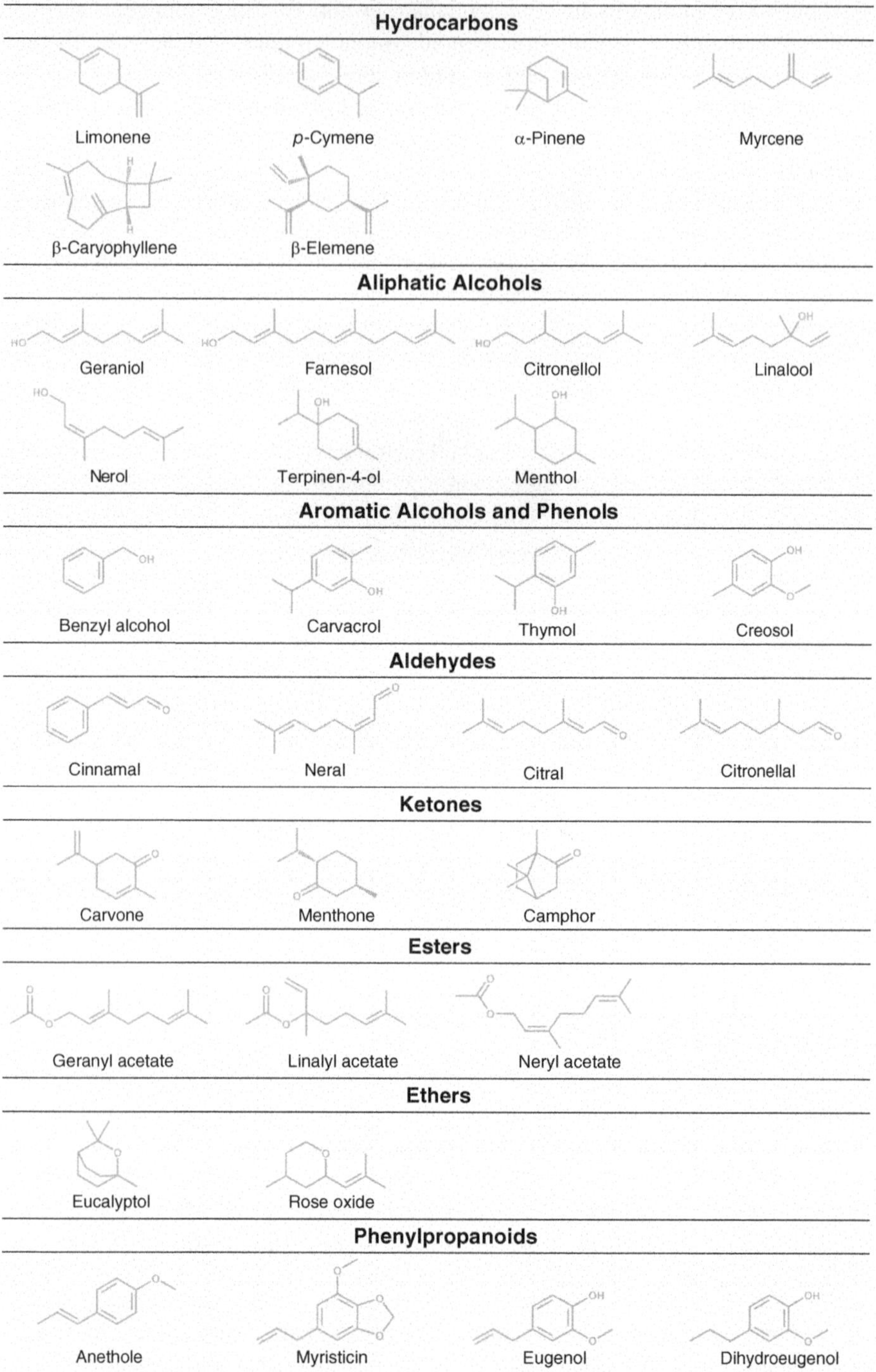

Fig. 16.1 Examples of commonly used fragrances and their classification into functional groups. For substances with multiple functional groups, the classification was made according to the dominant structural feature

isoprene units [$(C_5H_8)_n$] present in their structure. A distinction is made between hemiterpenes (C5), monoterpenes (C10), sesquiterpenes (C15) and diterpenes (C20). The term terpene refers to structures that are strictly hydrocarbons, whereas terpenoids contain additional functional groups. Terpenoids and phenylpropanoids are generated through different biosynthetic routes, while terpenes have a common precursor. Monoterpenes are the most abundant in essential oils (about 90%) with a great variety of structures. Geraniol/nerol, linalool, citronellol, citronellal and citral are the most important substances of this family and are widely used. Other well characterized phenolic agents such as eugenol are present in oils of cloverleaf.

Constituting an array of many lipophilic and highly volatile components derived from a great range of different chemical groups, essential oil components are known to be susceptible to conversion into each other by oxidation, isomerization, cyclization, or dehydrogenation reactions and degradation reactions. Such oxidative and polymerization processes may also result in a loss of quality and new properties. This has been extensively studied with thermolabile terpenoids that may be easily oxidized or hydrolyzed depending on their respective structure. Furthermore, many studies found that fragrance materials of pure orange oil, lavender oil and other oils have very low skin sensitizing potential, while the oxidized sample was shown to be highly sensitizing and allergenic [6].

Pharmacology of Fragrances

Fragrances interact with the olfactory pathway, which is a key sensory system which influences human well-being [7]. The loss of smell can indicate various neurodegenerative processes including effects by infections such as corona disease and influences an affected person's quality of life. The effects of fragrances are mediated by olfactory receptors which belong to the family of G protein-coupled receptor proteins. More than 900 olfactory receptors have been found in humans and are expressed not only in the nasal mucosa but in many other organs including skin, cardiovascular system, immune system, lung, GIT and others [8]. They are involved in many cellular functions such as cell-cell recognition, migration, apoptosis, or exocytosis, or proliferation e.g. the olfactory receptor OR2AT4 is involved in the regulation of human hair growth [9].

Adverse Effects of Fragrances

The ubiquitous use of fragrances leads to unavoidable exposures. Hence, possible adverse effects need to be evaluated. The main adverse effect is allergic contact dermatitis which will be primarily discussed in this chapter. Other unwanted side effects include contact urticaria, photosensitivity, and depigmentation (benzyl alcohol, cinnamal). Examples for photosensitivity include coumarin, eugenol and musk ambrette. Reactions to coumarin and musk ambrette can be very severe reactions and result in long-lasting hyperpigmentation [10]. Additional contact to fragrances is through smokeless tobacco pouches, so called "snuffs". For instance, patients with oral lichenoid lesions showed positive responses to carvone, one of several oxidation products of limonene. In line, the above-mentioned patients additionally reacted to hydroperoxides of limonene upon patch testing [11].

As fragrances are volatile, exposure may lead to effects on eyes and the naso-respiratory tract; leading to dry, itchy or watery eyes, nasal irritation including congestion and sneezing, and may worsen respiratory problems and boost asthma attacks. However, many studies have shown that these effects are mediated through irritancy of fragrance chemicals and are not an allergic reaction in contrast to allergic contact dermatitis [12]. However, the most common reaction to fragrance exposure is contact allergy and allergic contact dermatitis [13]. Until today, fragrance substances have been a frequent cause of contact allergy world-wide [14].

Allergic Contact Dermatitis and Role of Culprit Products in Fragrance-Induced Adaptive Immune Responses

Allergic contact dermatitis is a typical example of a delayed-type hypersensitivity reaction meaning that inflammatory symptoms develop approximately 12 h after exposure and peak after 24–72 h. In Europe, the conservatively estimated prevalence of fragrance contact allergy in the general population to Fragrance Mix (FM) I was 2.6% (95% confidence interval 2.1–3.2) and 1.9% (95% confidence interval 1.5–2.5) to FM II (for composition of FM see Sect. 1.5.2). Further, prevalence rates to fragrances in women are about twice those in men [15]. In addition, allergic contact dermatitis is a major cause of occupational skin diseases including fragrances as causative allergens. Examples include hairdressers, geriatric and nursing care, masseurs, physiotherapists, cleaners, housekeeping and food processing professions [16, 17].

The pathophysiology of allergic contact dermatitis is divided into two main phases, namely sensitization and elicitation. During the sensitizing phase (afferent phase) allergens (mostly low molecular weight compounds, <1000 Dalton) penetrate skin, where they act as haptens through stabile—many times covalently—binding to carrier proteins (protein haptenation) to become immunogenic [18, 19]. Many chemicals require activation prior interacting with proteins [20]. Activation of chemicals includes spontaneous oxidation or photo-oxidation (so-called prehaptens) or is mediated by enzymes (prohaptens) such as Cytochrome P450 (CYP) enzymes.

Patch test responses to air-oxidized terpene fragrances (prehaptens) such as limonene, linalool and citronellol are frequently observed [19]. Limonene and linalool were detected in around 30% of 2044 cosmetic products [21]. Limonene, linalool and citronellol are no strong sensitizers but they form potent sensitizing derivatives when exposed to air, and it has been shown that 2–3% of consecutive dermatitis patients are allergic to oxidized limonene or the hydroperoxide fraction of the oxidation mixture [22, 23]. Overall, prevalences of contact allergy to the different hydroperoxides of terpene fragrances are high, varying between 2.6% and 8.9%, in dependence of centers and countries [19].

The reactivity of the fairly stable hydroperoxides is initiated via radical mechanisms starting with the cleavage of the O-O bond, giving rise to unstable alkoxyl (RO•) and peroxyl (ROO•) radicals [24]. These radicals either react directly with a protein or rearrange into haptens that react as electrophiles. One example is 15-hydroperoxyabietate (15-HPA), a reactive intermediate of abietic acid, a component found in coniferous plants. Experimental studies showed that 15-HPA may react with skin proteins via an epoxide or via a radical mechanism [25]. Furthermore, due to the instability of alkoxyl and peroxyl radicals and the presence of double bonds in the terpene structure, these radicals may undergo additional radical rearrangements such as intramolecular cyclisation, allylic hydrogen abstraction or even a β-scission, and form more stable R• carbon radicals with a longer half-life. Thus, several reactive radical intermediates can derive from terpene fragrances depending on their chemical structure, and different chemical modifications of skin proteins may lead to sensitization [24]. Air-oxidation studies and testing the sensitizing potency of the individual oxidation products of terpene fragrances established that formed hydroperoxides are the strongest sensitizers among varying oxidations products characterized. For example, the naturally occurring hydroperoxides of limonene identified so far are limonene-1-hydroperoxide and limonene-2-hydroperoxide [22, 23]. Little is known about the location of hydroperoxides' activation and generation of antigenic structures and danger signals. Spatial reactivity of cumene hydroperoxide was found after topical application on reconstructed human skin. Explicitly, higher amounts of radicals and damage of keratinocytes were observed in deeper epidermal layers, namely at the epidermal-dermal junction zone, where proliferating keratinocytes are dominating and antigen-presenting dendritic cells are present [26]. In line, studies evaluating activation of monocyte-derived dendritic cells (MoDC) in coculture with human keratinocytes found for several hydroperoxides, especially for limonene-1 hydroperoxide, that donor variations in keratinocytes influenced even more pronounced DC activation than variations arising from MoDC donors [27].

In addition, prehaptens may also act as prohaptens. In general, the cytochrome P450 isoenzymes, particularly the four enzyme families P450 1,2, 3 and 4, are involved in the metabolism of chemicals and resulting metabolites may react with proteins and/or DNA to become immunogenic and/or genotoxic, respectively. For instance, geraniol is a well-studied fragrance acting as pre-and prohapten [28]. Geraniol was shown to be a substrate of CYP-isoenzymes [29]. In detail, the derivative 2,3-epoxygeraniol can be generated by CYP1B1 and CYP2E1, that are both expressed in skin. Furthermore, expression of CYP1B1 was detected in monocytes and MoDC [30, 31]. Many other fragrance chemicals may as well act as prohaptens. For example, cinnamic alcohol is converted to the aldehyde via the action of alcohol dehydrogenases in mice [32] and human epidermis [33]. The transformation of eugenol and isoeugenol by P450 enzymes into reactive haptens was shown using cytochrome P450 1A1 knock-out mice [34]. In line, activation of the aryl hydrocarbon receptor (AhR) and AhR-mediated expression of cytochromes in immortalized human HaCaT keratinocytes was demonstrated for eugenol and isoeugenol [35]. Also, transport of chemicals by efflux proteins may influence metabolism, sensitization and allergic contact dermatitis. Specifically, a role of multidrug resistance related proteins (MRP) in metabolism of eugenol was shown in human MoDC, suggesting a functional role of MRPs in the sensitization process of contact allergens [36]. Application of newer technologies such as the HR-MAS NMR (High Resolution Magic Angle Spinning Nuclear Magnetic Resonance) spectroscopy allowed the localization of chemical interactions of creosol with proteins e.g., in reconstructed human epidermis. Creosol, structurally related to eugenol and oxidized via CYPs, was demonstrated to form a 1,2 benzoquinone-protein adduct in the upper epidermis and its derivative formaldehyde was identified in the dermis [37, 38]. An impact of cutaneous CYPs on activation of Nrf2, a cellular sensor of oxidative and electrophilic stress induced by sensitizers [39], was found when HaCaT keratinocytes were exposed to creosol [38]. These studies show that epidermal enzymes are involved in generation of danger signals and formation of nominative antigens from fragrance chemicals. Furthermore, these and other studies indicate that the activation of fragrance chemicals and related prohaptens occurs in the living epidermis and not in stratum corneum, which consists out of dead cells [40, 41].

Studies investigating the interactions of electrophilic species with proteins in more detail demonstrated binding (covalently in many cases) to side chains of nucleophilic amino acids, typically Cys, Lys, His, Arg, and Tyr [42], and a set of mechanisms including first-order nucleophilic substitutions (SN1), second-order nucleophilic substitutions (SN2), nucleophilic substitution aromatic (SNAr), acylation (A), Schiff base formation (SB), and Michael acceptors (MA) have been established [20, 43]. Commonly, three of these mechanisms (A, SB and MA) are considered relevant to explain skin sensitization by many fragrances [44].

Antigen-presenting dendritic cells such as Langerhans cells are processing antigens and transport hapten-carrier complexes to the regional lymph nodes, where they interact with naïve T cells during acquisition of sensitization. In the additional presence of sufficient co-stimulatory molecules on DC they prime and expand allergen-specific naïve $CD8^+$ and $CD4^+$ T cells through the presentation of the haptenized peptides on MHC class I and II molecules, respectively [45]. The sensitization phase is normally symptom free but results in the generation of long-lived memory T cells. Upon renewed contact, specific effector T-cells, present at or attracted to the site of application, are stimulated by antigenic complexes (eliciting phase). They induce a cascade of inflammatory events, causing erythema, edema and vesiculation of the skin [46]. Interestingly, allergen-dependent differences in T-cell subsets generated in response to fragrances compared to metals were shown. Using RT-PCR, gene arrays, and immunohistochemistry a strong TH2 bias and some TH22 polarization by fragrances was observed [47]. Furthermore, contact allergy to fragrances seems more frequent in atopic patients, whereas contact allergy to other contact sensitizers is decreased in atopic patients [48]. To tackle the cause of fragrance allergies and to relate it to a certain product is challenging, as exposure typically occurs at the same time to many fragrance chemicals [10]. This may lead to an increased susceptibility to further products emphasizing the importance of tracking the responsible sensitizers.

Diagnosis of Fragrance Allergy

To diagnose e.g. an allergic response to fragrance materials patch testing is performed. Patch testing is the standard procedure used to detect contact allergy [49]. Most often is Fragrance Mix (FM) I used. FM I is a standardized blend and contains 1% (w/w) of eight common fragrances in petrolatum (α-amyl cinnamic aldehyde, cinnamic alcohol, cinnamic aldehyde, eugenol, geraniol, hydroxycitronellal, isoeugenol, oak moss absolute), plus an emulsifier (sorbitan sesquioleate, around 5%). In most surveys of patch test results during the last years the FM I is usually the second most often observed allergen after nickel sulfate in most countries, reflecting the relevance of allergic contact dermatitis due to fragrance materials [10]. Overall, more than 150 fragrance materials have been confirmed by in vivo or in vitro studies to be able to sensitize skin [10]. Substances such as Balsam of Peru, colophonium or sesquiterpene lactone as well as Compositae mix II can be used as additional fragrance markers besides the two established fragrance mixes (I and II). MF II contains six fragrances, typically formulated at a total concentration of 14% in petrolatum. FM II contains citral (1%), citronellol (0.5%), coumarin (2.5%), farnesol (2.5%), α-hexyl cinnamic aldehyde (5.0%), and 2.5% hydroxyisohexyl 3-cyclohexene carboxaldehyde (commonly known as HICC or Lyral). Patch-testing represents a reliable and easy method to test many components at the same time. However, discrepancies may occur when reactions to the mix and its constituents are compared. In some studies, only 40% to 60% of fragrance mix positive patients showed positive reactions to one or more of the tested single components of the mix [50]. These differences may have several reasons. One reason might be that there are interactions as well as cross-reactions between the fragrances in the mix. Second, the single compounds are typically tested with the same concentration that is used in the mix, although experimental studies found that the highest sensitivity is achieved with a 2% of the single fragrance compared to 1% present in the fragrance mixture [51]. Independently, patch test results may not always correlate with the clinical symptoms or history of the patient. Under clinical conditions this discrepancy can be controlled by the rapid open application test [17].

Lymphocyte Transformation Test to Identify Fragrance Allergy Ex Vivo

An in vitro approach to identify the causative allergen of allergic contact dermatitis can be the lymphocyte transformation test (LTT). In general, the uptake of the radiolabeled base analogue 3H-thymidine [52] or the non-radioactive 5'-Bromo-2-deoxy-uridine [53] into proliferating cells correlates well with lymphocyte proliferation, and represents one possibility to quantitate mitogenic or antigen-specific induced transformation. Also, the expression and production of cytokines and interleukins can be measured as an endpoint of this reaction. The LTT was repeatedly successful to detect type IV (delayed-type) hypersensitivity reactions, particularly to metal allergens, urushiol, *p*-phenylenediamine and drugs [54–56]. For an overview see Popple et al. [57] and Sachs et al. [58]. Specific application to fragrance allergens has been explored, though it remains less standardized compared to other allergens. The use of LTT to detect sensitization to common fragrances has been explored, but the results have been somewhat controversial and variable. A study involving 32 fragrance-allergic patients demonstrated significant T cell proliferation in response to eight fragrances, including eugenol, isoeugenol, geraniol, and cinnamic aldehyde [59]. Stimulation indices ranged from 2.1 to 21.8, indicating varying degrees of sensitization. The somewhat low response rate may be based on technical issues. Many fragrance chemicals are lipophilic and may have limited solubility in aqueous culture systems, potentially affecting test sensitivity and accuracy. Also, some fragrance substances can be cytotoxic to lymphocytes at higher concentrations, complicating the interpretation of LTT results. Furthermore, several studies indicate that combinations of fragrance allergens used for patch testing (FM I, FM II) can have additive or synergistic effects, leading to increased T cell proliferation compared to individual components [60]. The before mentioned study [59] found that the addition of human liver microsomes (CYP450) or recombinant CYP1A1 to lymphocytes enhanced responses of eugenol and isoeugenol in five of seven cases, suggesting that metabolic activation can influence allergenicity. This highlights the complexity of assessing sensitization to fragrance and fragrance mixtures. While the LTT can detect T cell-mediated sensitization to certain fragrance allergens, its application in this context is limited by methodological challenges and a lack of standardization.

Elucidation of the Pathogenesis of Fragrance-Induced Contact Allergy

The essential pathophysiological feature of allergic contact dermatitis is the presence of allergen-specific immune hypersensitivity reactions. Diagnosis relies on identifying the specific allergens to which a patient has been exposed, but skin reactions to fragrance materials are sometimes difficult to interpret and to distinguish from irritant responses. The identification and analysis of fragrance-specific T cell *ex vivo* have demonstrated that the hypersensitivity reaction to fragrances is a T-cell mediated, antigen-specific phenomenon rather than a non-specific irritative response. Further analysis of T cell clones has improved our understanding of immunological mechanisms underlying fragrance allergy. Accordingly, studies have successfully isolated T cells and established 18 T cell clones in vitro from lesional skin of fragrance-sensitized patients. Phenotypic analysis revealed that 83% of these clones expressed $CD3^+$, $CD4^+$, and $HLA\text{-}DR^+$, while 17% were $CD8^+$. Functional assays demonstrated that a subset of $CD4^+$ clones secreted significant amounts of IL-2 and IFN-γ but not IL-4 or IL-5, indicating a TH1-type response [59]. The findings suggest that both $CD4^+$ and $CD8^+$ T cells are involved in an allergic response to fragrances. As mentioned above, follow-up in vivo profiling of skin biopsies from fragrance-allergic patients has indicated that fragrances can induce a distinct pattern of T cell polarization—characterized by a strong TH2 bias, some TH22 polarization, and lesser TH1/TH17 contributions—in contrast to other clinically relevant allergens in allergic contact dermatitis [47]. Additionally, more recent studies have shown that CD1a, an abundant MHC I–like protein in human skin, can mediate recognition of certain compounds in fragrance oils. Subsequent screening structurally related compounds with CD1a-autoreactive human α/β T cell clones has identified additional stimulatory substances, including the hydrophobic farnesol [61].

Prediction of Sensitizing Chemicals Without Animal Experiments

Many times, the prediction of a test chemical to be a sensitizer is derived from a single animal-based test method. Newer methods aim to provide ethical and efficient alternatives to animal testing. There is a common agreement that as of today, one single non-animal test method is not sufficient to fully recapitulate the complexity of skin sensitization. This agreement is driven by data showing that contact allergens react via very different mechanisms [43]. Thus, several non-animal methods are being developed along four defined key events (KE 1–4) of a defined Adverse Outcome Pathway for Skin Sensitization (AOP) [62]. For some of the methods validated test protocols are already provided by the Organization for Economic Co-operation and Development (OECD, guideline 442C, D, E, 2024. https://www.oecd-library.org/environment/test-no-442). The first key event (KE 1) is the binding to nucleophilic centers of skin proteins, and validated test methods evaluate the relative reactivity of substances with synthetic model peptides containing cysteine and/or lysine (Direct Peptide Reactivity Assay, DPRA; kinetic DPRA, kDPRA). Other methods are using single amino acid derivatives instead of model peptides (Amino Acid Derivative Reactivity Assay, ADRA). Methods addressing the activation of keratinocytes (KE 2) are measuring the chemical-induced changes in expression of a marker gene in genetically modified HaCaT keratinocytes (KeratinoSens™, LuSens) or gene expression of markers in human reconstructed epidermis (EpiSensA). Maturation of DC (KE 3) is evaluated by measuring cell surface expression of specific markers on monocytic THP-1 or U937 cell lines (Human Cell Line Activation Test, h-CLAT; U937 cell line activation Test, U-SENS™), cytokines (Interleukin-8 Reporter Gene Assay, IL-8 Luc assay) or expression of a set of marker genes (GARD™skin). Validated methods to study the potential of a chemical to activate naïve T cells (KE 4) are still under development. Furthermore, strategies to combine individual results of testing KE 1–3, as well as in silico data of a given chemical into an outcome were developed [63]. For example, one strategy ("2 out of 3" approach) was shown to have a high accuracy (89%) to predict human skin sensitization hazard. This accuracy is already comparable to the predicted accuracy of the golden in vivo assay, namely the Local Lymph Node Assay (82%, [63]). Nevertheless, methods and integration strategies continue to be developed and refined [64].

Prediction of Sensitizing Fragrances In Vitro

Several studies have specifically explored the use of DC to predict the sensitizing potential of fragrances. Investigators were using mouse fetal skin-derived DC or human $CD34^+$ progenitor-derived DC assays to analyze gene expression and intracellular signaling to identify sensitizing fragrances and other sensitizers [65]. Other groups developed methods based on MoDC [66]. By optimizing conditions such as cytokine concentrations and incubation times, the assays achieved stable and reproducible results, demonstrating that fragrances induce DC activation and maturation. Also, the U-SENS™ assays were used to evaluate the activation of DC by measuring CD54 and/or CD86 on cell surface upon exposure to fragrances. Testing of fragrance chemicals with sufficient historical human and animal data to determine their sensitization potential was done with the U-SENS™ assay. Within the set of 61 sensitizers, the method correctly identified 50 fragrances while the remaining 11 gave false negative results. However, when the results of the U-SENS™ assay were combined with results of other assays like the DPRA and KeratinoSens™, the predictive accuracy improved, highlighting the benefit of integrated testing approaches [44]. Given that reconstructed human skin has been shown to possess metabolic enzymes that are like those found in normal human epidermis [67]), researchers combined DC with epidermis models to evaluate fragrances. This allows for topical application of lipophilic fragrances on the surface of reconstructed human epidermis [68]. The COCAT method involves coculturing monocytic THP-1 cells (surrogates of dendritic cells) with HaCaT keratinocytes to assess DC activation via CD86 and CD54 markers [69–71]. Among 27 fragrance chemicals tested with COCAT, CD86 proved to be a more sensitive marker. The system effectively identified sensitizers, including pre/prohaptens, demonstrating good reproducibility [72]. Overall, in vitro assays utilizing DC or surrogate of DC offer promising alternatives to animal testing for assessing the sensitizing potential of fragrance compounds. These methods, especially when integrated, provide reliable and ethical approaches for hazard identification and possibly potency assessment in skin sensitization.

Conclusions

In conclusion, fragrance materials (natural fragrances, synthetic fragrances, natural essential oils, fragrance mixtures) are ubiquitously used to create perfumes, refine cosmetic, hygiene and present in products such as soaps, shampoos, lotions, facial and toilet tissues, air fresheners, disinfectants, vaporizers, household cleansers and detergents. In this context, fragrances play also a considerable role in masking undesirable smells arising from fatty acids, oils and surfactants. The ubiquitous use of fragrances leads to unavoidable exposures. The most common adverse effect of fragrance exposure is allergic contact dermatitis. Overall, more than 150 fragrance materials have been confirmed by in vivo or in vitro studies to be able to sensitize skin. Many times, the fragrance chemicals are not sensitizing but they may form allergenic compounds upon spontaneous oxidation or photo-oxidation (prehaptens) or mediated by enzymes (prohaptens) such as Cytochrome P450 (CYP) enzymes. In addition, some fragrance chemicals act as prehapten and prohapten. In addition, transporter molecules may be involved in the formation of the nominative antigens. The identification and analysis of fragrance-specific T cell *ex vivo* have demonstrated that the hypersensitivity reaction to fragrances is an allergen-specific T-cell mediated Type IV hypersensitivity response. Several studies have specifically explored the development of non-animal-based methods to predict the human sensitizing potential of fragrances and other sensitizers. These methods, especially when integrated, may provide reliable and ethical approaches for hazard identification and possibly potency assessment in skin sensitization.

References

1. Sharmeen JB, Mahomoodally FM, Zengin G, Maggi F. Essential oils as natural sources of fragrance compounds for cosmetics and cosmeceuticals. Molecules. 2021;26(3):666.
2. Mallock-Ohnesorg N, Rinaldi S, Malke S, Dreiack N, Pieper E, Laux P, et al. Oral nicotine pouches with an aftertaste? Part 1: screening and initial toxicological assessment of flavorings and other ingredients. Arch Toxicol. 2023;97(9):2357–69.
3. Angulo Milhem S, Verriele M, Nicolas M, Thevenet F. Does the ubiquitous use of essential oil-based products promote indoor air quality? A critical literature review. Environ Sci Pollut Res Int. 2020;27(13):14365–411.
4. Guzmán E, Lucia A. Essential oils and their individual components in cosmetic products. Cosmetics. 2021;8(4):114.
5. Lin Z, Huang B, Ouyang L, Zheng L. Synthesis of cyclic fragrances via transformations of alkenes, alkynes and Enynes: strategies and recent Progress. Molecules. 2022;27(11):3576.
6. Karlberg AT, Bergstrom MA, Borje A, Luthman K, Nilsson JL. Allergic contact dermatitis-formation, structural requirements, and reactivity of skin sensitizers. Chem Res Toxicol. 2008;21(1):53–69.
7. Bratman GN, Bembibre C, Daily GC, Doty RL, Hummel T, Jacobs LF, et al. Nature and human Well-being: the olfactory pathway. Sci Adv. 2024;10(20):eadn3028.
8. Maßberg D, Hatt H. Human olfactory receptors: novel cellular functions outside of the nose. Physiol Rev. 2018;98(3):1739–63.
9. Cheret J, Bertolini M, Ponce L, Lehmann J, Tsai T, Alam M, et al. Olfactory receptor OR2AT4 regulates human hair growth. Nat Commun. 2018;9(1):3624.
10. de Groot AC. Fragrances: contact allergy and other adverse effects. Dermatitis. 2020;31(1):13–35.
11. Adwa U, Antelmi A, Sukakul T, Dahlin J, Bruze M, Svedman C. Oral lichenoid lesions in two snuff users with contact allergy to carvone. Contact Derm. 2024;90(1):74–8.

12. Basketter DA, Huggard J, Kimber I. Fragrance inhalation and adverse health effects: the question of causation. Regul Toxicol Pharmacol. 2019;104:151–6.
13. De Groot AC, Frosch PJ. Adverse reactions to fragrances. Contact Derm. 1997;36:57–86.
14. Botvid S, Bennike NH, Simonsen AB, Johansen JD, Uter W. Contact sensitization to fragrance mix I and fragrance mix II among European dermatitis patients: a systematic review. Contact Derm. 2024;91(3):177–85.
15. Diepgen TL, Ofenloch R, Bruze M, Cazzaniga S, Coenraads PJ, Elsner P, et al. Prevalence of fragrance contact allergy in the general population of five European countries: a cross-sectional study. Br J Dermatol. 2015;173(6):1411–9.
16. Montgomery RL, Agius R, Wilkinson SM, Carder M. UK trends of allergic occupational skin disease attributed to fragrances 1996-2015. Contact Derm. 2018;78(1):33–40.
17. Frosch P. Duftstoffe—Aufschlüsselung der Mixe, deklarationspflichtige Duftstoffe und ätherische Öle, pp. 186–191. In: Frosch P, Schnuch A, Uter W, editors. Kontaktdermatitis – Ein Leitfaden für die Praxis unter besonderer Berücksichtigung von Berufsdermatosen. Dustri-Verlag; 2014. p. 398.
18. Landsteiner K, Jacobs JL. Studies on the sensitization of animals with simple chemicals II. J Exp Med. 1936;64:625–39.
19. Johansen JD, Bonefeld CM, Schwensen JFB, Thyssen JP, Uter W. Novel insights into contact dermatitis. J Allergy Clin Immunol. 2022;149(4):1162–71.
20. Aleksic M, Meng X. Protein Haptenation and its role in allergy. Chem Res Toxicol. 2024;37(6):850–72.
21. Sukakul T, Bruze M, Mowitz M, Antelmi A, Bergendorff O, Bjork J, et al. Contact allergy to oxidized linalool and oxidized limonene: patch testing in consecutive patients with dermatitis. Contact Derm. 2022;86(1):15–24.
22. Karlberg AT. Oxidation products and the skin – the effect of hydroperoxides. Contact Derm. 2017;76(2):63–6.
23. Karlberg AT, Lepoittevin JP. One hundred years of allergic contact dermatitis due to oxidized terpenes: what we can learn from old research on turpentine allergy. Contact Derm. 2021;85(6):627–36.
24. Vileno B, Port-Lougarre Y, Gimenez-Arnau E. Electron paramagnetic resonance and spin trapping to detect free radicals from allergenic hydroperoxides in contact with the skin: from the molecule to the tissue. Contact Derm. 2022;86(4):241–53.
25. Gafvert E, Shao LP, Karlberg AT, Nilsson U, Nilsson JL. Contact allergy to resin acid hydroperoxides. Hapten binding via free radicals and epoxides. Chem Res Toxicol. 1994;7(2):260–6.
26. Soeur J, Eilstein J, Lereaux G, Jones C, Marrot L. Skin resistance to oxidative stress induced by resveratrol: from Nrf2 activation to GSH biosynthesis. Free Radic Biol Med. 2015;78:213–23.
27. Lichter J, Silva ESM, Peter N, Sahli F, Vileno B, Kuresepi S, et al. Skin sensitization to fragrance hydroperoxides: interplay between dendritic cells, keratinocytes and free radicals. Br J Dermatol. 2021;184(6):1143–52.
28. Hagvall L, Baron JM, Borje A, Weidolf L, Merk H, Karlberg AT. Cytochrome P450-mediated activation of the fragrance compound geraniol forms potent contact allergens. Toxicol Appl Pharmacol. 2008;233(2):308–13.
29. Stok JE, Giang PD, Wong SH, De Voss JJ. Exploring the substrate specificity of cytochrome P450(cin). Arch Biochem Biophys. 2019;672:108060.
30. Sieben S, Baron JM, Blömeke B, Merk HF. Multiple cytochrome P450-isoenzymes mRNA are expressed in dendritic cells. Int Arch Allergy Immunol. 1999;118(2–4):358–61.
31. Ott H, Bergström MA, Heise R, Skazik C, Zwadlo-Klarwasser G, Merk HF, et al. Cutaneous metabolic activation of Carvoxime, a self-activating, Skin-Sensitizing Prohapten. Chem Res Toxicol. 2009;22(2):399–405.
32. Basketter DA. Skin sensitization to cinnamic alcohol: the role of skin metabolism. Acta Derm Venereol. 1992;72(4):264–5.

33. Ndreu L, Carlsson J, Ponting DJ, Niklasson IB, Steen EJL, McHugh L, et al. Bioactivation of cinnamic alcohol in a reconstructed human epidermis model and evaluation of sensitizing potency of the identified metabolites. Front Toxicol. 2024;6:1398852.
34. Basketter DA, Pendlington RU, Sarll A, Scholes E. The role of P450 1A in the activation of prophaptens in skin sensitization. J Invest Dermatol. 1996;106(4):935.
35. Kalmes M, Neumeyer A, Rio P, Hanenberg H, Fritsche E, Blömeke B. Impact of the arylhydrocarbon receptor on eugenol- and isoeugenol-induced cell cycle arrest in human immortalized keratinocytes (HaCaT). Biol Chem. 2006;387(9):1201–7.
36. Skazik C, Heise R, Ott H, Czaja K, Marquardt Y, Merk HF, et al. Active transport of contact allergens in human monocyte-derived dendritic cells is mediated by multidrug resistance related proteins. Arch Biochem Biophys. 2011;508(2):212–6.
37. Elbayed K, Berl V, Debeuckelaere C, Moussallieh F-M, Piotto M, Namer I-J, et al. HR-MAS NMR spectroscopy of reconstructed human epidermis: potential for the in situ investigation of the chemical interactions between skin allergens and nucleophilic amino acids. Chem Res Toxicol. 2013;26(1):136–45.
38. Huth L, Moss E, Skazik C, Huth S, Lepoittevin J, Baron J, et al. 285 skin cytochrome P450 dependent activation of creosol (C) to a complete antigen. J Invest Dermatol. 2017;137(5):S49.
39. Natsch A. The Nrf2-Keap1-ARE toxicity pathway as a cellular sensor for skin sensitizers -functional relevance and a hypothesis on innate reactions to skin sensitizers. Toxicol Sci. 2010;113(2):284–92.
40. Kao J, Patterson FK, Hall J. Skin penetration and metabolism of topically applied chemicals in six mammalian species, including man: an in vitro study with benzo[a]pyrene and testosterone. Toxicol Appl Pharmacol. 1985;81(3 Pt 1):502–16.
41. Hoath SB, Leahy DG. The organization of human epidermis: functional epidermal units and phi proportionality. J Invest Dermatol. 2003;121(6):1440–6.
42. Parkinson E, Aleksic M, Kukic P, Bailey A, Cubberley R, Skipp P. Proteomic analysis of the cellular response to a potent sensitiser unveils the dynamics of haptenation in living cells. Toxicology. 2020;445:152603.
43. Roberts DW, Aptula AO, Patlewicz G. Electrophilic chemistry related to skin sensitization. Reaction mechanistic applicability domain classification for a published data set of 106 chemicals tested in the mouse local lymph node assay. Chem Res Toxicol. 2007;20(1):44–60.
44. Lee I, Na M, O'Brien D, Parakhia R, Alepee N, Westerink W, et al. Assessment of the skin sensitization potential of fragrance ingredients using the U-SENS assay. Toxicol In Vitro. 2022;79:105298.
45. Steinman RM. Decisions about dendritic cells: past, present, and future. Annu Rev Immunol. 2012;30:1–22.
46. Kaplan DH, Igyártó BZ, Gaspari AA. Early immune events in the induction of allergic contact dermatitis. Nat Rev Immunol. 2012;12(2):114–24.
47. Dhingra N, Shemer A, Correa da Rosa J, Rozenblit M, Fuentes-Duculan J, Gittler JK, et al. Molecular profiling of contact dermatitis skin identifies allergen-dependent differences in immune response. J Allergy Clin Immunol. 2014;134(2):362–72.
48. Correa da Rosa J, Malajian D, Shemer A, Rozenblit M, Dhingra N, Czarnowicki T, et al. Patients with atopic dermatitis have attenuated and distinct contact hypersensitivity responses to common allergens in skin. J Allergy Clin Immunol. 2015;135(3):712–20.
49. Sukakul T, Bruze M, Svedman C. Fragrance contact allergy – a review focusing on patch testing. Acta Derm Venereol. 2024;104:adv40332.
50. Enders F, Przybilla B, Ring J. Patch testing with fragrance-mix and its constituents: discrepancies are largely due to the presence or absence of sorbitan sesquioleate. Contact Derm. 1991;24(3):238–9.
51. Frosch PJ, Rastogi SC, Pirker C, Brinkmeier T, Andersen KE, Bruze M, et al. Patch testing with a new fragrance mix – reactivity to the individual constituents and chemical detection in relevant cosmetic products. Contact Derm. 2005;52(4):216–25.

52. Caron GA, Sarkany I, Williams HS, Todd AP. Roadioactive method for the measurement of lymphocyte transformation in vitro. Lancet. 1965;II:1266–8.
53. Magaud J-P, Sargent I, Mason DY. Detection of human white cell proliferative responses by immunoenzymatic measurement of bromodeoxyuridine uptake. J Immunol Methods. 1988;106:95–100.
54. Nyfeler B, Pichler WJ. The lymphocyte transformation test for the diagnosis of drug allergy: sensitivity and specificity. Clin Exp Allergy. 1997;27(2):175–81.
55. Pichler WJ, Schnyder B, Zanni M. Case 26-1996: hypersensitivity to carbamazepine. N Engl J Med. 1997;336(5):377.
56. Räsänen L, Tuomi M-L. Diagnostic value of the lymphocyte proliferation test in nickel contact allergy and provocation in occupational coin dermatitis. Contact Derm. 1992;27:250–4.
57. Popple A, Williams J, Maxwell G, Gellatly N, Dearman RJ, Kimber I. The lymphocyte transformation test in allergic contact dermatitis: new opportunities. J Immunotoxicol. 2016;13(1):84–91.
58. Sachs B, Fatangare A, Sickmann A, Glässner A. Lymphocyte transformation test: history and current approaches. J Immunol Methods. 2021;493:113036.
59. Sieben S, Hertl M, Al Masaoudi T, Merk HF, Blömeke B. Characterization of T cell responses to fragrances. Toxicol Appl Pharmacol. 2001;172(3):172–8.
60. Bonefeld CM, Geisler C, Gimenez-Arnau E, Lepoittevin JP, Uter W, Johansen JD. Immunological, chemical and clinical aspects of exposure to mixtures of contact allergens. Contact Derm. 2017;77(3):133–42.
61. Nicolai S, Wegrecki M, Cheng TY, Bourgeois EA, Cotton RN, Mayfield JA, et al. Human T cell response to CD1a and contact dermatitis allergens in botanical extracts and commercial skin care products. Sci Immunol. 2020;5(43):eaax5430.
62. OECD. The adverse outcome pathway for skin sensitisation initiated by covalent binding to proteins, OECD Series on Testing and Assessment 168. OECD; 2014.
63. OECD. Guideline No. 497: Guideline on defined approaches for skin sensitization. In: Chemicals OGfTo, editor.: Organisation for Economic Co-operation and Development; Paris 2021.
64. Kolle SN, Natsch A, Gerberick GF, Landsiedel R. A review of substances found positive in 1 of 3 in vitro tests for skin sensitization. Regul Toxicol Pharmacol. 2019;106:352–68.
65. Neves BM, Goncalo M, Figueiredo A, Duarte CB, Lopes MC, Cruz MT. Signal transduction profile of chemical sensitisers in dendritic cells: an endpoint to be included in a cell-based in vitro alternative approach to hazard identification? Toxicol Appl Pharmacol. 2011;250(2):87–95.
66. Reuter H, Gerlach S, Spieker J, Ryan C, Bauch C, Mangez C, et al. Evaluation of an optimized protocol using human peripheral blood monocyte derived dendritic cells for the *in vitro* detection of sensitizers: results of a ring study in five laboratories. Toxicol In Vitro. 2015;29(5):976–86.
67. Netzlaff F, Lehr C-M, Wertz P, Schaefer U. The human epidermis models EpiSkin®, SkinEthic® and EpiDerm®: an evaluation of morphology and their suitability for testing phototoxicity, irritancy, corrosivity, and substance transport. Eur J Pharm Biopharm. 2005;60(2):167–78.
68. Schellenberger MT, Bock U, Hennen J, Groeber-Becker F, Walles H, Blömeke B. A coculture system composed of THP-1 cells and 3D reconstructed human epidermis to assess activation of dendritic cells by sensitizing chemicals after topical exposure. Toxicol In Vitro. 2019;57:62–6.
69. Hennen J, Aeby P, Goebel C, Schettgen T, Oberli A, Kalmes M, et al. Cross talk between keratinocytes and dendritic cells: impact on the prediction of sensitization. Toxicol Sci. 2011;123(2):501–10.
70. Hennen J, Blömeke B. Keratinocytes improve prediction of sensitization potential and potency of chemicals with THP-1 cells. ALTEX. 2017;34(2):279–88.

71. Eskes C, Hennen J, Schellenberger MT, Hoffmann S, Frey S, Goldinger-Oggier D, et al. The HaCaT/THP-1 Cocultured activation test (COCAT) for skin sensitization: a study of intra-lab reproducibility and predictivity. ALTEX. 2019;36(4):613–22.
72. Peter N, Lichter J, Hagvall L, Bock U, Blömeke B. Common fragrance chemicals activate dendritic cells in coculture with keratinocytes. Contact Derm. 2023;89(1):1–15.

Chapter 17
Photoreactions

N. J. Neumann and H. W. Vohr

Definitions

When a chemical interacts with ultraviolet and/or visible light in the skin, photoreactions can occur. A chemical that absorbs UV radiation or visible light and causes a biological reaction is called a photosensitizer. As far as the reactions between exogenous chemicals, UV light, and the human skin are concerned, the term "photosensitization" includes both phototoxic and photoallergic reactions.

Phototoxic reactions are defined as reactions caused by a single exposure to a photoreactive chemical plus UV irradiation or visible light and occurring immediately or delayed (up to 48 h) after irradiation. Phototoxic reactions from topically applied substances are also called photo-irritant reactions. Photoallergic reactions are defined as immunologically mediated reactions. Unlike phototoxic reactions, there are no detectable skin reactions after initial exposure to a photoallergen and UV light. Only after an induction period of approximately 1 week, the second exposure results in a typical delayed skin reaction.

Since this article refers to UV-induced short-term skin reactions, genotoxic effects, e. g. photomutagenicity and photocarcinogenicity, will not be characterized.

N. J. Neumann (✉)
Department of Dermatology, Heinrich-Heine-University, Duesseldorf, Germany
e-mail: neumannt@uni-duesseldorf.de

H. W. Vohr
Department of Toxicology, Bayer AG, Leverkusen, Germany

P. Elsner et al. (eds.), *Cosmetics*, https://doi.org/10.1007/978-3-032-14644-1_17

Epidemiology and Pathogenesis

Based on clinical experience, phototoxic reactions are much more common than photoallergic reactions, but precise data on the incidence and prevalence of photoreactions are not available.

Jung and Maurer classified 4% of all photo reactions they observed in their dermatological center between 1960 and 1965 as photoallergic reactions [27–30, 52, 53].

In 1966 only 1% of all contact reactions were diagnosed as photoallergic reactions. Taken into account a presumed overall prevalence of 1% for contact allergic reactions in a given population, the prevalence of photoallergy, therefore, could be predicted as 0.01% (1 case out of 10.000 people).

The evaluation of our own data from 1984–1994 revealed 6402 positive epicutaneous test reactions (clinically relevant contact allergies) and 82 positive photopatch test reactions (photoallergies). Thus, 1.3% of all relevant test reactions were classified as photoallergic. Although this rate is in accordance with other reports, an incidence of photoallergy of 1% remains questionable. In contrast to the standardized epicutaneous test, which is widely used by dermatologists worldwide, the photopatch test is a specialized procedure that is only performed in a few dermatology centers [24, 36, 74].

Therefore, it seems reasonable to assume that the incidence of photoallergy is less than 0.01%.

From 1964–1971 Magnus (in [52]) retrospectively analyzed photoreactions caused by systemically applied drugs. According to his results, one out of 212.000 prescriptions led to a photoreaction. Focusing on the subgroups of protriptylin, desmethylchlortetracylin, and nalidixin acid, out of 14.000 prescriptions one photoreaction was observed. These photoreactions were predominantly classified as phototoxic. Many photosensitizers are capable of causing both [22, 57] phototoxic and photoallergic reactions, and often an accurate clinical and histopathological assessment is not possible.

Photoallergy is considered to be a T-cell mediated delayed hypersensitivity reaction.

Via complex interactions, UV-light modifies a prohapten to become a hapten. Afterwards, the hapten reacts with skin proteins building a hapten-protein conjugate. Langerhans cells take up this complex, mature and migrate to local draining lymph nodes. There, relevant antigen determinants are presented via MHC-molecules (signal 1) to T-cells and to co-stimulatory molecules (ICAM-1, B7-1,87-2) and induce T-cell proliferation and memory T-cell formation [10]. In contrast to contact dermatitis, additional UV radiation, mainly in the UVA range, is a prerequisite for triggering photoallergies.

Phototoxic reactions are based on a non-immunological (non-antigen-specific) inflammatory skin reaction. Phototoxic substances are inactive in the absence of UV light. Thus, only the combination of the phototoxic substance and UV light (subsequently applied) may provoke a phototoxic reaction. Therefore, a possible mechanism could be the absorption of a photon leading to a short-lived, now electronically excited photosensitizer in a singlet or mainly in a triplet state [6]. In general, phototoxicity is elicited in two different ways:

(a) Free radicals built by electron or hydrogen transfer (type I)
(b) Singlet oxygen species built by energy transfer (type II)

The chemical structure of the photosensitizer and the substrate conditions determine the phototoxic reaction. However, both types of reaction can cause cytotoxic damage to keratinocytes and Langerhans cells. In addition, phototoxicity induces proinflammatory cytokines in keratinocytes [54], which in turn may activate Langerhans cells, macrophages, and T cells. Furthermore, a markedly increased expression of ICAM-I on endothelial cells and keratinocytes has been reported during chemically induced phototoxicity. Furthermore, TNF-a can induce differentiation, proliferation and degranulation of mast cells.

Clinical Characteristics

Similar to contact dermatitis, (after an induction phase), photoallergic reactions exhibit the typical symptoms of eczema. After the starting with erythema and infiltration, papulovesicles or even bullae develop on areas of UV exposed skin [57]. After prolonged exposure to a photoallergen and UV radiation, chronic actinic dermatitis with lichenoid scaly dermatitis can also develop diffusely beyond the edge of the irradiated skin. Both acute and chronic photoallergic dermatitis are often associated with severe pruritus. Occasionally distinguishing between an airborne contact dermatitis (e. g., caused by compositae) and a photoallergic dermatitis may be a problem. In these cases, dermatitis-free areas behind the ears, under the chin and in the folds of the neck [less sunlight-exposed skin areas] may be helpful in supporting the diagnosis of a photoallergy. (Fig. 17.1).

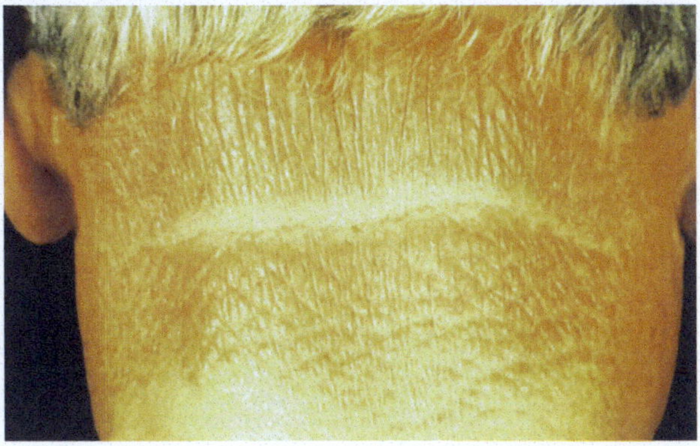

Fig. 17.1 Olaquindox-induced photoallergy. Wrinkles around in the neck-area are free of dermatitis

The clinical manifestations of phototoxic reactions depend on the type and concentration of the photosensitizer, as well as the intensity, wavelength, and duration of irradiation. Predominantly, the phototoxic reaction appears as an exaggerated sunburn dermatitis (Fig. 17.2) consisting of erythema, edema (infiltration) and burning pain up to 24 h after UV-irradiation, followed by persistent hyperpigmentation. This type of reaction is most commonly induced by tar, dyes, benaxoprofen, and amidodarone in combination with relative high doses of UVA light.

Psoralen [contained in several plants, e. g. amni majus, (phytophotocontact dermatitis, Fig. 17.3)] or bergaptene [contained in diverse perfumes (berloque

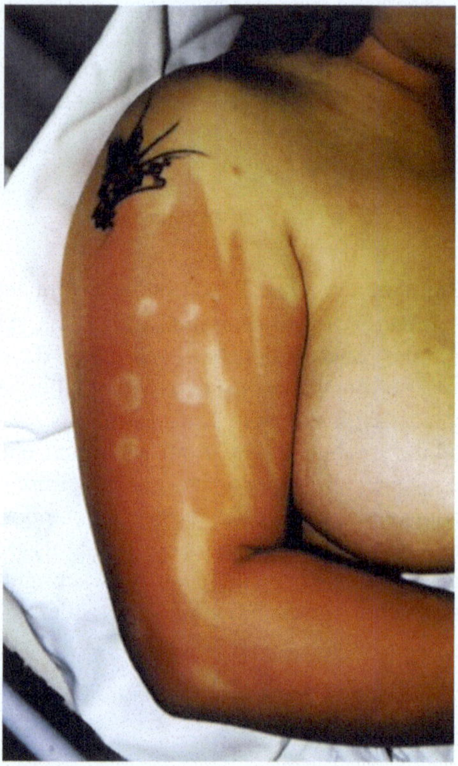

Fig. 17.2 Phototoxic reaction after topically applied 8-MOP followed by an overdosed UVA irradiation

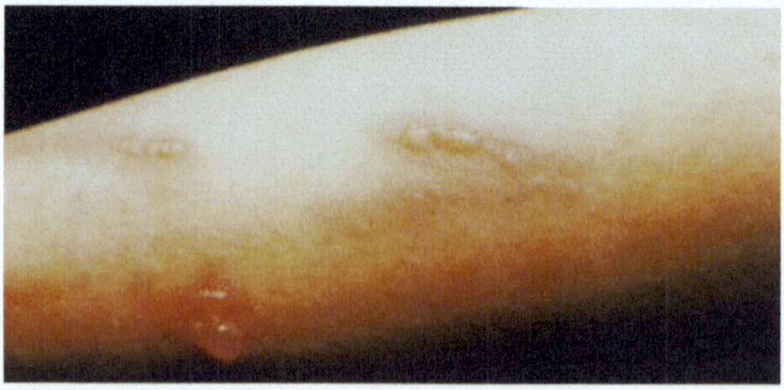

Fig. 17.3 Phytophotodermatitis. Erythema with marked bullae

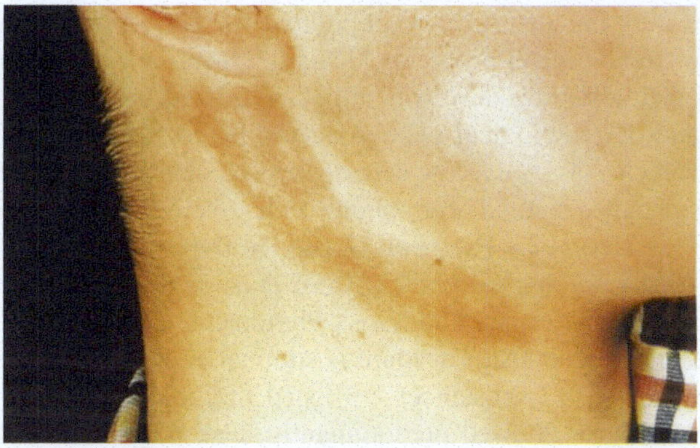

Fig. 17.4 Berloque dermatitis, often followed by a long-lasting hyperpigmentation

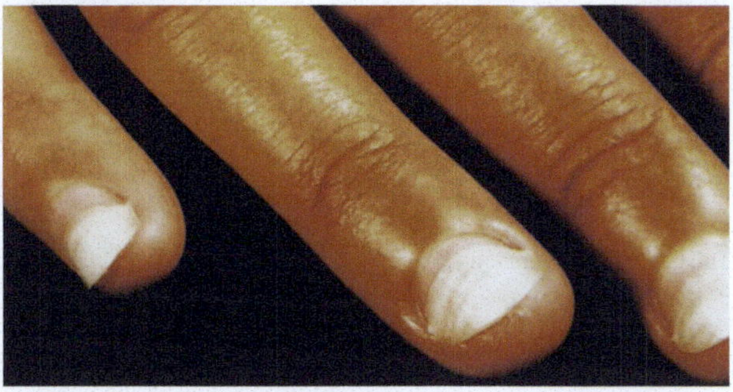

Fig. 17.5 Photooncholysis after oral administration of tetracycline and subsequent exposure to sunlight

dermatitis, (Fig. 17.4)] lead to a typical delayed painful erythema often observed with additional bullae. Later on, an intensive long-lasting hyperpigmentation was observed frequently [81].

A special form of phototoxic reactions is photoonycholysis which has been described repeatedly after systemic application of 8-methoxypsoralen, benoxaprofen, tetracycline or after photodynamic therapy [21], and more recently during treatments with vandetanib, a tyrosine kinase inhibitor [63].

Photoonycholysis (Fig. 17.5) begins in the distal part of the nail bed, especially after prolonged exposure to UV light, and patients with porphyria cutanea tarda characteristically develop additional bullae with clear fluid, milia and pain from easily traumatised and fragile skin, especially on the fingers. In contrast, erythropoietic protoporphyria (EPP) induces acute phototoxic symptoms such as burning pain associated with erythema and edema shortly after UV irradiation. Cumulative phototoxic skin damage may cause hyalinosis cutis-like lesions typical for juvenile EPP patients [42].

Diagnostic Procedures

The diagnosis of photosensitivity is based on the history, the clinical and histopathological findings and, in particular, on photodiagnostic test procedures [23, 32, 34–41]. Early on, Stephan Epstein emphasized the eminent role of the photopatch test for the identification of photosensitizers, followed by numerous publications on methodological problems [11–14]. Nevertheless, until the early 1980s, the photopatch test procedure was not standardized and varied between different countries and dermatological centers according to the test tray, substance concentrations, vehicles, as well as the assessment and classification of test reactions [22]. The first standard method for photopatch testing was defined by the Scandinavian Photodermatitis Research Group (SPDRG) in 1982 [26]. Inspired by the SPDRG, 45 dermatological centers from Austria, Germany and Switzerland founded the Austrian, German and Swiss Photopatch Test Group (DAPT) in 1984. Their new standardized test procedure is summarized in Tables 17.1, 17.2, and 17.3. In addition, the test substances are listed in Tables 17.4 and 17.5. Systemically applied substances showed predominantly false negative photopatch test results, because metabolites rather than topically applied test substances are likely to be the relevant photosensitizers.

Before initial irradiation of the test areas (preferably on the back), the suspected photoallergic drug should be administered orally, preferably at twice the usual dose. Taking into account pharmacokinetics, additional areas of skin should be exposed to 10 J/cm^2 UVA, e.g., at 1, 2, 3, 5, 8 and 12 h after drug administration. Readings

Table 17.1 Photopatch test

Application of test substances in Finn-Chambers
24 h occlusive to the back
Irradiation 10 J/cm^2 UVA (320–400 nm)
Controls: Unirradiated patch test site and UVA-irradiated skin without patch-test

Table 17.2 Photopatch test gradings

0	No reaction
1+	Erythema
2+	Erythema and infiltrate
3+	Erythema and papulovesicles
4+	Erythema bullae or erosions

Table 17.3 Classification of test reactions

Contact reaction
Every positive reaction in the control area without 1+ immediately after removal of the test tray
Phototoxic reaction
1+ or 2+, immediate or delayed, as decrescendo reaction
Photoallergic reaction
3+ or 4+, delayed, as crescendo reaction as well as the reaction pattern
0, 1+. 2+,3+

Table 17.4 List of substances: photopatch test 1985–1990

1. Tetrachlorosalicylanilide	0,10	17. • Fragrance Mix	8.00
2. Monobromsalicylchloranilide	1,00	18. • 6-Methylcumarine	1,00
3. Tribromsalicylanilide	1,00	19. Paraaminobenzoic acid	5,00
4. Buclosamide	5,00	20. Hydrochlorothiazide	1,00
5. Fenticlor	1,00	21. • Furosemide	1,00
6. Hexachlorophen	1,00	22. 2.hydroxymethoxybenzophenone	2.00
7. Bithionol	1,00	23. 3-(4-methylbenzyliden)-Campher	5,00
8. Triclosan	2,00	24. 4-isopropyldibenzoylmethane	5,00
9. Sulfanilamide	5,00	25. • Cyclamate	1,25
10. Chlorpromazine	0,10	26. • Saccharin	0,40
11. Promethazine	0,10	27. Wood tar	3,00
12. Carprofen	5,00	28. Colophony	20,00
13. Tiaprofenic acid	5,00	29. Balsam of Peru	25.00
14. Quinidine	1,00	30. Compositae Mix	6,50
15. Moschus Ambrette	5,00	31. •Tolbutamid	5,00
16. Moschus Mix	5,00	32. Thiourea	0,10

• Substances were removed from the test tray in 1990 because they caused no or only a few photoreactions or a photoallergy was triggered for the first time during the photopatch test by tested substance itself.

Table 17.5 List of substances: photopatch test 1991–1997

1. Tetrachlorosalicylanilide	0.10	14. Moschus Ambrette	5,00
2. Monobromsalicylchloranilide	1,00	15. Hydrochlorothiazide	1,00
3. Tribromsalicylanilide	1,00	16. Balsam of Peru	25,00
4. Buclosamid	5,00	17. Compositae mix	6,50
5. Fenticlor	1,00	18. Paraaminobenzoic acid	5,00
6. Hexachlorophene	1,00	19. 2-hydroxy-4-methoxybenzophenone	2,00
7. Bithionol	1,00	20. 3-(4-methylbenzyliden)-Campher	5,00
8. Triclosan	2,00	21. 4-isopropyldibenzoylmethane	10,00
9. Chlorpromazine	0,10	22. • 4-tert-butyl-4-methoxydibenzoylmethane	10,00
10. Promethazine	0,10	23. • 2-ethylhexyl-p-methoxycinnarnate	10,00
11. Carprofen	5.00	24. • Phenylbenzimidazolsulphonic acid	10,00
12. Chinidinsulfat	5,00	25. •p-methoxy-isoamyl-cinnamate	10,00

• Substances newly integrated in the test tray in 1991

should be taken immediately and at 24, 48 and 72 h after the first exposure. An example of a positive photoreaction (after systemic application of quinidine) is shown in Fig. 17.6 [70, 71].

Although photoallergies may be a rare phenomenon, the diagnosis of chemically induced photoallergies is very important to prevent severe forms of chronic actinic dermatitis and to detect new photosensitizers. The increasing use of cosmetics and toiletries as well as the topical or systemic application of newly developed pharmaceutical products [3, 5, 21, 63] determine the potential risk for consumers to be

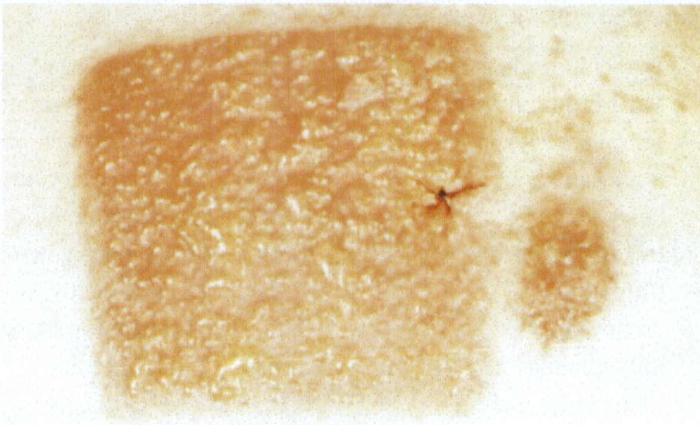

Fig. 17.6 Quinidine induced photoallergy (positive test reaction after systemic photoprovocation)

Table 17.6 Ranking list of phototoxic reactions (1985–1990)

Substances	Frequencies (%)	Substances	Frequencies (%)
1. Tiaprofenic acid	30,41	Wood tar	5,16
2. Promethazine	21,33	Hexachlorophene	4,36
3. Carprofen	8,50	Balsam of Peru	3,38
4. Chlorpromazine	8,00	Fenticlor	3,29
5. Fragrance Mix	5,54	Triclosan	2,93

Table 17.7 Ranking list of photoallergic reactions (1985–1990)

Substances		Frequencies (%)	Substances		Frequencies (%)
1.	Tiaprofenic acid	3,15	6.	Promethazine	0,54
2.	Fenticlor	1,60	7.	Tetrachlorosalicylanilde	0,54
3.	Carprofen	1,34	8.	Moschus Ambrette	0,54
4.	4-isopropyldibenzoylmethane	0,89	9.	Fragrance Mix	0,37
5.	2-hydroxy-4-methoxybenzophenone	0,71	10.	Moschus Mix	0,36

exposed to unknown photosensitizers. A prominent example was the epidemic of photoallergy to tetrachlorosalicylanilide (TCSA), which was used as a disinfectant in soaps and other toiletries in England between 1960 and 1993. In addition, moschus ambrette, a synthetic fragrance and preservative used in cosmetic products worldwide, has been shown to be an important photosensitizer. According to the results of a Scandinavian multicenter study [74], moschus ambrette caused the highest rate of photosensitization of all substances tested. Restrictive guidelines issued by the International Fragrance Association in 1985 regarding the use of moschus ambrette in cosmetics led to a remarkable decrease in the photosensitization rate. Therefore, afterwards published photopatch test kits include moschus ambrette only as a "historical photoallergen" [68].

The DAPT studies revealed that non-steroidal anti-inflammatory drugs, disinfectants, sunscreens, phenothiazines and fragrances are currently the most relevant photosensitizers (Tables 17.6 and 17.7).

Based on a consensus agreed in 2012, a retrospective analysis of 116 patients tested with the European Photopatch test series between 2014 and 2016 was performed by the European Photopatch Test group [20]. Nonsteroidal anti-inflammatory drugs (ketoprofen, dexketoprofen, etofenomat) followed by organic UV absorbers (benozophenone-3 and octocrylene) provoked the most photopatch test reactions [73]. Thus, their results are nearly comparable to the photoallergic reactions published by the DAPT.

Meanwhile, some of the identified and proven photosensitizers, including tetracycline derivatives and certain non-steroidal anti-inflammatory drugs, are being withdrawn from the market.

In addition to these synthetic photosensitizers, there are also exogenous or endogenous natural phototoxic substances e. g. in plants: leguminaceae, moraceae, rotaceae and umbiliferae. Furthermore, porphyrins are important photosensitizers, which accumulate in various tissues and cells in case of distinct enzymatic defects, leading to clinically relevant phototoxic skin reactions if irradiated with UV light [42, 61].

Predictive Test Procedures

Several test systems (e.g., Buehler's test [4], guinea pig test [45–47, 77], mouse ear swelling test [16], local lymph node assay [25, 44]) have been recommended by the OECD for the risk assessment of contact allergic or contact irritant reactions [64]. Although precise final guidelines for the risk assessment of the photoallergic potency of newly developed substances are still lacking, the European Community in 1997[1] required procedures to determine the potential photoallergic and phototoxic risk of skin care products. Because UV absorbing filters can cause severe phototoxic and photoallergic reactions (when applied to the skin and subsequently exposed to UV light), the authorities have specifically required safety assessment procedures for sunscreen products. At almost the same time, they called for an end to animal testing. A variety of biological systems were employed to evaluate phototoxicity. In general, phototoxic effects can be investigated by in vitro or in vivo test procedures (Table 17.8).

In 1900, the first studies of photosensitizers were performed by Raab using freshwater ciliates (paramecia) [66]. Since then, this model has been used by numerous investigators. The paramecia assay is inexpensive and relatively simple to perform, and therefore may serve as a phototoxicity model for large series of tests. Another phototoxicity test procedure based on Candida albicans was introduced by Daniels in 1965 [7]. He exposed Candida albicans on Sabouraud's medium to a photosensitizer and UVA as a screening model for phototoxicity. Based on

[1] Commission of the European Communities, Scientific Committee on Cosmetology, sixth Amendment to the Cosmetics Directive (EC); Guidelines for Safety Assessment of a Cosmetic Product 1997.

Table 17.8 In vitro test systems for phototoxicity

Photohemolysis-test with erythrocytes
Photo-basophils-histamin-releasing test
Fibroblasts-indol-red-uptake test
Candida albicans-inhibition test
Paramecium aurelia-lethality test
Photo hen's egg test
3T3 neutral red uptake (NRU) phototoxicity test
Human 3D epidermis model

phototoxic growth inhibition, the Candida albicans test is a very simple, inexpensive, and effective method that has been particularly useful in testing the phototoxic properties of psoralen [19, 35]. However, the well-known phototoxic agents sulfanilamide and demethylchlortetracycline did not induce phototoxic reactions in the Candida inhibition test system.

In 1909, Hasselbach studied photohemolysis using dyes. Erythrocytes are cells without a nucleus or cytoplasmic organelles. Thus, erythrocytes provide the opportunity to study cell membrane damage caused by phototoxicity [31]. The experimental conditions are inexpensive and easy to perform. An induction of photohemolysis of 5% indicates a phototoxic reaction. Erythrocytes obtained from only one individual and exposed to a phototoxic agent showed a wide range of different results. Therefore, pooled erythrocytes from different individuals are required for testing. However, known potent phototoxic substances (e.g., psoralen) did not elicit an adequate phototoxic response in this test system.

Other in vitro test systems are based on cell cultures to test phototoxic agents [15, 50, 65]. For example, fibroblasts must be obtained from healthy skin samples and cultured to confluence, or keratinocytes until multilayers are formed. The highest non-toxic concentration of a test chemical must be added to the cell cultures for an incubation period of 24 h. Cell cultures incubated with the test chemical alone, without additional UVA irradiation, and cell cultures irradiated with UVA light alone are used as controls. After an incubation period of 24 h, the morphological changes of the cells are analyzed microscopically and cell viability can be determined, e.g., by the uptake of vital dyes [48].

The 3 T3 Neutral Red Uptake (NRU) Phototoxicity-Test

The 3 T3 Neutral Red Uptake (NRU) phototoxicity assay has been developed on the basis of immortalized mouse fibroblast cell lines (Balb/c 3 T3). This method is used to determine the photocytotoxicity of a test substance that is irradiated with a non-cytotoxic dose of ultraviolet (UV) light (solar simulator). A non-irradiated but otherwise similarly treated cell culture serves as a control [1]. As a measure of UV-induced cytotoxicity, the concentration-dependent reduction in the uptake of

Table 17.9 3 T3 NRU phototoxicity-test procedure

Cell suspension (Balb/c) in two 96-well culture plates
96-wells exposed to the test compounds
First 96-well (+Irr): application of a non-toxic UV-dose
Second 96-well (−Irr): no application of any light
24 h later determination of the neutral red uptake
Calculation of the photo-irritation-factor

the vital dye neutral red is determined 24 h after application of the test substance and subsequent UV irradiation. This is because a potentially phototoxic test substance in combination with UV radiation can change the cell surface in such a way that the uptake capacity or binding capacity of the vital dye is reduced (Table 17.9). A spectrophotometer can then be used to differentiate between viable, damaged or dead cells and thus prove whether a given test substance have phototoxic potential or not.

Using the 3 T3-NRU-PT, the phototoxic properties of a test substance can be detected with a sensitivity of 100%. This test method is therefore ideally suited to reliably rule out a suspected phototoxic potential. However, it cannot detect photoallergic or even differentiate between phototoxic and photoallergic reactions. In addition, positive results in the 3 T3-NRU-PT are often not associated with an actually clinically detectable phototoxicity risk. Nevertheless, in combination with the results of other in vitro test methods, the 3 T3 NRU PT can at least help to reduce the number of animal tests required for the phototoxicity assessment. Due to its relatively strong reliability and practicability this method has found its way into guidelines, i.e. OCED Test No. 432.

As mentioned before a positive result in a 3 T3-NRU assay should trigger subsequent investigations for possible photoallergic properties of the relevant test compound, for example by the modified UV-dependent LLNA as described below. Ideally, such investigations should be carried out before a compound comes into first contact with humans (for example before phase I of clinical drug development), but this is up to now not strictly required by authorities at this early stage, only before or during phase III (ICH guideline S10, 2015).

The Human 3D Epidermis Model

A 3D reconstructed epidermal model has been investigated for use in phototoxicity testing to overcome the limitations of cell-based in vitro methods. Human keratinocyte cultures on collagen substrate containing human dermal fibroblasts were used as the basis for this in vitro human skin model. Such 3D skin equivalents are physiologically similar to natural human skin due to their epidermal stratification and epidermal-dermal interaction, and results of tested chemicals may be more reliable and reproducible compared to 2D test models. A notable advantage of such 3D skin models is the ability to distinguish between effects induced by topical or systemic (liquid) applications. On the other hand, the determination of photoallergic reactions is still difficult due to the lack of different types of immune cells present in natural skin.

Lelievre et al. investigated with a human reconstructed epidermis model (EPA: EpiSkin phototoxicity assay) the phototoxic potency of topically or systemically applied chemicals. Using the EPA, they were able to differentiate phototoxic from non-phototoxic test substances with a sensitivity of 92.3%, specificity of 100%, and overall accuracy of 94.1% [43].

Since a number of cytokines can be determined based on 3D skin models and histological examinations are possible, the test results may also be useful for estimating the photoallergenicity of tested compounds. However, to ensure reproducibility and comparability of results, the implementation of standardized protocols for the creation of 3D skin models is critical and overall, this method is more expensive and labor intensive than the 3 T3-NRU assay.

The Photo Hen's Egg Test

In the search for photobiological test systems that are more advanced than cell cultures [16] but can replace animal models, Neumann et al. developed the extraembryonic vasculature of the incubated chicken egg in combination with UV-irradiation as a screening model for testing the phototoxic or photoprotective potential of various chemicals [56, 58–62] and as an alternative to the Draize test [8] (rabbit eye test). A similar test, but without irradiation, was originally introduced by toxicologists as a screening model for mucocutaneous toxicity [9, 67].

First, a non-toxic level of the test substance and a non-toxic dose of UVA have to be defined. Therefore, the first step of the photo hen's egg test (PHET) is similar to the classical hen's egg test. Preliminary studies have shown that 5 J/cm^2 UVA does not induce any visible pathological effects on the yolk sac vasculature (YS).

The second part of the PHET has a 2 × 2 factorial design with the factors "irradiation" and "substance application" and the levels "yes" and "no".

The following parameters were evaluated over a period of 24 h: embryo-lethality, membrane discoloration and haemorrhages (Figs. 17.7, 17.8 and 17.9, Table 17.10).

Fertile white Leghorn eggs (Shaver Starcross 288 A, Lohmann, Cuxhaven, Germany) were incubated in a commercial incubator at 37.5 degrees Celsius and 65% relative humidity in a horizontal position [58]. All eggs were candled to discard any defective eggs after 3 days of incubation. Without damaging the shell, a hole was drilled in the shell through which 5 ml of egg white was aspirated to lower the embryo and the surrounding YS. Afterwards a 1.5 × 2.5 cm window then was cut out of the shell.

The eggs were covered with a wax sheet and returned into the incubator. At day 4 of incubation, only eggs with normally developed embryos and blood vascular systems were used for testing. Since we are interested in plain phototoxic reactions, in the PHET the embryo's yolk sac blood vessel system is exposed to a proven

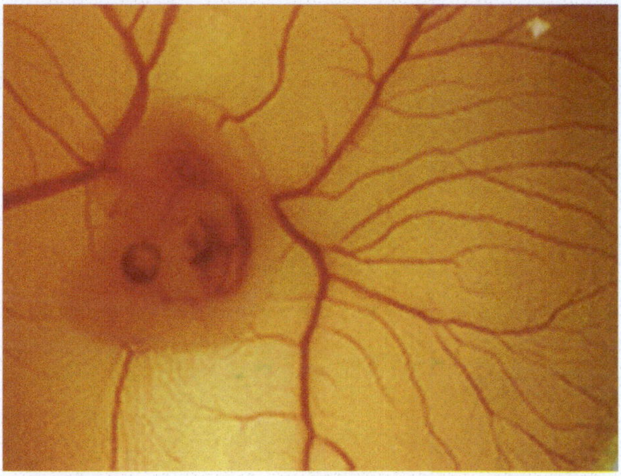

Fig. 17.7 Photo hen's egg test. Normal yolk sac blood vessel system (YS) at day 3 of incubation

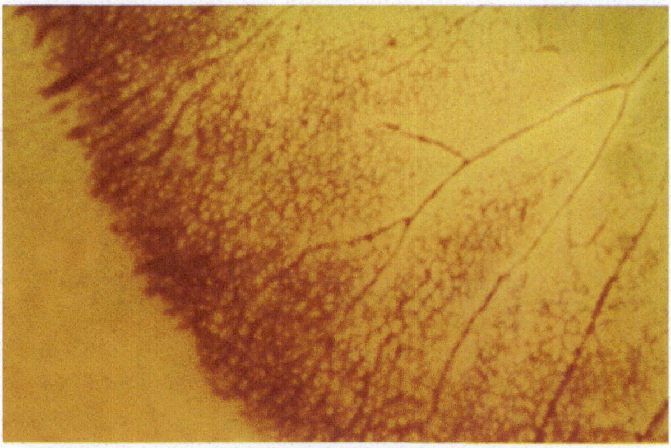

Fig. 17.8 Photo hen's egg test. Severe hemorrhage 24 h after application of 8-MOP and 5 J/cm^2 UVA irradiation

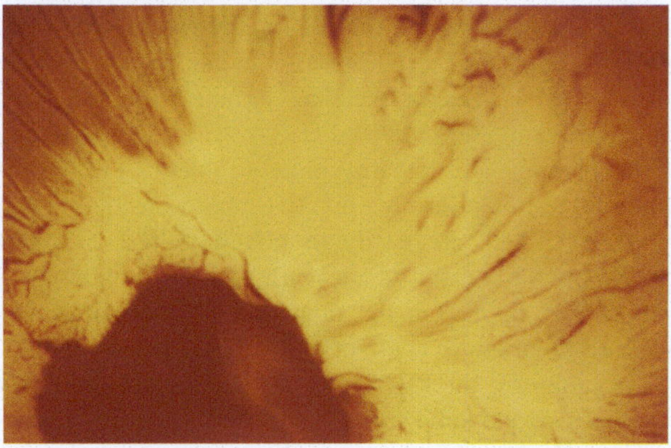

Fig. 17.9 Photo hen's egg test. Membrane discoloration 24 h after application of promethazine and 5 J/cm^2 UVA irradiation

Table 17.10 Photo hen's egg test classification of membrane discoloration (MD) and hemorrhage (HE)

No Level 0 (no)	No visible MD or HE
Level 1 (slight)	Just visible MD or HE
Level 2 (moderate)	Visible MD or HE, structures are covered partially
Level 3 (severe)	Visible MD or HE, structures are covered totally

Table 17.11 Photo hen's egg test factors

Relative lethality factors	Lethality rate of the interaction group (L_i) minus the average lethality rate of controls $L_C = (I_{C1} + I_{C2} + I_{C3})/3$
	Rel. lethality factor $L = L_i - L_C$
	$\text{Rel. lethality factor } L(\%) = \frac{L \times 100}{12}$
Relative morphology factors	Sum of the morphological gradings (m + h) from the interaction group (M_i) minus the sum of the average morphological gradings (m + h) of controls (M_C)
	$Mc = [(mc1 + hc1) + (mc2+ hc2) + (mc3 + hxc3)]/3$
	Rel. morphology factor $M = M_i - M_C$
	$\text{Rel. morphology factor } M(\%) = \frac{M \times 100}{12}$

non-toxic concentration of a test substance and subsequently to a non-toxic UVA dose. Therefore, at day 4 of the incubation period, group 1 (12 eggs per group) is exposed to a test substance, immediately followed by an irradiation with 5 J/cm^2 UVA (320–400 nm, Philips TL 09/40 W, Hamburg, Germany). Isotonic sodium chloride (NaCl) solution is usually used as the vehicle. Two additional groups serve as controls and are exposed to NaCI and 5 J/cm^2 UVA, and to NaCl and the test substance alone, respectively. Measurements are made 24 h after exposure. During this observation period, morphological parameters such as membrane discoloration (MD), hemorrhage (HR) [monitored and graded on a four-point scale using a macroscope (M 420, Leitz, Wetzlar, Germany)], and the embryo lethality are evaluated. The test parameters MD and HR as well as embryo lethality can be summarized in a morphology and lethality index (Table 17.11). Using these indices, the relative phototoxic potential of a putative photosensitizer compared to other well-known photosensitizers are easily to obtain. 8-Methoxypsoralen (8-MOP), a classical potent phototoxic substance (with no known photoallergic potential) is the leading phototoxic agent. On the other hand, olaquindox, a well-known photoallergen, showed no phototoxic effect in the PHET (Table 17.12).

In summary, the PHET is a simple and rapid test procedure that provides a new, inexpensive and valid screening model for phototoxicity and helps to reduce animal testing. However, focusing on the immunological sensitizing properties of photosensitizers, we assumed that animal testing cannot be completely replaced. Therefore, the UV-dependent lymph node assay (UV-LLNA) has proven to be an excellent test method.

Table 17.12 Photoxicity ranking list (based on the photo hen's egg testing)

Substances	Rel. Lethality factor (%)	Rel. Morphology factor (%)
1. 8-MOP	100,00	67,60
2. Promethazine	94,50	54,64
3. Protoporphyrine IX	94,50	64,82
4. Sparfloxacin	58,33	50,90
5. Acridine	58,33	49,54
6. TCSA	44,50	32,42
7. Hematoporphyrine	41,67	58,81
8. Lomefloxacin	30,58	35,67
9. Ciprofloxacin	0,00	62,50
10. Tetracyclin	0,00	2,79
11. Olaquindox	0	0

To study the photoallergenicity of chemicals, erythema tests with an induction and challenge phase (in vivo test systems) were developed in the 1960s [78]. The erythema tests were later improved with special pretreatments that resulted in increased penetration rates, higher immunological reactivity and better photosensitivity of the skin. These pretreatments included: mechanical skin irritation (brushing), injection of an adjuvant (e.g., freund's adjuvant), or application of irritants (e.g, sodium laurylsulfate). Even very weak photoallergens have been detected with these improved test systems. On the other hand, these techniques are very laborious, time-consuming (up to 63 days) and expensive [49, 51]. In addition, large numbers of animals are required and subjective criteria are used to classify the test reactions (erythema scores). The first test system based on objective criteria was the mouse ear swelling test (MEST) [16–18]. A relatively short test period (8 days), a low number of animals and an objective test parameter (ear thickness) are major advantages of the MEST. Unfortunately, the ear swelling test is nonspecific and does not allow differentiation between phototoxic and photoallergic reactions.

The UV-dependent Lymph-Node Assay

The Local Lymph Node Assay (LLNA) is a predictive test for identifying the contact sensitizing potential of chemicals in mice (OECD Test No. 429, 2010). It is a rapid and cost-effective alternative to the widely used Buehler's occluded patch test and other guinea pig tests. Compared to these tests, the LLNA is capable of detecting at least moderate to strong contact sensitizers. The LLNA is distinct from the guinea pig model and the mouse ear swelling test (MEST) in that it detects a primary immune response through auricular lymph node activation after topical application of chemicals to the dorsal surface of the ear. The measurement of in vivo 3[H]-thymidine incorporation has been primarily used to assess LNC proliferation and activation. Vohr et al. proposed a modified Local Lymph Node Assay (LLNA) that detects increases in lymph node weight and cell count. This alternative to the original LLNA does not use radioactive materials. The authors also introduced UVA irradiation to identify photoreactive compounds [79, 80]. Although the LLNA was originally described to selectively detect allergic skin immune responses, recent studies have shown that (photo)irritant test compounds also induce lymph node cell proliferation in vivo [55, 69, 72, 78].

Previous studies have shown that optimal sensitization and hapten-induced activation of skin-draining lymph node cells are achieved after three consecutive days of sensitizing treatment [16, 33, 78]. Therefore, five female NMRI mice per group were treated topically on the dorsal surfaces of both ears with 25 μl of photoallergic (e.g., TCSA) or phototoxic (e.g., 8-MOP) standards or vehicle alone on three consecutive days. To induce photocontact allergies and photoirritanies, mice were irradiated with 10 J/cm^2 UVA immediately after topical treatment. On day 0 and day 3, ear thickness was measured with a spring-loaded micrometer (Oditest; Kroeplin, Schluechtern, Germany) and mean ear swelling was calculated. In addition, mice were sacrificed and the auricular lymph nodes were removed from each animal on day 3 and pooled (for each individual mouse). Lymph node cell proliferation was determined by automated counting of lymph node cells per mouse (Coulter Counter ZM, Coulter, Heidelberg, Germany) and calculation of lymph node cell count indices. Lymph node cell count indices (LN indices) were defined as the ratio of the mean lymph node cell counts of mice treated with the test compound to the corresponding results of vehicle-treated control groups. Positive responses were defined as either significant ear swelling or a significant increase in lymph node cell counts [2, 75, 76, 79].

The main findings regarding the differentiation of photoallergic and phototoxic skin reactions are as follows:

1. Photocontact allergens as well as photoirritants induce skin-draining lymph node cell activation.
2. Photoirritants predominantly induce skin inflammation, which in turn induces proliferation of draining lymph nodes.
3. Induction of photocontact allergies causes only marginal skin inflammation but strong activation of skin draining lymph nodes.

Regarding the mechanisms of phototoxic and photoallergic skin reactions, the results of the LLNA show that the development of an integrated model may provide accurate criteria to distinguish between phototoxic and photoallergic potential of a compound by comparing local draining lymph node activation with skin inflammation. In this context, validation studies with both LLNA and MEST have led to recognition by the OECD. These tests have been classified as suitable for screening chemicals for sensitizing activity as the first step in an assessment process. Chemicals may be designated as potential photosensitizers if a positive response is recorded in these tests (Fig. 17.10).

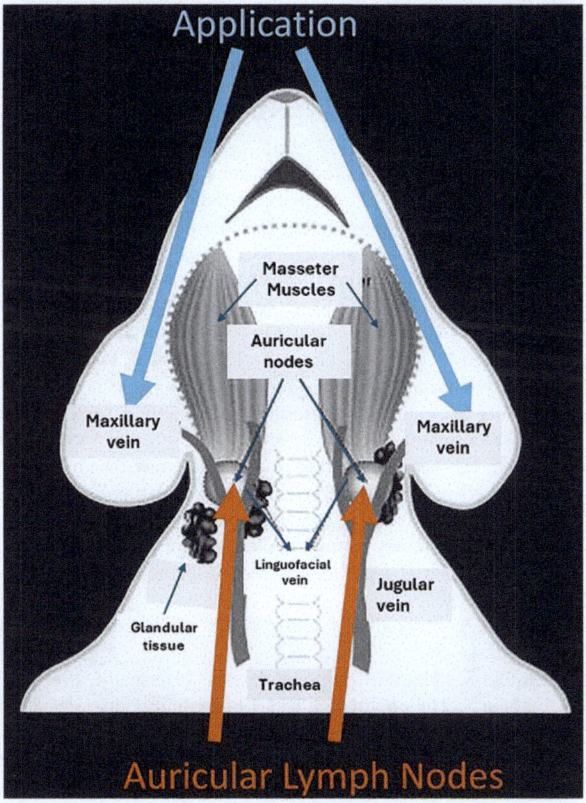

Fig. 17.10 UV-dependent Lymph-Node Essay (taken and modified from the ICCVAM protocol of 1999

In conclusion, the modified LLNA provides a non-radioactive method for differentiating between chemical-induced allergic and irritant skin reactions. Compared to guinea pig tests, this model is objective and measures immunologically relevant endpoints, is significantly less expensive, requires less vivarium space, is shorter in duration (4 days), uses less test substance, and can test colored materials [16, 17, 33]. In addition, the monophasic treatment protocol offers the opportunity to skip the assessment of minimum phototoxic or maximum non-irritating doses of a test compound. The UV-dependent modified LLNA offers also the valuable possibility to verify a possible photoallergic reaction by booster experiments.

Acknowledgements We would like to pay tribute to our highly esteemed mentor and former co-author Prof. Dr. Percy Lehmann, who unfortunately left us all too soon and unexpectedly. Without his scientific work, his profound dermatological expertise, his critical but always collegial and benevolent support, modern dermatology would be missing not only essential knowledge but also numerous committed (photo)dermatologists. Although cost pressure, workload and not only "deadlines" in university medicine have constantly increased in recent years, Prof. Lehmann always knew how to keep the caring and humane treatment of patients in mind. May his exemplary manner live on in our thoughts and actions.

References

1. Anon. Statement on the scientific validity of the 3T3 NRU PT test (an in vitro test for phototoxic potential). ATLA. 1998;26:7–8.
2. Blotz A, Laurence M, Moysan A, Blümel J, Dubertret L, Ahr HJ, Vohr H-W. Analyses of cutanteous fluoroquinolones photoreactivity using the integrated model for the differentiation of skin reactions. J Photochem Photobiol. 2000;58:46.
3. Boudon SM, Plappert-Helbig U, Odermatt A, Bauer D. Characterization of vemurafenib phototoxicity in a mouse model. Toxicol Sci. 2014;137(1):259–67.
4. Buehler EV. Delayed contact hypersensitivity in the Guinea pig. Arch Dermatol. 1965;91:171.
5. Blakely KM, Drucker AM, Rosen CF. Drug-induced photosensitivity-an update: culprit drugs, prevention and management. Drug Saf. 2019;42(7):827–47.
6. Baptista MS, Cadet J, Greer A, Thomas AH. Photosensitization reactions of biomolecules: definition, targets and mechanisms. Photochem Photobiol. 2021;97(6):1456–83.
7. Daniels F. A simple mikrobiological method for demonstrating phototoxic compounds. J Invest Dermatol. 1965;44:259–63.
8. Draize HJ. Lntracutaneous sensitization test on Guinea pigs. In: Apraisal of the safety of chemicals in food, drugs and cosmetics. Austin: Association of Food and Drug Officials of the United States; 1959.
9. Duffy PA. Irritancy testing-a cultured approach. Toxic In Vitro. 1989;3:157–8.
10. Enk AH, Katz SI. Contact sensitivity as a model for T-cell activation in skin. J Invest Dermatol. 1995;105:80.
11. Epstein S. Photoallergy and primary photosensitivity to sulfanilamide. J Invest Dermatol. 1939;2:43–51.
12. Epstein S. “Masked” photopatch tests. J Dermatol. 1963;41:369–70.
13. Epstein S. The photopatch test. Lts technique, manifestations, and significance. Ann Allergy. 1964;22:1–11.
14. Epstein S. Simplified photopatch testing. Arch Dermatol. 1966;93:216–20.
15. Freeman RG, Murtishaw W, Knox 1M. Tissue culture techniques in the study of cell photobiology and phototoxicity. J Invest Dermatol. 1970;54:164–9.
16. Gad SC. The mouse ear swelling test (MEST) in the 1990s. Toxicology. 1994;93:33.
17. Gad SC, Dunn BI, Dobbs DW, Reilly C, Walsh RD. Development and validation of an alternative dermal sensitization test: the mouse ear swelling test (MEST). Toxicol Appl Pharmacol. 1986;l84:93.
18. Gerberick GF, Ryan CA. A predictive mouse ear swelling model for investigating topical photoallergy. Food Chem Toxicol. 1990;28(5):361.
19. Gibbs NK. All adaption of the Candida albicans phototoxicity test to demonstrate photosensitizer action spectra. Photo-Dermatology. 1987;4:312–6.
20. Goncalo M, Ferguson GM, Bonevalle A, Bruyznzeel DP, Gimenez-Arnau A, Goosens A, Kerr A, Lech M, Neumann N, Niklasson B, Pigatto P, Rhodes LE, Rustemeyer T, Sarkany R, Thomas P, Wilkinson M. Photopatch testing: recommendations for a European photopatch test baseline series. Contact Dermat. 2013;68(4):239–43.
21. Hanneken S, Wessendorf U, Neumann NJ. Photodynamic onycholysis: first report of photo-onycholysis after photodynamic therapy. Clin Exp Dermatol. 2008;33(5):659–60.
22. Hoelzle E, Neumann N, Hausen B, Przybilla B, Schaudcr S, Hoenigsmann H, Bircher A, Plewig G. Photopatch testing: the 5-year experience of the German, Austrian, and Swiss Photopatch Test Group. J Am Acad Dermatol. 1991;25:59–68.
23. Hoelzle E, Plewig G, Hofmann C, Braun-Falco O. Photopatch testing. Results of a survey on testprocedures and experimental findings. Zbl Hautkr. 1985;151:361–6.
24. Hoelzle E, Plewig G, Lehmann P. Photodermatoses – diagnostic procedures and their interpretation. Photodermatol Photoimmunol Photomed. 1987;4:109–14.
25. Ikarashi Y, Tsukamoto Y, Tsuchiya T, Nakamura A. Influence of irritants on lymph node cell proliferation and the detection of contact sensitivity to metal salts in the murine local lymph node assay. Contact Derm. 1993;29:128.

26. Jansen CT, Wennerstein G, Rystedt I, Thune P, Brodthagen H. The Scandinavian standard photopatch test procedure. Contact Derm. 1982;8:155–8.
27. Jung EG. Die photoallergische Testung. Ther Umsch. 1974;31:313–6.
28. Jung EG. In vitro-Untersuchungen zur Chlorpromazin (CPZ)-Photoallergie. Arch Klin Exp Dermatol. 1979;237:501–l6.
29. Jung EG. Photoallergien. Zbl Hautkr. 1980;144:169–76.
30. Jung EG. Die belichtete Epikutantestung. Akt Dermalol. 1981:163–165.
31. Kahn G, Fleischaker B. Evaluation of phototoxicity of salicylanilides and similar compounds by photohemolysis. J Invest Dermatol. 1971;56:91–7.
32. Kaidbey KH, Kligman AM. Photomaximization test for identifying photoallergic contact sensitizers. Contact Derm. 1980;6:161–9.
33. Kimber I, Dearman RI, Scholes EW, Basketter DA. The local lymph node assay: developments and applications. Toxicology. l994;93:13.
34. Kimber I, Weisenberger C. A murine local lymph node assay for the identification of contact allergenes. Assay development and results of initial validation study. Arch Toxicol. 1989;163:274.
35. Knudson EA. The Candida phototoxicity test. The sensitivity of different strains of Candida, standardization attempts and analysis of the dose-response curves for 5- and 8-methoxypsoralen. Photo-Dermatology. 1985;2:80–5.
36. Lehmann P. Die deutschsprachige Arheitsgemeinschaft Photopatch-Test (DAPT). Hautarzt. 1990;41:295–7.
37. Lehmann P. Photodiagnostische Testverfahren in der Dermatologie. In: Macher E, Kolde G, Brücker B, editors. Jahrbuch der Dermatologie 19921993. Zuelpich: Biermann Verlag; 1992. p. 81–100.
38. Lehmann P. Principles of photo testing and photopatch testing: a European perspective. Retinoids Today and Tomorrow. 1993;31:36–42.
39. Lehmann P. Principles of photo testing and photopatch testing. In: Altmeyer P, Hoffmann K, Stuecker M, editors. Skin cancer and UV radiation. Berlin Heidelberg: Springer-Verlag; 1997.
40. Lehmann P, Hoelzle E, Plewig G. Photoallergie auf Neotri mit Kreuzreaktion auf Teneretic Nachweis durch systemische Photoprovokation. Hautarzt. 1988;39:38–41.
41. Lehmann P, Hoelzle E, von Kries R, Plewig G. Uebersicht – Neue Konzepte. Lichtdiagnostische Verfahren bei Patienten mit Verdacht auf Photodermatosen. Zbl Hautkr. 1986;152:667–82.
42. Lehmann P, Scharfetter K, Kind P, Goerz G. Erythropoetische Protoporphyrie; synopsis von 20 Patienten. Hautarzt. 1991;42:570–4.
43. Lelièvre D, Justine P, Christiaens F, Bonaventure N, Coutet J, Marrot L, Cotovio J. The EpiSkin phototoxicity assay (EPA): development of an in vitro tiered strategy using 17 reference chemicals to predict phototoxic potency. Toxicol In Vitro. 2007;21(6):977–95.
44. Maeda Y, Hirosaki H, Yamanaka H, Takeyoshi H. New approach to predict photoallergic potentials of chemicals based on murine local lymph node assay. J Appl Toxicol. 2018;38(10):1316–22.
45. Magnusson B, Kligman AM. The identification of contact allergens by animal assay. The Guinea pig maximization test. J Invest Dermatol. 1969;52:268.
46. Maguire HC. The bioassay of contact allergens in the Guinea pig. J Soc Cosmet Chem. 1973;24:51.
47. Maguire HC Jr, Chase MW. Studies of the sensitization of animals with simple chemical compounds. 13. Sensitization of Guinea pigs with picric acid. J Exp Med. 1972;135:357.
48. Maier K, Schmitt-Landgraf R, Siegmund B. Development of an in vitro test system with human skin cells for evaluation of phototoxicity. Toxicol In Vitro. 1991;5(6):457–61.
49. Maurer T. Experimentelle Modelle des photoallergischen Ekzems. Allergologie. 1986;9:3–7.
50. Maurer T. Pholotoxicity testing – in vivo and in vitro. Food Chem Toxicol. 1987;25:407–14.
51. Maurer T, Thomann P, Weirich EG, Hess R. The optimization test in the Guinea pig. Agents Actions. 1975;5:174.
52. Maurer T, Weirich EG, Hess R. The optimization lest in the Guinea pig in relation to other predictive sensitization methods. Toxicology. 1980;15(3):163–71.

53. Maurer T, Weirich EG, Hess R. Photokontallergie. Zur Epidemiologie und praediktiven tierexperimentellen Erfassung. Derm Beruf Umwelt. 1980;28:70–81.
54. McKenzie RC, Sauder DN. The role of keratinocyte cytokines in inflammation and immunity. J Invest Dermatol. 1991;95:105.
55. Yu MP, Cl ZM. Lymphocyte chemotactic activity of human interleukin- I. J Immunol. 1984;133:2007.
56. Neumann NJ, Fritsch C, Goerz G, Ruzicka T, Lehmann P. D-Aminolevulinic acid in the photo hen's egg test. Arch Dermatol Res. 1997;289(supp):A49.
57. Neumann NJ, Hoelzle E, Lehmann P, Benedikter S, Tapernoux B, Plewig G. Pattern analysis of photopatch test reactions. Photodermatol Photoimmunol Photomed. 1994;10(2):65–73.
58. Neumann NJ, Hoelzle E, Lehmann P, Rosenbruch M, Klaucic A, Plewig G. Photo hen's egg test: a model for phototoxicity. Br J Dermatol. 1997;136:326–30.
59. Neumann NJ, Klaucic A, Hoelzle E, Lehmann P. Evaluation of the phototoxic potential of ciprofloxacin in the photo hen's egg test. Arch Dermatol Res. 1995;287:384.
60. Neumann NJ, Hoelzle E, Wallerand M, Vierbaum S, Ruzicka T, Lehmann P. The photoprotective effect of ascorbic acid, and indomethacin evaluated by the photo hen's egg test. Photodermatol Photoimmunol Photomed. 1999;15(5):166–70.
61. Neumann NJ, Hanneken S, Ruzicka T, Lehmann P. Phototoxicity of exogenous protoporphyrin IX and delta-aminolevulinic acid in the photo hen's egg test. Photodermatol Photoimmunol Photomed. 2004;20(5):224–9.
62. Neumann NJ, Blotz A, Wasinska-Kempka G, Rosenbruch M, Lehmann P, Ahr HJ, Vohr HW. Evaluation of phototoxic and photoallergic potentials of 13 compounds by different in vitro and in vivo methods. Photochem Photobiol B. 2005;79(1):25–34.
63. Negulescu M, Zerdoud S, Boulinguez S, Tournier E, Delord JP, Baran R, Sibaud V. Development of Photoonycholysis with Vandetanib Therapy. Skin Appendage Disord. 2017;2(3–4):146–51.
64. OECD (Organisation for Economic Cooperation and Development) (1992) Guideline 406 for testing chemicals. Adopted 1992.
65. Przybilla B, Schwab-Przybilla U, Ruzicka T, Ring J. Photoxicity of non-steroidal antiinflammatory drugs demonstrated in vitro by a photo-basophil-histamine-release test. Photo-Dermatology. 1987;4:73–8.
66. Raab O. Ueber die Wirkung flourescierender Stoffe auf Infusorien. Z Biol. 1900;39:524–46.
67. Rosenbruch M. Toxizitaetsuntersuchungen am bebrueteten Huehnerei. Derm Beruf Umwelt. 1990;38:5–11.
68. Ruenger TM, Lehmann P, Neumann NJ, Matthies C, Schauder S, Ortel B, Muenzberger C, Hoelzle E. Empfehlung einer Photopatch-Test Standardreihe durch die deutschsprachige Arbeitsgruppe "Photopatch-Test". Hautarzt. 1995;46:240–3.
69. Schilling C, Homey B, Ruzicka T, Lehmann P, Schuppe HC, Vohr HW. Characterization of the induction phase of contact hypersensitivity in murine epidermal and local draining lymph node cells. J Eur Acad Dermatol Venerol. 1996;7:A37.
70. Schuerer NY, Hoelzle E, Plewig G, Lehmann P. Photosensitivity induced by quinidine sulfate: experimental reproduction of skin lesions. Photodermatol Photoimmunol Photomed. 1992;9:78–82.
71. Schuerer NY, Lehmann P, Plewig G. Chinidininduzierte Photollergie. Eine klinische und experimentelle Studie. Hautarzt. 1991;42:158–61.
72. Shivji GM, Gupta AK, Suder DR (1994) Role of cytokines in irritant contact dermatitis. In: Alternative methods in toxicology series, volume 10: in vitro skin toxicology: irritation phototoxicity, sensitization. A. Rougier, A.M. Goldberg, H.I. Maibach, eds. Mary Ann Liebert, Inc., Publishers, New York, NY, 13-21.
73. Subiabre-Ferrer D, Esteve-Martinez, Blasco-Encinas R, Sierra-Talamantes C, Perez-Ferriols, Zaragoza-Ninet. European photopatch test baseline series: a 3-year experience. Contact Dermat. 2019;80(1):5–8.
74. Thune A, Jansen C, Wennersten G, Rystedt I, Brodthagen H, McFadden N. The Scandinavian multicenter photopatch study 1980–1985: final report. Photodermatology. 1988;5:261–9.

75. Ulrich P, Homey B, Vohr H-W. A modified murine local lymph node assay for the differentiation of contact photoallergy from phototoxicity by analysis of cytokine expression in skin-draining lymph node cells. Toxicology. 1998;125:140.
76. Ulrich P, Vohr H-W. Local lymph node assay (IMDS) modifications. In: Encyclopedia of immunotoxicology. 2nd ed. Springer; 2015.
77. Vinson LJ, Borselli VF. A Guinea pig assay of photosensitizing potential of topical germicides. J Soc Cosmet Chem. 1966;17:123.
78. Vinson LJ, Borselli VF, Singer EF. Realistic methods for determining photosenzitation potential of topical agents. Am Perfumer Cosmet. 1968;83:37.
79. Vohr H-W, Blümel J, Blotz A, Homey B, Ahr HJ. An intra-laboratory validation of the Integrated Model for the Differentiation of Skin Reactions (IMDS): discrimination between (photo)allergic and (photo)irritant skin reaction in mice. Regul Toxicol. 2000;73:501.
80. Vohr HW, Homey B, Schuppe HC, Kind P. Detection of photoreactivity demonstrated in a modified local lymph node assay in mice. Photodermatol Photoimmunol Photomed. 1994;10:57–64.
81. Zaynoun ST, Aftimos BA, Tenekjian KK, Kurban AK. Berloque dermatitis – a continuing cosmetic problem. Contact Derm. 1981;7(2):111–6.

Chapter 18
Genotoxicity

Tetyana Kobets and A. Wallace Hayes

Abbreviations

BER	Base excision repair
CA	Chromosomal aberration
CIR	Cosmetic Ingredient Review
CPCP	Cosmetics and personal care product
CPSR	Cosmetic Product Safety Report
CYP	Cytochrome P450
DDR	DNA damage response
DL	Dominant lethal
EC	European Commission
EU	European Union
FD&C	Federal Food, Drug, and Cosmetic Act
FDA	Food and Drug Administration
FEMA	Flavor Extract Manufacturers Association
GMP	Good manufacturing practices
GPI	Glycosylphosphatidylinositol
HPRT	Hypoxanthine phosphoribosyl transferase
HR	Homologous recombination
ICCR	Cooperation on Cosmetics Regulation
ICH	International Conference on Harmonisation of Chemicals

T. Kobets (✉)
Department of Pathology, Microbiology and Immunology, New York Medical College, Valhalla, NY, USA
e-mail: Tetyana_Kobets@nymc.edu

A. W. Hayes
University of South Florida College of Public Health, Tampa, Florida, and Institute of Integrative Toxicology, Michigan State University, East Lansing, MI, USA

P. Elsner et al. (eds.), *Cosmetics*, https://doi.org/10.1007/978-3-032-14644-1_18

IPCS	International Programme on Chemical Safety
ISO	International Organization for Standardization
MLA	Mouse lymphoma assay
MMR	Mismatch repair
MN	Micronucleus
MoA	Mode of action
MoCRA	Modernization of Cosmetics Regulation Act
MoE	Margin of Exposure
MoS	Margin of Safety
mRNA	Messenger RNA
NAM	New approach methodology
NER	Nucleotide excision repair
NHEJ	Non-homologous end joining
NHP	Natural health product
NMPA	National Medical Products Administration
OECD	Organization for Economic Co-operation and Development
OTC	Over-the-counter
PPD	para-Phenylenediamine
QSAR	Quantitative Structure-Activity Relationship
REACH	Registration, Evaluation, Authorization and Restriction of Chemicals
RIFM	Research Institute for Fragrance Materials
SCCS	Scientific Committee on Consumer Safety
TGR	Transgenic rodent
TK	Thymidine kinase
TTC	Threshold of Toxicological Concern
UV	Ultraviolet
WoE	Weight of Evidence
XPRT	Xanthine phosphoribosyl transferase

Introduction

Genotoxicity refers to a chemical's ability to directly alter a genetic material of a cell (i.e., produce direct DNA damage), potentially leading to genomic instability and disruption of normal cellular functions [129, 131]. This term encompasses permanent changes in DNA sequence (*mutagenicity*) and structural and/or numerical chromosomal abnormalities (*clastogenicity/aneugenicity*, respectively). Such alterations in somatic cells have been linked to the development of various adverse effects, including neoplasia [82, 85, 129, 166, 167], accelerated aging [3, 64], immune dysfunction [42], and neurodegenerative diseases [2]. Meanwhile, in germ cells, genetic damage most often results in reproductive failure (e.g., infertility and spontaneous abortion) [46]. While mutations have been implicated in the pathogenesis of numerous diseases [21], the primary emphasis of genetic toxicology has been directed at assessing its link to cancer risk [38, 59, 99].

Mechanisms of Genotoxicity

Mechanisms of genotoxicity can be broadly categorized based on the type of DNA damage produced by a chemical (Fig. 18.1). These include modifications of the physical and/or chemical structure of DNA. Specifically, genotoxic (i.e., *DNA-reactive*) compound, either in its parent form or after biotransformation by metabolic enzymes, is capable of forming reactive electrophiles that can (1) covalently bind to DNA base(s) forming *DNA adducts* or (2) to multiple sites on DNA on the same or opposite strands creating *inter- and intrastrand DNA crosslinks,* (3) get inserted between base pairs on both DNA strands, a process referred to as *intercalation,* or (4) disrupt the continuity of DNA helix resulting in *single or double DNA strand break(s)* [19, 82, 85, 131, 138].

DNA binding occurs when an electron-deficient (*electrophilic*) functional group of a chemical forms a covalent bond with an electron-rich (*nucleophilic*) site on DNA [68, 85]. Types of DNA adducts depend on various factors, including the chemical structure and the ability of a chemical to intercalate with DNA as well as steric factors (i.e., accessibility of nucleophilic sites). DNA binding is usually more extensive in the transcriptionally active DNA due to open chromatin structure [128]. The most common sites for DNA binding are the N3 and N7 positions of the guanine or adenine due to their high nucleophilicity [68]. However, some chemical

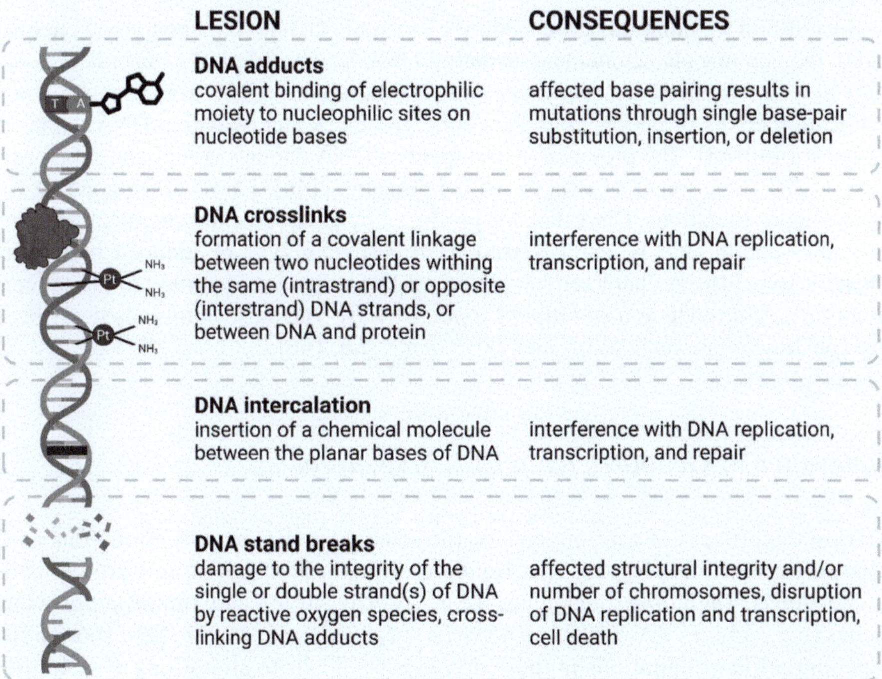

Fig. 18.1 Types of DNA damage produced by genotoxic carcinogens. (Created in BioRender)

entities, in particular aryl amines and heterocyclic aromatic amines, favor C8 atoms of these DNA bases [8, 31, 68, 127].

DNA lesions are often mutagenic and can become fixed in the genome if not repaired properly. For example, DNA adducts can lead to aberrant base pairing and incorporation of incorrect nucleotides into the opposite strand. If left unrepaired, a subsequent round of DNA replication will convert this mismatch into a permanent point mutation (e.g., replacing a G:C base pair with an A:T base pair). In addition to base pair substitutions, mutations can also arise through base pair insertions or deletions [131, 136]. Mutations can potentially disrupt the accurate translation of messenger RNA (mRNA) into functional proteins. Agents that are capable of altering the nucleotide sequence are referred to as *mutagens*.

Large-scale damage to chromosomal DNA can result in deviation in chromosome structure (breaks, deletions, rearrangements) [131] or number such as gain or loss of individual chromosomes (*aneuploidy*) or multiple entire sets of chromosomes (*polyploidy*) [91, 140, 144]. Agents classified as *clastogens* generate acentric chromosomal fragments through direct DNA breaks, while *aneugens* affect the segregation of chromosomes during mitosis or meiosis [34]. Either of these events can lead to the induction of micronuclei (MNs), structures composed of chromosomal fragments, or whole chromosome(s) that did not incorporate into the nucleus during cell division [149]. Functionally, chromosomal aberrations can lead to changes in the expression of one or more genes by amplification, deletion, or translocation mechanisms.

In addition to mutations produced by exogenous factors (e.g., genotoxic chemicals), the genome also contains preexisting DNA lesions referred to as either *spontaneous* or *background mutations*. These alterations arise from spontaneous replication errors or endogenous metabolic processes and oxidative DNA damage [19, 96, 146, 163]. The presence of endogenous DNA damage complicates the process of risk assessment of exogenous carcinogens [146]. However, in contrast to spontaneous mutations, DNA damage produced by environmental chemicals is usually site-specific and is characterized by a particular type of induced base pair changes [66, 146]. A characteristic pattern of DNA damage identified in the cancer genome is referred to as a *mutational signature* [60]. The most commonly described are specific mutations in *K-ras* and *TP53* genes [66, 146].

Relevance of Genotoxicity to Carcinogenesis

During the process of carcinogenesis, the affected cell(s) acquire mutations and altered expressions of genes that regulate critical processes of cell growth and homeostasis, including oncogenes (e.g., *H-Ras*, *Myc*) and tumor-suppressor genes (e.g., *p53*, *PTEN*, *Cdk2A*, *RASSF1A*) [7, 32, 59, 82, 89, 97, 125, 166–168]. Accumulation of mutations in these driver genes leads to alterations of genomic pathways and an abnormal activation of molecules involved in signal transduction. This, in turn, disrupts processes of telomere maintenance, chromatin remodeling, cell cycle regulation, apoptosis, and cell differentiation [94, 95]. As a result, an initiated cell undergoes transformation into a cell with a neoplastic phenotype with specific characteristics that enable cancer development and progression. These properties, also referred to as *hallmarks of cancer*, include acquisition of genome instability, capabilities for sustaining proliferative signaling, evasion of growth suppressors, resistance to cell death, enabled replicative immortality, activation of angiogenesis, ability to invade and metastasize, deregulated cellular metabolism, avoidance of immune destruction, unlocked phenotypic plasticity and non-mutational epigenetic reprogramming, cellular senescence, presence of tumor-promoting inflammation, and polymorphic microbiomes [56–58].

DNA reactivity is the defining characteristic of genotoxic carcinogens [82, 85]. Since carcinogens of this type can produce adverse effects at low dosages and/or after a short-term exposure, the general assumption is that they do not exhibit thresholds [11, 114]. This implies that such chemicals are assumed to pose a cancer risk regardless of the administered dose. However, a growing body of evidence supports the possibility of thresholds for DNA-reactive carcinogens [45, 81, 157, 164].

In addition to genotoxicity, the mode of action (MoA) of DNA-reactive carcinogens can encompass other effects [82, 85, 138] such as cytotoxicity [13, 23, 110], epigenetic alterations (e.g., DNA methylation or histone modifications) [126] or induction of oxidative DNA damage [78]. These effects can enhance fixation of mutations by, for example, increasing cell proliferation [22, 165]. Overall, MoAs of chemical carcinogens depend on various factors, including dose and conditions of exposure [38, 59], as well as individual susceptibility of a host, including their ability to bioactivate and detoxify the substance or to repair induced DNA damage [69, 79].

Principles of Genotoxicity as Applied to Cosmetics

Several factors should be considered when evaluating the potential genotoxicity of cosmetics and personal care products (CPCPs). These include the conditions of exposure, the characteristics of the contact site, and the formulation of the product. As mentioned above, individual susceptibility might also play a role.

Factors Influencing Genotoxic Risk of CPCPs

The widespread use of CPCPs by the general population often daily leads to frequent but typically low-concentration exposures [63]. The application of CPCPs mainly results in their direct contact with the skin and mucous membranes; however, other routes of exposure (e.g., inhalation of aerosolized products or ingestion of lipstick) are possible. Thus, it is important to consider the ability of a compound to be absorbed by the skin or to be photoactivated by ultraviolet (UV) light. The skin is the largest organ in the body with a variety of functions, including its important role as a protective barrier. The capacity of a chemical to penetrate the epidermis and dermis depends on its physico-chemical properties, including molecular weight, lipophilicity, etc. [12, 28]. Additionally, factors such as the metabolic competency and sensitivity of the skin, as well as its capacity to repair DNA damage, must be considered when evaluating the potential risks associated with consumer exposures to CPCPs.

Many chemicals require bioactivation with xenobiotic enzymes to become DNA-reactive and exhibit genotoxicity [31, 85, 160]. These reactions occur predominantly in the liver. The phase I metabolic reactions introduce a reactive polar group to the parent compound, thus converting it into an electrophile or free radical capable of covalent binding to DNA [119]. Meanwhile, the phase II conjugation reactions enhance excretion of a metabolite by increasing its polarity due to added endogenous hydrophilic groups [116]. Cells composing mammalian skin (e.g., keratinocytes of the epidermis) have been shown to possess major metabolic enzymes, which participate in the first-pass metabolism of xenobiotics administered by the dermal route [48, 102, 117]. However, the activity of these enzymes is relatively limited compared to other organs with metabolic capabilities, especially the liver [35, 161]. Thus, the expression of phase I bioactivation enzymes, including cytochrome P450 (CYP) enzymes, in particular the CYP1 family, has been detected in the skin, mainly in the epidermis and sebaceous glands [48, 72, 113, 117]. Human skin also possesses other enzymes involved in phase I metabolism, including flavin-dependent monooxygenases, alcohol and aldehyde dehydrogenases, esterases/amidases, and epoxide hydrolases; however, their specific activity in skin is less than 10% of that in the liver.

The ability of the skin to bioactivate certain genotoxic compounds into DNA-reactive intermediates is evident by the detection of DNA adducts following the administration of several carcinogens of this type, including coal tar [49], tamoxifen [17], and benzo[a]pyrene [50].

The major phase II detoxification enzymes, such as glutathione S-transferases, sulfotransferases, N-acetyltransferases, and UDP-glucuronosyltransferases, in the skin are generally expressed at much higher levels compared to phase I enzymes [48, 72, 100, 117, 161]. Such higher expression of phase II enzymes is essential for the protective function of the skin. Absorption and metabolism of xenobiotics by the skin can be affected by various conditions (e.g., psoriasis, dermatitis, aging), which compromise the integrity or thickness of the skin.

The skin is frequently exposed to a plethora of environmental stressors capable of producing DNA damage and oxidative stress, including UV radiation and chemical carcinogens [103, 108, 145]. As such, it requires a robust capacity for DNA repair to maintain homeostasis and integrity. DNA damage, including that caused by genotoxic chemicals, usually activates lesion-specific sensor proteins, which initiate the DNA damage response (DDR) pathway. This complex cellular signaling cascade can promote cell-cycle arrest and cell death or stimulate various DNA repair mechanisms, including direct repair, base excision repair (BER), nucleotide excision repair (NER), mismatch repair (MMR), non-homologous end joining (NHEJ), and homologous recombination (HR) [19, 55, 65]. Specific DNA lesions are usually repaired by certain DNA repair mechanisms, although overlap may occur. Thus, BER usually fixes small lesions that do not distort the DNA helix, such as oxidative bases and abasic sites, NER repairs bulky DNA adducts, MMR corrects errors that occur during DNA replication, while NHEJ and HR are key mechanisms for repairing double-strand DNA breaks and crosslinks.

Defects in the DDR and DNA repair pathways can lead to the accumulation of unrepaired DNA damage, increasing the risk of mutations and genomic instability. Accordingly, certain deficits in DNA repair mechanisms are linked to various skin disorders [67], with the most common example being xeroderma pigmentosum in patients with a deficient NER pathway [124]. Individuals with compromised DNA repair may be especially vulnerable to potential genotoxic effects from CPCPs.

Another, less explored factor that might also contribute to the effects of CPCPs is their interplay with the skin microbiome, which is composed of diverse populations of bacteria, viruses, and fungi [16, 20, 137, 139]. Microorganisms can metabolize cosmetic ingredients, influencing their genotoxic potential. In turn, xenobiotics can disrupt the normal microflora of the skin, altering its homeostasis and immune response and increasing susceptibility to exogenous stressors.

The composition of CPCPs typically consists of a mixture of ingredients; as such, safety evaluation should involve the assessment of individual components as well as the final product [63]. Moreover, consumers often use multiple CPCPs concurrently; thus, it is also important to understand the effects of combined exposures [90]. It is widely recognized that the same chemical can be used in different CPCPs at varying concentrations depending on its intended function, which also can affect the associated risks.

Genotoxicity Assessment of Ingredients in CPCPs

Genotoxicity is the primary MoA of the majority of animal and human carcinogens [59, 82, 85, 129]. Moreover, regulatory agencies generally consider genotoxic carcinogens to have no safe levels of exposure (i.e., thresholds) [11, 59, 114]. This necessitates that manufacturers demonstrate that their CPCPs do not possess the properties of a genotoxicant.

The traditional paradigm of genotoxicity assessment involves *hazard identification* (qualitative assessment of genotoxic potential) and *characterization* (quantitative evaluation of the relationship between the dose and an adverse (genotoxic) response), as well as *risk characterization* (risk associated with consumer exposure) [106].

Standard Genotoxicity Assays

A variety of *in vitro* and *in vivo* assays have been developed and approved globally for the assessment of genotoxicity (Table 18.1); however, only a few are regulatory acceptable for cosmetic ingredients. The regulatory battery of genotoxicity assays is

Table 18.1 Summary of genotoxicity endpoints and testing strategies for their assessment

Endpoint	Assay	OECD test guideline
In vitro		
Mutagenicity	Bacterial reverse mutation assay (Ames test) Mammalian cell gene mutation test using the hypoxanthine phosphoribosyl transferase (HPRT) and xanthine phosphoribosyl transferase (XPRT) genes	471[a] 476[b]
Mutagenicity and clastogenicity	Mammalian cell gene mutation test using the thymidine kinase (TK) gene/Mouse lymphoma assay (MLA)	490[c]
Clastogenicity and aneugenicity	Mammalian chromosomal aberration (CA) assay Mammalian cell micronucleus (MN) assay	473[d] 487[e]
In vivo		
Mutagenicity	Mammalian erythrocyte Pig-A gene mutation assay Transgenic rodent (TGR) somatic and germ cell gene mutation assay	470[f] 488[g]
Mutagenicity and clastogenicity in germ cells	Rodent dominant lethal (DL) test	478[h]
Clastogenicity and aneugenicity	Mammalian erythrocyte MN assay Mammalian bone marrow CA assay	474[i] 475[j]
DNA damage	Mammalian alkaline comet assay	489[k]

Notes: commonly used mammalian cells: mouse lymphoma (L5178Y) cells, Chinese hamster ovary (CHO) or lung (V79) cells, Syrian hamster embryo (SHE) cells, human peripheral blood lymphocytes, or TK6 lymphoblasts

Examples of TGR: lacZ or cII bacteriophage mouse (Muta™Mouse); lacZ plasmid mouse; gpt delta (gpt and Spi−) mouse and rat; lacI or cII bacteriophage mouse and rat (Big Blue®)

Links to the Organization for Economic Co-operation and Development (OECD) guidelines:

[a]https://www.oecd.org/en/publications/test-no-471-bacterial-reverse-mutation-test_9789264071247-en.html

[b]https://www.oecd.org/en/publications/test-no-476-in-vitro-mammalian-cell-gene-mutation-tests-using-the-hprt-and-xprt-genes_9789264264809-en.html

[c]https://www.oecd.org/en/publications/2016/07/test-no-490-in-vitro-mammalian-cell-gene-mutation-tests-using-the-thymidine-kinase-gene_g1g6fb2e.html

[d]https://www.oecd.org/en/publications/2016/07/test-no-473-in-vitro-mammalian-chromosomal-aberration-test_g1g6ed0e.html

[e]https://www.oecd.org/en/publications/2023/07/test-no-487-in-vitro-mammalian-cell-micronucleus-test_g1g6fb2a.html

[f]https://www.oecd.org/en/publications/2022/06/test-no-470-mammalian-erythrocyte-pig-a-gene-mutation-assay_8d5eb84f.html

[g]https://www.oecd.org/en/publications/2022/06/test-no-488-transgenic-rodent-somatic-and-germ-cell-gene-mutation-assays_g1g3404a.html

[h]https://www.oecd.org/en/publications/2016/07/test-no-478-rodent-dominant-lethal-test_g1g6fb1c.html

[i]https://www.oecd.org/en/publications/2016/07/test-no-474-mammalian-erythrocyte-micronucleus-test_g1g6fb16.html

[j]https://www.oecd.org/en/publications/2016/07/test-no-475-mammalian-bone-marrow-chromosomal-aberration-test_g1g6fb18.html

[k]https://www.oecd.org/en/publications/2016/07/test-no-489-in-vivo-mammalian-alkaline-comet-assay_g1g6fb2c.html

designed to evaluate several genotoxic endpoints, including mutagenicity, as well as clastogenicity and aneugenicity [26, 76, 106, 131, 166–169].

The main principles of the most commonly used genotoxicity assays listed in Table 18.1 are briefly summarized below:

A. *In vitro* assays:

- *The bacterial reverse mutation assay (Ames test)* evaluates the ability of a test substance to induce mutations in bacterial strains, *Salmonella typhimurium* (*S. typhimurium*) and *Escherichia coli (E. coli)*, which lack the ability to synthesize histidine or tryptophan, respectively. Mutations induced by a genotoxic substance allow the bacteria to regain its ability to grow in histidine- or tryptophan-deficient media. The test is required to be performed in at least five specific tester strains, including *S. typhimurium TA98*, *TA100*, *TA1537*, *TA102*, *TA7/TA97a*, and *E. coli* WP2*uvrA* or WP2*uvrA*/pKM101, each covering a wide range of mutational events and showing specificity to mutagens that cause base-pair substitutions or frame-shift mutations.
- *Mammalian cell (HPRT/XPRT) gene mutation assay* examines gene mutations at specific loci, hypoxanthine phosphoribosyl transferase (HPRT) and xanthine phosphoribosyl transferase (XPRT) genes, in mammalian cells. Cells with HPRT mutations acquire resistance to the effects of cytotoxic agents (e.g., 6-thioguanine). Since HPRT gene is located on the X-chromosome, only cells with one functional X-chromosome are used for the assay (e.g., cell lines derived from male Chinese hamsters).
- *Mouse lymphoma assay (MLA)* assesses point mutations and chromosomal aberrations at the thymidine kinase (TK) gene locus in L5178Y mouse lymphoma cells. Mutant cells lose sensitivity to the cytotoxicity of trifluorothymidine and continue to grow in a selective medium. The size of the mutant colony can indicate which type of genetic damage occurred. Large colony mutants usually possess small base changes (i.e., point mutations), while small colony mutants harbor large chromosomal mutations or rearrangements.

B. *In vivo* assays:

- *Mammalian erythrocyte Pig-A gene mutation assay* detects gene mutations in the Pig-A gene, which is located on the X-chromosome and encodes a protein involved in glycosylphosphatidylinositol (GPI) anchor synthesis. Functional mutations in this gene lead to the loss of GPI-anchored proteins (e.g., CD59), which can be detected by flow cytometry.
- *Transgenic rodent (TGR) gene mutation assay* evaluates chemical-induced gene mutations in various tissues of transgenic rodents carrying a bacterial reporter gene (e.g., lacZ or cII) that acts as a mutational target. Upon cessation of dosing, the shuttle vector is recovered and introduced into a bacterial host (e.g. *E. coli*). Mutation frequency is then scored by analyzing formation of the mutant colonies in a selective medium.
- *Rodent dominant lethal (DL) test* assesses genotoxic potential of a chemical in sperm cells of male rodents across different stages of germ cell develop-

ment. DL effects are primarily associated with chromosomal damage, although mutagenic events cannot be excluded. Heritable DL mutations manifest as an increase in early embryonic or fetal mortality or a reduction in the rate of successful implantations.

C. *In vitro/in vivo* assays:

- *Chromosomal aberration (CA) assay* detects structural chromosomal abnormalities in cultured mammalian cells or in the bone marrow of rodents following exposure to a test substance. Cells are examined microscopically for breaks, deletions, or rearrangements of chromosomes.
- *MN assay* measures the induction of MN formation in nucleated cells (primarily lymphocyte cell cultures or bone marrow tissue), which is indicative of either chromosome breakage (clastogenicity) or interference with the mitotic spindle (aneugenicity).
- *Alkaline comet (single-cell gel electrophoresis) assay* detects DNA single-strand breaks by measuring DNA migration patterns in cells subjected to electrophoresis under alkaline conditions. Any cell or tissue type can be used in this assay.

Since the majority of DNA-reactive chemicals require metabolic activation to become genotoxic [31, 85], *in vitro* tests are required to be performed in the absence and presence of metabolic activation [93]. Metabolic competence is usually achieved by the addition of the rat-or hamster-induced liver S9 fraction or microsomes.

The extent of testing is determined by the intended use of a material (e.g., pharmaceuticals, cosmetic ingredients, food additives) and its annual production or import volume (tonnage). In some cases, for example, with flavor and fragrance materials [4], the prediction of chemical hazard and determination of the priority for testing is done using a data-driven approach (*read-across*) or *in silico* computationally-driven predictive models (e.g., Quantitative Structure-Activity Relationship (QSAR) models) [1, 147]. These models detect the presence of structural alerts predictive of genotoxic potential by comparing the compound of interest to structurally similar substances with available toxicity data.

Chemicals are then tested in the *in vitro* genotoxicity battery with and without metabolic activation. Usually, two tests, which include the detection of mutagenicity in the Ames assay and clastogenicity/aneugenicity in the MN or CA assays using mammalian cells (Table 18.1), are recommended [76]. Most compounds that yielded positive results *in vitro* should be further evaluated for the positive endpoints in the higher tier *in vivo* assays [106, 131, 166, 167]. However, due to ethical concerns regarding animal testing, *in vivo* follow-up studies for cosmetic ingredients are prohibited within the European Union (EU) and Canada [37, 51]. Hence, regulatory decisions for this group of compounds are often based on the *in vitro* data alone.

While *in vitro* tests have high sensitivity when predicting *in vivo* genotoxicity and carcinogenicity outcomes, their specificity, or ability to predict negative outcomes *in vivo*, is rather low [26, 43, 74–77, 120, 158]. False positive outcomes *in vitro* can often result from high doses of chemicals used in these assays, which are not relevant to actual human intakes, or from limited detoxification capabilities due to a lack of phase II metabolizing enzymes in the exogenous liver subcellular preparations for bioactivation (S9). Limitations of the *in vitro* battery are recognized by the regulatory bodies; however, their recommendations are targeted towards improving the assay protocols and better interpretation of the outcomes, rather than replacing the existing testing strategy [36].

While *in vivo* tests are designed to reduce false positive outcomes, they still maintain a certain level of uncertainty [107, 152, 153]. Since no single assay can simultaneously assess all of the genotoxic endpoints, several assays should be conducted in combination to improve the sensitivity of the *in vivo* battery [134, 173]. Various test guideline programs and organizations such as the Organization for Economic Co-operation and Development (OECD) (https://www.oecd.org/en.html), the International Programme on Chemical Safety (IPCS) (https://www.inchem.org/#/), the International Conference on Harmonisation of Chemicals (ICH) (https://www.ich.org/), and the EU's Registration, Evaluation, Authorization and Restriction of Chemicals (REACH) (https://www.trade.gov/eu-reach), have detailed standard approaches for genotoxicity testing to minimize the artifacts and evaluate potential alternative models.

The Interpretation of Outcomes in Genotoxicity Assays

The evaluation of outcomes of regulatory genotoxicity assays is often dichotomous, i.e., positive or negative; however, the interpretation of results can be challenging and requires expert knowledge [98, 106]. The major challenge is often the lack of consensus between the outcomes in various assays for a single material. In addition, the endpoints assessed in the regulatory battery do not include testing for mechanisms other than direct DNA damage and mutagenicity, which limits early detection of chemical carcinogens with a non-genotoxic or epigenetic mode of action.

Compounds that yield negative results in the testing battery are considered non-genotoxic, although the absence of genotoxicity does not necessarily imply the lack of carcinogenicity [82, 85]. Negative genotoxicity findings *in vitro* for compounds with low production volumes (i.e., less than 100 tons per year) are considered sufficient to ensure a lack of genotoxic risk, and thereby, these materials do not require further testing *in vivo*. Studies with equivocal outcomes should be repeated. Compounds that yielded positive results are assumed to be potentially mutagenic and/or carcinogenic in humans. Positive outcomes in a genotoxicity testing battery can be a basis for restricted use or prohibition of a chemical. Nevertheless, positive outcomes in one or more assays can be addressed using several approaches [33, 106]. The weight of evidence (WoE) approach can be used to suggest a lack of genotoxic hazard by evaluating the biological relevance of the available data. Positive results can also be satisfactorily explained by the mechanism of action of a chemical. Additional testing that can contribute to the WoE or mechanism of action clarification can also be conducted.

Many efforts have been made to design a more insightful approach to chemical hazard assessment and risk characterization. Application of principles such as the

Threshold of Toxicological Concern (TTC) [15, 92, 172] or Margin of Exposure (MoE) and Margin of Safety (MoS) [10, 73] enhances scientifically informed and refined risk assessment that is more relevant to human exposures. The TTC approach can be applied to chemicals with known chemical structures but which lack comprehensive toxicological data and are expected to have minimal human exposure [61, 172]. Threshold values are typically based on experimental data on both cancer and non-cancer toxicity endpoints and represent the maximum level of exposure to a substance below which no significant adverse effects on human health are expected. MoE and MoS represent the ratio between the experimentally derived no-observed-adverse-effect level or benchmark dose and the predicted or estimated human exposure level to an ingredient. These concepts are particularly applicable to substances for which no health-based guidance values can be established (e.g., genotoxic carcinogens).

Advances in the understanding of the process of tumor development have identified alternative endpoints that can be investigated as part of safety assessment [44, 45, 80].

New Approach Methodologies (NAMs)

The growing focus on the principles of replacement, reduction, and refinement (i.e., the 3Rs) of animal research has stimulated the development of non-animal models and new approach methodologies (NAMs), in particular for the safety assessment of cosmetic products [6, 30, 118, 120–122, 141]. Three-dimensional (3D) cell culture models, such as organotypic models (organoids) and spheroids, show the most promise [9, 62, 122, 123, 130]. Compared to two-dimensional (2D) monolayer cell cultures, 3D models more accurately resemble intact organs and represent a physiologically relevant approach with relevant exposure sites for many chemicals. Reconstructed human skin consists of a multilayered, fully differentiated human epidermis, and as such, can be used to assess toxic effects and transdermal absorption of compounds administered mainly by the dermal route, e.g., topical ointments and cosmetics [112, 122]. Hence, the use of MN or comet assays in the reconstructed skin models has been validated for cosmetic ingredients [121–123]. Moreover, human reconstructed skin has been shown to possess an inherent complement of phase I and II enzymes [161].

The avian egg-based (*in ovo*) models, including the Chicken and Turkey Egg Genotoxicity Assays (CEGA and TEGA), were developed as screening NAMs to potentially replace *in vivo* genotoxicity assays for chemicals that are positive *in vitro* [83, 84, 86–88, 150, 166, 167]. Both models utilize metabolically competent avian fetal livers to evaluate endpoints indicative of nuclear DNA damage, including the formation of DNA adducts and single-strand breaks. Another *in ovo* model, the Hen Egg Micronucleus assay, has been successfully utilized to assess chemically-induced formation of MNs in the red blood cells of chicken embryos [133, 170, 171]. Overall, *in ovo* models demonstrated reasonably high reliability

Table 18.2 Summary of alternative techniques and New Approach Methodologies (NAMs) for genotoxicity testing

Endpoint	Example of technique/assay
DNA damage and repair, genomic instability	Hepatocyte DNA damage assay Unscheduled DNA synthesis (UDS) assay Host cell reactivation (HCR) assay The excision assay Enzyme-linked immunosorbent assay (ELISA) Spectral karyotyping (SKY), karyotyping Single-cell or Next generation sequencing Error-corrected next generation sequencing (e.g., Duplex sequencing)
Direct DNA binding	Nucleotide ^{32}P-postlabeling (NPL) assay Immunoassay/immunohistochemistry (IHC)-based assays Gas or liquid chromatography/mass spectrometry (GC/MS or LC/MS)-based assays
Short-term genotoxicity	Green Screen® and Gadd45-Gluc BlueScreen HC reporter gene assays 3D skin model (comet and micronucleus assay) MiniAmes assay γH2AX phosphorylation reporter assay ToxTracker® assay MicroFlow® and MultiFlow® assays CometChip® assay Chicken or Turkey egg genotoxicity assay Hen egg micronucleus assay

in detecting the genotoxic potential of chemicals. An avian embryo is a complex, intact, non-animal organism with genetic and morphologic resemblance to mammals. Hence, other endpoints, including histopathology and genomic profiling, can be evaluated.

A variety of techniques can also be used to investigate the ability of a chemical to induce direct DNA damage and repair (Table 18.2), providing critical insights into its genotoxic potential. These methods include traditional assays as well as advanced molecular techniques. The integration of high-throughput "-omics" approaches (e.g., transcriptomics, proteomics, metabolomics), in addition to facilitating hazard identification, also allows for potential elucidation of MoAs, which is of particular value for data-poor compounds [14, 41, 101].

Regulatory Framework and Guidelines for CPCPs

The global revenue from the cosmetics market in 2023 was estimated at 295.95 billion US dollars [52]. With a projected 6% annual growth by 2030, the cosmetics industry is facing increasing regulatory attention. Each major market has a set of regulatory frameworks and legislations (Table 18.3 and Fig. 18.2) that aims to ensure the safety, efficacy, and quality of products.

Table 18.3 CPCPs regulations in selected major markets.

Country/region	Regulatory authority	Legislation
European Union (EU)	European Commission (EC) Scientific Committee on Consumer Safety (SCCS)	Cosmetic Regulation (EC) No. 1223/2009 Regulation (EC) No 1907/2006 for Registration, Evaluation, Authorisation and Restriction of Chemicals (REACH)
United States (US)	US Food and Drug Administration (US FDA)	US Federal Food, Drug, and Cosmetics (FD&C) Act US FDA Code of Federal Regulations (CFR) Title 21 Modernization of Cosmetics Regulation Act of 2022 (MoCRA) Fair Packaging and Labelling Act (FPLA)
Canada	Health Canada	Food and Drugs (F&D) Act Cosmetic Regulations (C.R.C., c.869) Canadian Environmental Cosmetic Act (CEPA) Consumer Packaging and Labelling Act (CPLA)
China	National Medical Products Administration (NMPA) State Administration for Market Regulation (SAMR)	Cosmetics Supervision and Administration Regulations (CSAR) Administrative Measures on Cosmetics Labelling
South Korea	Ministry of Food & Drug Safety (MFDS)	Cosmetics Act Enforcement Decree of the Cosmetics Act Enforcement Rule of the Cosmetics Act
India	Ministry of Health and Family Welfare's Central Drugs Standard Control Organization (CDSCO) Bureau of Indian Standards (BIS)	Drugs and Cosmetics Act of 1940 Cosmetic Rules of 2020 BIS Labelling Declarations
Association of Southeast Asian Nations (ASEAN)[a]	National Regulatory Authorities (NRA) of member states	ASEAN Cosmetic Directive (ACD)
Japan	Ministry of Health, Labor and Welfare's (MHLW) Pharmaceutical and Medical Devices Agency	Pharmaceutical and Medical Devices (PMD) Act
Australia	Australian Industrial Chemicals Introduction Scheme (AICIS) Australian Competition and Consumer Commission (ACCC) Therapeutic Goods Administration (TGA)	Industrial Chemicals Act 2019 Consumer Goods (Cosmetics) Information Standard 2020

(continued)

Table 18.3 (continued)

Country/region	Regulatory authority	Legislation
New Zealand	Environmental Protection Authority (EPA)	Cosmetic Products Group Standard Medicines Act 1981 Hazardous Substances and New Organisms (HSNO) Act 1996
Brazil	Brazilian Health Regulatory Agency (ANVISA)	Collegiate Board Resolution (RDC) 907/2024 RDC 894/2024 RDC 752/2022 RDC 806/2023

Notes: [a]ASEAN includes 10 member countries: Brunei Darussalam, Cambodia, Indonesia, Malaysia, Myanmar, Lao PDR, Philippines, Singapore, Thailand, and Vietnam

Fig. 18.2 QR codes for assessing web pages with major cosmetic legislations worldwide

Internet sites that host relevant policies can be accessed using the QR codes provided in Fig. 18.2.

Regulations and requirements of CPCPs usually depend upon the activity of ingredients and product claims. Thus, products applied for cleaning, beautifying, or altering appearance, which do not permanently affect the physical structure or physiological functions of the body, are classified as CPCPs. In contrast, products that make claims related to disease prevention or treatment can be designated as over-the-counter (OTC) drugs, dietary supplements, natural health products (NHPs), or prescription drugs [39, 63, 115]. The distinction between these categories is not always clear, and certain products (e.g., anti-dandruff shampoo or fluoride toothpaste) may be classified by some regulations as both, CPCP and OTC medicine. Moreover, a particular product might be categorized differently in some countries. For example, sunscreens are classified as cosmetics in the EU, Brazil, Japan, and China, while in the US and Canada, they are regulated respectively as OTC drugs or NHPs [39].

Focusing on the three largest markets for cosmetics, North Asia (China), North America (US and Canada), and Europe (EU), each region has a different set of standards and guidelines for manufacturing, marketing, and sales of CPCPs ranging from ingredient approval and animal testing policies to pre-market assessments and claims substantiation (Tables 18.3 and 18.4) [39, 63]. Nevertheless, their common goal is to ensure that the products introduced to consumers are safe and their ingredients fall within the safe usage limits.

Depending on the region, obtaining pre-market approval for CPCPs is usually not required (Table 18.4). In contrast, the fundamental process for safety verification remains consistent worldwide. While the regulatory agencies monitor compliance with the regulatory standards, manufacturers are ultimately responsible for ensuring their products and ingredients are safe for consumers [63]. The safety of CPCPs is maintained through several strategies, including using ingredients with an established safe use, adhering to good manufacturing practices (GMP), regularly testing ingredients for potential risks, and offering consumers clear guidance on proper use to maintain safe exposure levels.

The steady growth and innovation of the cosmetics sector and consumer demands for "clean" and sustainable products drive many regulatory changes. For example, the US Food and Drug Administration (FDA) has amended the Federal Food, Drug, and Cosmetic (FD&C) Act of 1938 with the Modernization of Cosmetics Regulation Act of 2022 (MoCRA) (https://www.fda.gov/cosmetics/cosmetics-laws-regulations/modernization-cosmetics-regulation-act-2022-mocra), which grants the FDA a more extensive oversight of cosmetics manufacturers and processors. Thus, while in the past, the FDA relied primarily on voluntary compliance, with limited pre-market approval, new provisions require mandatory facility and product registration for all cosmetics manufacturers, regardless of their location, as well as adequate safety substantiations prior to a product being sold in the US.

Canada follows a similar regulatory structure through Health Canada under the Food and Drugs Act, with the Cosmetic Regulations establishing requirements for safety, ingredient disclosure, and labeling. Health Canada also conducts some pre-market assessments, particularly for products making certain claims.

The National Medical Products Administration (NMPA) is in charge of overseeing China's cosmetics regulations. According to NMPA regulations, cosmetics must comply with rigorous safety assessments and stringent ingredient regulations. Products are also subject to registration before they can be marketed in China.

The EU has one of the most stringent cosmetic regulatory frameworks, governed by Regulation (EC) No 1223/2009. This regulation ensures that all cosmetics products placed on the EU market are safe for human health, with specific requirements for product safety assessments, good manufacturing practices, and labeling. Importantly, the EU implemented a comprehensive ban on the sale of cosmetics and

Table 18.4 Regulations and Safety Testing Approaches to CPCPs in the EU, US, Canada, and China

Regulation	US	Canada	EU	China
Pre-market approval	Not required, unless specific products or claims	Not required	Not required	Mandatory only for certain, mainly imported, products
Notification of products	Product listing required by the Modernization of Cosmetics Regulation Act of 2022 (MoCRA)	Required Cosmetic Notification Form (CNF)	Required through the Cosmetic Products Notification Portal (CPNP)	Registration for special-use products; notification for general cosmetics
Data on product safety and efficacy	Safety must be assessed	Safety must be assessed	Safety must be assessed by a qualified safety assessor, provided in the Cosmetic Product Safety Report (CPSR) and Product Information File (PIF)	Product dossier provided to authorities
Testing requirements	No formal requirements	No formal requirements	Scientific Committee on Consumer Safety (SCCS) guidelines	National Medical Products Administration (NMPA) guidelines
Animal testing	Allowed, not mandatory	Banned for most cosmetics since 2023	Banned for cosmetics since 2013	Required for most imported cosmetic products
Responsible party for product safety	Manufacturer	Manufacturer	Manufacturer	Manufacturer
Adherence to Good Manufacturing Practice (GMP)	Required under MoCRA	Not required but encouraged	Mandatory	Mandatory
Labeling and packaging requirements	Must include product name, ingredients, and specific claims	Must include product name, ingredients, and specific claims	Must include product name, ingredients, and specific claims	Must include product name, ingredients, and specific claims
List of banned ingredients	11 ingredients in Prohibited & Restricted Ingredients in Cosmetics	573 ingredients in the Cosmetic Ingredient Hotlist,	1722 ingredients in Annex II Cosmetic Regulation (EC) No 1223/2009	Hygienic Standard for Cosmetics, over 1200 ingredients

(continued)

Table 18.4 (continued)

Regulation	US	Canada	EU	China
Positive list	Color additives	N/A	Colorants, UV filters, preservatives	Colorants, hair dyes, UV filters, preservatives
Adverse event reporting	Required for serious adverse events	Required for serious adverse events	Required for serious adverse events	Required for serious adverse events
Post-market surveillance	US Food and Drug Administration (FDA)	Health Canada	Platform of European market surveillance authorities for cosmetics (PEMSAC)	NMPA

cosmetic ingredients that were tested in animal safety studies. Additionally, the EU requires a Cosmetic Product Safety Report (CPSR) for each product, which includes a detailed evaluation of the product's safety based on its ingredients, formulation, and intended use.

As the global cosmetic market becomes more interconnected, companies face difficulties in complying with multiple, sometimes conflicting, standards across different countries. Several international organizations, including the OECD (https://www.oecd.org/en/about.html), the International Cooperation on Cosmetics Regulation (ICCR) (https://www.iccr-cosmetics.org/about-us), and the International Organization for Standardization (ISO) (https://www.iso.org/committee/54974.html), have been formed to streamline development of harmonized standards and guidelines for the cosmetics industry [39]. In addition to regulatory bodies, voluntary expert committees have been established via industry or government support to advise on the safety of ingredients and standards. These include Expert Panels of the Cosmetic Ingredient Review (CIR) (https://www.cir-safety.org/), the Research Institute for Fragrance Materials (RIFM) (https://rifm.org/), the Flavor Extract Manufacturers Association (FEMA) (https://www.femaflavor.org/), and the Scientific Committee on Consumer Safety (SCCS) (https://health.ec.europa.eu/scientific-committees/scientific-committee-consumer-safety-sccs_en), [63].

Cosmetic Ingredients of Concern

Most legislations provide strict control over the inclusion of ingredients with hazard properties (i.e., *chemicals of concern*) in CPCP formulations (Table 18.4). For example, Annex II (https://ec.europa.eu/growth/tools-databases/cosing/reference/annexes/list/II) of the European Cosmetic Regulation 1223/2009 [24] currently lists over 1700 chemicals that are prohibited from use in CPCPs. Many of these substances are contaminants, including polyaromatic hydrocarbons and mercury compounds. However, the list also features ingredients that can be hazardous but are considered safe when used in appropriate concentrations, including preservatives such as chlorhexidine and formaldehyde precursors. Annex III (https://ec.europa.eu/growth/tools-databases/cosing/reference/annexes/list/III) lists close to 400 restricted substances that can only be used under specified conditions or applications set out in the legislation. Annex XVII of Regulation (EU) No 1907/2006 (REACH) (https://echa.europa.eu/documents/10162/3bfef8a3-8c97-4d85-ae0b-ac6827de49a9) also prohibits the marketing of the genotoxic chemicals, either as a single compound or in a mixture, to the general public. However, in certain cases, exceptions may apply.

In the US, in addition to sunscreens in cosmetics, the FDA prohibits 10 substances or chemical classes based on identified safety concerns [155]. These include bithional, chlorofluorocarbon propellants, chloroform, halogenated salicylanilides (di-, tri-, metabromsalan and tetrachlorosalicylanilide), hexachlorophene, mercury compounds, methylene chloride, prohibited cattle materials, vinyl chloride, and zirconium-containing complexes. For some ingredients with special functions (colorant, preservative, or UV filter), manufacturers can only use permitted ingredients that are listed on *'positive lists'* (Table 18.4). Moreover, several states, including California, New York, and Washington, passed legislations that either limit or prohibit manufacturing or distribution of cosmetics that contain some of the specific ingredients of concern on a state level [18, 111, 159] (chart-state-laws-banning-the-use-of-ingredients-in-cosmetic-products.pdf).

Historic Perspectives

Prior to the implementation of the FD&C Act by the US Congress in 1938 [143], the cosmetics industry lacked any formal regulatory framework. Accordingly, manufacturers were not required to ensure the safety of their marketed product(s). Such absence of oversight allowed several CPCPs with harmful properties to enter the market, resulting in severe adverse health effects among consumers. Several notable examples of dangerous products that played a major role in driving regulatory actions are discussed below.

Koremlu was marketed as a cream for the permanent removal of facial hair. In the late 1920s, many Koremlu consumers suffered severe side effects ranging from the loss of body hair and baldness to paralysis and optic nerve damage [53, 71]. These effects were primarily attributed to thallium acetate (Fig. 18.3), an active ingredient in Koremlu [53], which was also commonly used as a rodenticide [47]. The legal actions brought against the manufacturing company in 1932 ultimately led to its bankruptcy, resulting in the product's removal from the market. Due to its toxicity, thallium acetate has been banned for use as a pesticide in the US since 1970, although thallium compounds are still used in various industrial applications [154].

Lash Lure was manufactured in 1933 as a mascara and eyebrow dye. In many users, it caused severe allergic reactions, including dermatitis and vesicular rash of the eyelids and surrounding skin, as well as keratitis, corneal ulceration, and necrosis

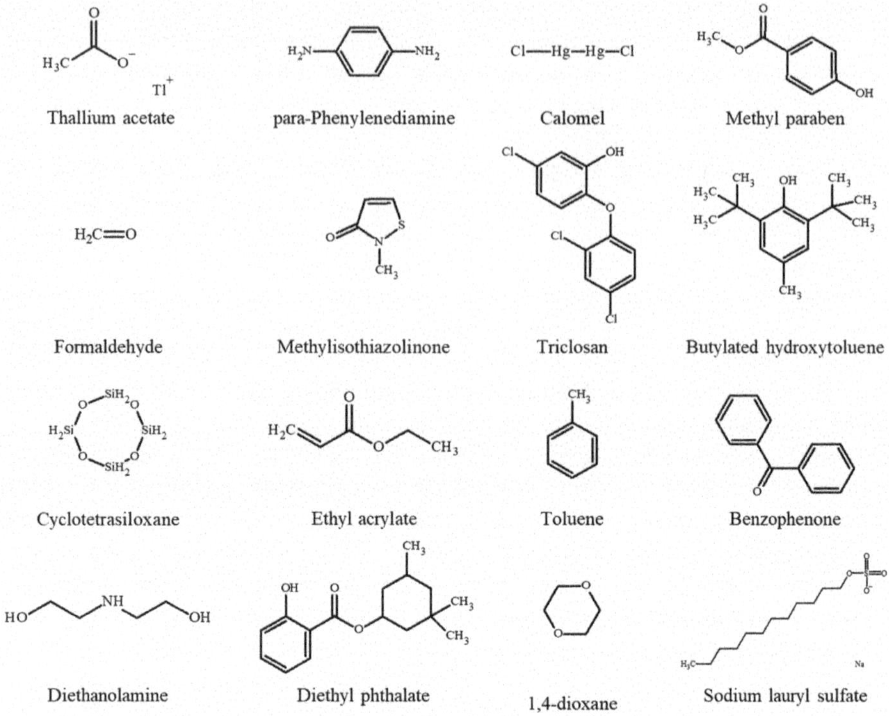

Fig. 18.3 Chemical structure of selected compounds of concern in CPCPs

[54, 70, 71, 104]. One documented fatality occurred in a woman who, shortly after applying Lash Lure to a recently plucked eyebrow, developed severe dermatitis with ulceration of the eyelid and palpebral conjunctiva [40]. She passed away within 48 hours, presumably due to a secondary bacterial infection. Acute toxicity of Lash Lure was attributed to an aniline derivative, para-phenylenediamine (PPD) (Fig. 18.3), which is an established contact allergen [109, 148, 156]. Lash Lure became the first CPCP to be withdrawn from the market following the passage of the FD&C Act [71]. Presently, PPD is the most common component of many hair dyes [151].

Gouraud's Oriental Cream, for several decades, was marketed as a popular anti-blemish product. However, its prolonged use was associated with symptoms of mercury poisoning, including bluish discoloration of the gums and loss of teeth. These adverse effects were attributed to the primary constituent of Gouraud's Cream, calomel (i.e., mercury chloride) (Fig. 18.3) [27]. In response to health concerns, the formulation of the cream was modified in 1936 to remove calomel from the product. Presently, certain skin-lightening creams (mainly imported or sold online) may contain inorganic mercury salts at concentrations above 1000 ppm [25, 105].

Ruth deForest Lamb, the first Chief Educational Officer at the US FDA, was instrumental in the passage of the FD&C Act. Her 1936 book "American Chamber of Horrors: the truth about food and drugs" brought public awareness to the issues of dangerous marketed products, which, at the time, were not regulated by the FDA. Prompted by growing public concern, the enactment of the FD&C Act granted the FDA the authority to oversee and regulate the production, sale, and distribution of cosmetics alongside food, drugs, and medical devices. Over the years, the Act was amended to address issues pertaining to labeling, safety testing, and post-marketing surveillance. The most comprehensive update to cosmetic regulation was the implementation of MocRA in 2022, which introduced stricter requirements for CPCPs' safety and manufacturing practices to enhance consumer protection.

Current Issues

Due to strict regulations and safety standards, most chemicals in CPCPs are generally regarded as safe. Nevertheless, potential adverse effects associated with exposure to certain ingredients and contaminants raise concerns among consumers. Common examples include preservatives (e.g., parabens, formaldehyde and formaldehyde-releasing compounds, methylisothiazolinone and methylchloroisothiazolinone, triclosan); stabilizers (e.g., butylated hydroxyanisole and butylated hydroxytoluene); polymers (e.g., siloxanes, acrylates); hair dyes and synthetic colors (e.g., toluene, polycyclic aromatic hydrocarbons); UV filters in sunscreens (e.g., benzophenone, homosalate); ethanolamines (e.g., diethanolamine); petroleum-derived ingredients (e.g., petrolatum); phthalates (e.g., diethyl phthalate, dibutyl phthalate); byproducts (e.g., 1,4-dioxane); emulsifiers (sodium lauryl sulfate and sodium laureth sulfate); heavy metals (e.g., lead); inorganic minerals (e.g., mica and asbestos) (Fig. 18.3). These compounds, albeit primarily under experimental conditions, have been linked to various effects ranging from acute reactions (e.g., irritation, allergic reactions) to chronic conditions (e.g., cancer, endocrine disruption, and reproductive toxicity) [5, 115, 135]. The relevance of these findings to human risk should be interpreted with caution, considering levels and frequency of exposure as well as route of administration, etc.

Growing public appeal of natural and/or organic products results in high demand for plant-based CPCPs. Botanical products are often perceived as safe due to a long history of use, although such claims can be misleading. Botanicals are complex mixtures composed of various ingredients, for which interactions and safety data are not always available. Additionally, different batches of a particular plant-derived product may have different compositions depending on various factors, including the part of the plant used to prepare the extract, location, climate, cultivation, and harvest environment, as well as manufacturing conditions, including extraction and purification which can introduce hazardous contaminants such as heavy metals [115, 142, 169]. Certain plant-derived ingredients can produce adverse reactions in the skin, including phototoxicity observed with St. John's Wort extract [162] or allergic contact dermatitis associated with the use of certain essential oils [29, 132], highlighting the potential risks when used in cosmetics.

The rise of e-commerce platforms and online promotions introduces additional regulatory challenges. Manufacturers are still expected to adhere to regulations and requirements specific to their product and target market(s) when selling online. Nevertheless, an abundance of CPCPs available on the digital market makes it increasingly difficult for authorities to monitor and enforce compliance with these regulations. This, in turn, increases the risk of counterfeit, adulterated, or misbranded products reaching consumers.

Conclusions

Genotoxicity, which arises from alterations to the physical and/or chemical structure of DNA, is associated with various adverse outcomes, including mutagenicity and carcinogenicity. Understanding the mechanisms underlying DNA-reactivity, their relevance to carcinogenesis, and factors that influence genotoxic potential provides critical insight into the potential risks posed by CPCPs and their ingredients to consumers. Standard genotoxicity assays, alongside emerging NAMs, offer useful tools for detecting, evaluating, and characterizing genotoxic risk. However, the interpretation of genotoxicity assay outcomes requires careful consideration, particularly regarding human relevance. Thus, integrated approaches such as WoE are crucial for a more informed hazard assessment process. Rigorous safety assessments and regulatory guidelines promote consumer safety by ensuring that products on the market meet established safety standards. Nevertheless, some challenges and concerns regarding CPCPs safety remain.

Questions

1. What are the key mechanisms by which chemicals can induce genotoxic effects? How does genotoxicity relate to carcinogenicity?
2. Which factors might play a role in determining the genotoxic potential of cosmetic ingredients? How?
3. What are the commonly accepted genotoxicity assays, and what type of genetic damage do they assess? Which challenges are pertinent to the safety assessment of CPCPs?
4. Which regulatory agencies oversee cosmetics in major markets, and how do their approaches differ (e.g., EU vs US vs China)?
5. What are some examples of cosmetic ingredients of concern? Why?

References

1. Alexander-White C, Bury D, Cronin M, Dent M, Hack E, Hewitt NJ, Kenna G, Naciff J, Ouedraogo G, Schepky A, Mahony C, Europe C. A 10-step framework for use of read-across (RAX) in next generation risk assessment (NGRA) for cosmetics safety assessment. Regul Toxicol Pharmacol. 2022;129:105094. https://doi.org/10.1016/j.yrtph.2021.105094.

2. Alonso-Gonzalez A, Rodriguez-Fontenla C, Carracedo A. *De novo* mutations (DNMS) in autism spectrum disorder (ASD): pathway and network analysis. Front Genet. 2018;9:406. https://doi.org/10.3389/fgene.2018.00406.
3. Ames BN. Endogenous DNA damage as related to cancer and aging. Mutat Res. 1989;214(1):41–6. https://doi.org/10.1016/0027-5107(89)90196-6.
4. Api AM, Belsito D, Bruze M, Cadby P, Calow P, Dagli ML, Dekant W, Ellis G, Fryer AD, Fukayama M, Griem P, Hickey C, Kromidas L, Lalko JF, Liebler DC, Miyachi Y, Politano VT, Renskers K, Ritacco G, Wilcox DK. Criteria for the Research Institute for Fragrance Materials, Inc. (RIFM) safety evaluation process for fragrance ingredients. Food Chem Toxicol. 2015;82:S1–S19. https://doi.org/10.1016/j.fct.2014.11.014.
5. Balwierz R, Biernat P, Jasińska-Balwierz A, Siodłak D, Kusakiewicz-Dawid A, Kurek-Górecka A, Olczyk P, Ochędzan-Siodłak W. Potential carcinogens in makeup cosmetics. Int J Environ Res Public Health. 2023;20(6) https://doi.org/10.3390/ijerph20064780.
6. Barthe M, Bavoux C, Finot F, Mouche I, Cuceu-Petrenci C, Forreryd A, Chérouvrier Hansson A, Johansson H, Lemkine GF, Thénot J-P, Osman-Ponchet H. Safety testing of cosmetic products: overview of established methods and new approach methodologies (NAMs). Cosmetics. 2021;8(2):50. https://www.mdpi.com/2079-9284/8/2/50
7. Basu AK. DNA damage, mutagenesis and cancer [Review]. Int J Mol Sci. 2018;19(4).
8. Beland FA, Kadlubar FF. Formation and persistence of arylamine DNA adducts in vivo. Environ Health Perspect. 1985;62:19–30. https://doi.org/10.1289/ehp.856219.
9. Bell CC, Hendriks DFG, Moro SML, Ellis E, Walsh J, Renblom A, Fredriksson Puigvert L, Dankers ACA, Jacobs F, Snoeys J, Sison-Young RL, Jenkins RE, Nordling Å, Mkrtchian S, Park BK, Kitteringham NR, Goldring CEP, Lauschke VM, Ingelman-Sundberg M. Characterization of primary human hepatocyte spheroids as a model system for drug-induced liver injury, liver function and disease. Sci Rep. 2016;6:25187. https://doi.org/10.1038/srep25187.
10. Benford D, Bolger PM, Carthew P, Coulet M, DiNovi M, Leblanc J-C, Renwick AG, Setzer W, Schlatter J, Smith B, Slob W, Williams G, Wildemann T. Application of the Margin of Exposure (MOE) approach to substances in food that are genotoxic and carcinogenic. Food Chem Toxicol. 2010;48:S2–S24. https://doi.org/10.1016/j.fct.2009.11.003.
11. Bevan RJ, Harrison PTC. Threshold and non-threshold chemical carcinogens: a survey of the present regulatory landscape. Regul Toxicol Pharmacol. 2017;88:291–302. https://doi.org/10.1016/j.yrtph.2017.01.003.
12. Bos JD, Meinardi MM. The 500 Dalton rule for the skin penetration of chemical compounds and drugs. Exp Dermatol. 2000;9(3):165–9. https://doi.org/10.1034/j.1600-0625.2000.009003165.x.
13. Bradley MO. Cytotoxicity as a mechanism of carcinogenesis. Basic Life Sci. 1985;34:99–109. https://doi.org/10.1007/978-1-4684-4976-1_9.
14. Buick JK, Williams A, Meier MJ, Swartz CD, Recio L, Gagné R, Ferguson SS, Engelward BP, Yauk CL. A modern genotoxicity testing paradigm: Integration of the high-throughput CometChip® and the TGx-DDI transcriptomic biomarker in human HepaRG™ cell cultures. Front Public Health. 2021;9:694834. https://doi.org/10.3389/fpubh.2021.694834.
15. Bury D, Head J, Keller D, Klaric M, Rose J. The Threshold of Toxicological Concern (TTC) is a pragmatic tool for the safety assessment: Case studies of cosmetic ingredients with low consumer exposure. Regul Toxicol Pharmacol. 2021;123:104964. https://doi.org/10.1016/j.yrtph.2021.104964.
16. Byrd AL, Belkaid Y, Segre JA. The human skin microbiome. Nat Rev Microbiol. 2018;16(3):143–55. https://doi.org/10.1038/nrmicro.2017.157.
17. Cai Q, Wei H. In vivo formation of DNA-adducts in mouse skin DNA by tamoxifen. Cancer Lett. 1995;92(2):187–92. https://doi.org/10.1016/0304-3835(95)03802-4.
18. California Legislature. Assembly Bill (AB) No. 496. Cosmetic safety. 2023. Retrieved from https://legiscan.com/CA/text/AB496/id/2686857/California-2023-AB496-Introduced.html

19. Chatterjee N, Walker GC. Mechanisms of DNA damage, repair, and mutagenesis. Environ Mol Mutagen. 2017;58(5):235–63. https://doi.org/10.1002/em.22087.
20. Chen YE, Tsao H. The skin microbiome: current perspectives and future challenges. J Am Acad Dermatol. 2013;69(1):143–55. https://doi.org/10.1016/j.jaad.2013.01.016.
21. Claussnitzer M, Cho JH, Collins R, Cox NJ, Dermitzakis ET, Hurles ME, Kathiresan S, Kenny EE, Lindgren CM, MacArthur DG, North KN, Plon SE, Rehm HL, Risch N, Rotimi CN, Shendure J, Soranzo N, McCarthy MI. A brief history of human disease genetics. Nature. 2020;577(7789):179–89. https://doi.org/10.1038/s41586-019-1879-7.
22. Cohen SM. Cell proliferation and carcinogenesis: an approach to screening for potential human carcinogens. Front Oncol. 2024;14:1394584. https://doi.org/10.3389/fonc.2024.1394584.
23. Cohen SM, Ellwein LB. Cell growth dynamics and DNA alterations in carcinogenesis. In: Scientific issues in quantitative cancer risk assessment. Boston: Birkhäuser; 1990. p. 116–35.
24. Commission Regulation, (EU). Restricted Substances: Annex III, Regulation 1223/2009/EC on Cosmetic Products, as amended by Regulation (EU) 2020/1683, 13 November 2020. 2020. Retrieved April 1 from https://echa.europa.eu/lv/cosmetics-restricted-substances
25. Copan L, Fowles J, Barreau T, McGee N. Mercury toxicity and contamination of households from the use of skin creams adulterated with mercurous chloride (calomel). Int J Environ Res Public Health. 2015;12(9):10943–54. https://doi.org/10.3390/ijerph120910943.
26. Corvi R, Madia F. In vitro genotoxicity testing – can the performance be enhanced? Food Chem Toxicol. 2017;106:600–8. https://doi.org/10.1016/j.fct.2016.08.024.
27. Council on Pharmacy and Chemistry. The propaganda for reform. J Am Med Assoc. 1913;61(8):615–6. https://doi.org/10.1001/jama.1913.04350080091022.
28. Cross SE, Magnusson BM, Winckle G, Anissimov Y, Roberts MS. Determination of the effect of lipophilicity on the in vitro permeability and tissue reservoir characteristics of topically applied solutes in human skin layers. J Invest Dermatol. 2003;120(5):759–64. https://doi.org/10.1046/j.1523-1747.2003.12131.x.
29. de Groot A, Schmidt E. Essential oils. Part V: Peppermint oil, lavender oil, and lemongrass oil. Dermatitis. 2016;27(6):325–32. https://doi.org/10.1097/der.0000000000000218.
30. Dent M, Amaral RT, Da Silva PA, Ansell J, Boisleve F, Hatao M, Hirose A, Kasai Y, Kern P, Kreiling R, Milstein S, Montemayor B, Oliveira J, Richarz A, Taalman R, Vaillancourt E, Verma R, Posada NVORC, Weiss C, Kojima H. Principles underpinning the use of new methodologies in the risk assessment of cosmetic ingredients. Comput Toxicol. 2018;7:20–6. https://doi.org/10.1016/j.comtox.2018.06.001.
31. Dipple A. DNA adducts of chemical carcinogens [Research Support, U S Gov't, P H S Review]. Carcinogenesis. 1995;16(3):437–41.
32. Dixon K, Kopras E. Genetic alterations and DNA repair in human carcinogenesis. Semin Cancer Biol. 2004;14(6):441–8. https://doi.org/10.1016/j.semcancer.2004.06.007.
33. EFSA Scientific Committee, Hardy A, Benford D, Halldorsson T, Jeger M, Knutsen HK, More S, Naegeli H, Noteborn H, Ockleford C, Ricci A, Rychen G, Silano V, Solecki R, Turck D, Younes M, Aquilina G, Crebelli R, Gürtler R, Schlatter J. Clarification of some aspects related to genotoxicity assessment. EFSA J. 2017;15(12):e05113. https://doi.org/10.2903/j.efsa.2017.5113.
34. EFSA Scientific Committee, More SJ, Bampidis V, Bragard C, Halldorsson TI, Hernández-Jerez AF, Hougaard Bennekou S, Koutsoumanis K, Lambré C, Machera K, Naegeli H, Nielsen SS, Schlatter J, Schrenk D, Turck D, Younes M, Aquilina G, Bignami M, Bolognesi C, Benford D. Guidance on aneugenicity assessment. EFSA J. 2021;19(8):e06770. https://doi.org/10.2903/j.efsa.2021.6770.
35. Eilstein J, Grégoire S, Fabre A, Arbey E, Géniès C, Duplan H, Rothe H, Ellison C, Cubberley R, Schepky A, Lange D, Klaric M, Hewitt NJ, Jacques-Jamin C. Use of human liver and EpiSkin™ S9 subcellular fractions as a screening assays to compare the in vitro hepatic and dermal metabolism of 47 cosmetics-relevant chemicals. J Appl Toxicol. 2020;40(3):416–33. https://doi.org/10.1002/jat.3914.

36. Elespuru RK, Agarwal R, Atrakchi AH, Bigger CAH, Heflich RH, Jagannath DR, Levy DD, Moore MM, Ouyang Y, Robison TW, Sotomayor RE, Cimino MC, Dearfield KL. Current and future application of genetic toxicity assays: the role and value of in vitro mammalian assays. Toxicol Sci. 2009;109(2):172–9. https://doi.org/10.1093/toxsci/kfp067.
37. European Commission, (EC). Executive summary of the impact assessment on the animal testing provisions in Regulatio (EC) 1223/2009 on cosmetics. Accompanying the document Communication from the Commission to the European Parliament and the Council on the animal testing and marketing ban and on the state of play in relation to alternative methods in the field of cosmetics. 2009. https://eur-lex.europa.eu/legal-content/EN/TXT/?uri=CELEX:52013SC0067
38. Felter SP, Bhat VS, Botham PA, Bussard DA, Casey W, Hayes AW, Hilton GM, Magurany KA, Sauer UG, Ohanian EV. Assessing chemical carcinogenicity: hazard identification, classification, and risk assessment. Insight from a Toxicology Forum state-of-the-science workshop. Crit Rev Toxicol. 2021;51(8):653–94. https://doi.org/10.1080/10408444.2021.2003295.
39. Ferreira M, Matos A, Couras A, Marto J, Ribeiro H. Overview of cosmetic regulatory frameworks around the world. Cosmetics. 2022;9:72. https://doi.org/10.3390/cosmetics9040072.
40. Forbes SB, Blake WC. Fatality resulting from the use of Lashlure on the eyebrow and eyelashes. J Am Med Assoc. 1934;103(19):1441–2. https://doi.org/10.1001/jama.1934.72750450002008a.
41. Fortin AV, Long AS, Williams A, Meier MJ, Cox J, Pinsonnault C, Yauk CL, White PA. Application of a new approach methodology (NAM)-based strategy for genotoxicity assessment of data-poor compounds. Front Toxicol. 2023;5:1098432. https://doi.org/10.3389/ftox.2023.1098432.
42. Fournier B, Mahlaoui N, Moshous D, de Villartay JP. Inborn errors of immunity caused by defects in the DNA damage response pathways: importance of minimizing treatment-related genotoxicity. Pediatr Allergy Immunol. 2022;33(6):e13820. https://doi.org/10.1111/pai.13820.
43. Fowler P, Smith R, Smith K, Young J, Jeffrey L, Kirkland D, Pfuhler S, Carmichael P. Reduction of misleading ("false") positive results in mammalian cell genotoxicity assays. II. Importance of accurate toxicity measurement. Mutat Res Genet Toxicol Environ Mutagen. 2012;747(1):104–17. https://doi.org/10.1016/j.mrgentox.2012.04.013.
44. Fukushima S, Kinoshita A, Puatanachokchai R, Kushida M, Wanibuchi H, Morimura K. Hormesis and dose–response-mediated mechanisms in carcinogenesis: evidence for a threshold in carcinogenicity of non-genotoxic carcinogens. Carcinogenesis. 2005;26(11):1835–45. https://doi.org/10.1093/carcin/bgi160.
45. Fukushima S, Gi M, Kakehashi A, Wanibuchi H. Qualitative and quantitative assessments on low-dose carcinogenicity of genotoxic hepatocarcinogens. In: Thresholds of genotoxic carcinogens. Elsevier; 2016. p. 1–17.
46. García-Rodríguez A, Gosálvez J, Agarwal A, Roy R, Johnston S. DNA damage and repair in human reproductive cells. Int J Mol Sci. 2018;20(1) https://doi.org/10.3390/ijms20010031.
47. Genchi G, Carocci A, Lauria G, Sinicropi MS, Catalano A. Thallium use, toxicity, and detoxification therapy: an overview. Appl Sci. 2021;11(18):8322. https://www.mdpi.com/2076-3417/11/18/8322
48. Gibbs S, van de Sandt JJ, Merk HF, Lockley DJ, Pendlington RU, Pease CK. Xenobiotic metabolism in human skin and 3D human skin reconstructs: a review. Curr Drug Metab. 2007;8(8):758–72. https://doi.org/10.2174/138920007782798225.
49. Godschalk RW, Ostertag JU, Moonen EJ, Neumann HA, Kleinjans JC, van Schooten FJ. Aromatic DNA adducts in human white blood cells and skin after dermal application of coal tar. Cancer Epidemiol Biomark Prev. 1998;7(9):767–73.
50. Godschalk RWL, Moonen EJC, Schilderman PAEL, Broekmans WMR, Kleinjans JCS, Van Schooten FJ. Exposure-route-dependent DNA adduct formation by polycyclic aromatic hydrocarbons. Carcinogenesis. 2000;21(1):87–92. https://doi.org/10.1093/carcin/21.1.87.

51. Goverment of Canada. Food and Drugs Act (R.S.C., 1985, c. F-27). 2024. Retrieved from https://laws-lois.justice.gc.ca/eng/acts/f-27/.
52. Grand View Research Inc. Cosmetics market size, share & trends analysis report by product (skin care, hair care), by end-user (men, women), by distribution channel (offline, online), by region (North America, Europe), and segment forecasts, 2024–2030. 2024. https://www.grandviewresearch.com/industry-analysis/cosmetics-market.
53. Greenbaum SS. Reports of thallium acetate poisoning following the use of Koremlu. J Am Med Assoc. 1931;96(22):1868. https://doi.org/10.1001/jama.1931.27220480003010a.
54. Greenbaum SS. Dermatoconjuctivitis due to Lash-Lure, an eyelash and eyebrow dye. J Am Med Assoc. 1933;101(5):363–4. https://doi.org/10.1001/jama.1933.27430300001010a.
55. Hakem R. DNA-damage repair; the good, the bad, and the ugly. EMBO J. 2008;27(4):589–605. https://doi.org/10.1038/emboj.2008.15.
56. Hanahan D. Hallmarks of cancer: new dimensions. Cancer Discov. 2022;12(1):31–46. https://doi.org/10.1158/2159-8290.Cd-21-1059.
57. Hanahan D, Weinberg RA. The hallmarks of cancer. Cell. 2000;100(1):57–70. https://doi.org/10.1016/s0092-8674(00)81683-9.
58. Hanahan D, Weinberg RA. Hallmarks of cancer: the next generation. Cell. 2011;144(5):646–74. https://doi.org/10.1016/j.cell.2011.02.013.
59. Hartwig A, Arand M, Epe B, Guth S, Jahnke G, Lampen A, Martus H-J, Monien B, Rietjens IMCM, Schmitz-Spanke S, Schriever-Schwemmer G, Steinberg P, Eisenbrand G. Mode of action-based risk assessment of genotoxic carcinogens. Arch Toxicol. 2020;94(6):1787–877. https://doi.org/10.1007/s00204-020-02733-2.
60. Helleday T, Eshtad S, Nik-Zainal S. Mechanisms underlying mutational signatures in human cancers. Nat Rev Genet. 2014;15(9):585–98. https://doi.org/10.1038/nrg3729.
61. Hennes EC. An overview of values for the threshold of toxicological concern. Toxicol Lett. 2012;211(3):296–303. https://doi.org/10.1016/j.toxlet.2012.03.795.
62. Hewitt NJ, Edwards RJ, Fritsche E, Goebel C, Aeby P, Scheel J, Reisinger K, Ouédraogo G, Duche D, Eilstein J, Latil A, Kenny J, Moore C, Kuehnl J, Barroso J, Fautz R, Pfuhler S. Use of human in vitro skin models for accurate and ethical risk assessment: metabolic considerations. Toxicol Sci. 2013;133(2):209–17. https://doi.org/10.1093/toxsci/kft080.
63. Hickey C, Juraimi SA, Hutchison L, Api AM, Smith B. Safety assessment of cosmetics and personal care products. In: H. A. W. a. K. T, editor. Hayes' principles and methods of toxicology, vol. 2. 7th ed. CRC Press; 2023. p. 831–53.
64. Hoeijmakers JH. DNA damage, aging, and cancer. N Engl J Med. 2009;361(15):1475–85.
65. Huang R, Zhou P-K. DNA damage repair: historical perspectives, mechanistic pathways and clinical translation for targeted cancer therapy. Signal Transduct Target Ther. 2021;6(1):254. https://doi.org/10.1038/s41392-021-00648-7.
66. Hussain SP, Harris CC. p53 biological network: at the crossroads of the cellular-stress response pathway and molecular carcinogenesis. J Nippon Med Sch. 2006;73(2):54–64. https://doi.org/10.1272/jnms.73.54.
67. Hussain M, Krishnamurthy S, Patel J, Kim E, Baptiste BA, Croteau DL, Bohr VA. Skin abnormalities in disorders with DNA repair defects, premature aging, and mitochondrial dysfunction. J Invest Dermatol. 2021;141(4s):968–75. https://doi.org/10.1016/j.jid.2020.10.019.
68. Hwa Yun B, Guo J, Bellamri M, Turesky RJ. DNA adducts: formation, biological effects, and new biospecimens for mass spectrometric measurements in humans. Mass Spectrom Rev. 2020;39(1–2):55–82. https://doi.org/10.1002/mas.21570.
69. Irigaray P, Belpomme D. Basic properties and molecular mechanisms of exogenous chemical carcinogens. Carcinogenesis. 2009;31(2):135–48. https://doi.org/10.1093/carcin/bgp252.
70. Jamieson RC. Eyelash dye (Lash-Lure) dermatitis with conjunctivitis. J Am Med Assoc. 1933;101(20):1560. https://doi.org/10.1001/jama.1933.27430450003009b.
71. Kay G. Dying to be beautiful: the fight for safe cosmetics. Am Hist Rev. 2005; https://doi.org/10.1086/ahr.111.4.1194a.

72. Kazem S, Linssen EC, Gibbs S. Skin metabolism phase I and phase II enzymes in native and reconstructed human skin: a short review. Drug Discov Today. 2019;24(9):1899–910. https://doi.org/10.1016/j.drudis.2019.06.002.
73. Kim S-T, Shao K, Oleschkewitz C, Hamilton R. Margin of exposure to free formaldehyde in personal care products containing formaldehyde-donor preservatives: evidence for consumer safety. Regul Toxicol Pharmacol. 2023;145:105519. https://doi.org/10.1016/j.yrtph.2023.105519.
74. Kirkland D, Aardema M, Henderson L, Müller L. Evaluation of the ability of a battery of three in vitro genotoxicity tests to discriminate rodent carcinogens and non-carcinogens: I. Sensitivity, specificity and relative predictivity. Mutat Res Genet Toxicol Environ Mutagen. 2005;584(1):1–256. https://doi.org/10.1016/j.mrgentox.2005.02.004.
75. Kirkland D, Pfuhler S, Tweats D, Aardema M, Corvi R, Darroudi F, Elhajouji A, Glatt H, Hastwell P, Hayashi M, Kasper P, Kirchner S, Lynch A, Marzin D, Maurici D, Meunier J-R, Müller L, Nohynek G, Parry J, White P. How to reduce false positive results when undertaking in vitro genotoxicity testing and thus avoid unnecessary follow-up animal tests: report of an ECVAM Workshop. Mutat Res Genet Toxicol Environ Mutagen. 2007;628(1):31–55. https://doi.org/10.1016/j.mrgentox.2006.11.008.
76. Kirkland D, Reeve L, Gatehouse D, Vanparys P. A core in vitro genotoxicity battery comprising the Ames test plus the in vitro micronucleus test is sufficient to detect rodent carcinogens and in vivo genotoxins. Mutat Res Genet Toxicol Environ Mutagen. 2011;721(1):27–73. https://doi.org/10.1016/j.mrgentox.2010.12.015.
77. Kirkland D, Zeiger E, Madia F, Gooderham N, Kasper P, Lynch A, Morita T, Ouedraogo G, Parra Morte JM, Pfuhler S, Rogiers V, Schulz M, Thybaud V, van Benthem J, Vanparys P, Worth A, Corvi R. Can in vitro mammalian cell genotoxicity test results be used to complement positive results in the Ames test and help predict carcinogenic or in vivo genotoxic activity? I. Reports of individual databases presented at an EURL ECVAM Workshop. Mutat Res Genet Toxicol Environ Mutagen. 2014;775–776:55–68. https://doi.org/10.1016/j.mrgentox.2014.10.005.
78. Klaunig JE, Kamendulis LM, Hocevar BA. Oxidative stress and oxidative damage in carcinogenesis. Toxicol Pathol. 2010;38(1):96–109. https://doi.org/10.1177/0192623309356453.
79. Knudsen LE, Loft SH, Autrup H. Risk assessment: the importance of genetic polymorphisms in man. Mutat Res Fundam Mol Mech Mutagen. 2001;482(1):83–8. https://doi.org/10.1016/S0027-5107(01)00213-5.
80. Kobets T, Williams GM. Thresholds for hepatocarcinogenicity of DNA-reactive compounds. In: Thresholds of genotoxic carcinogens. Chemico-Biological Interactions; 2016. p. 19–36.
81. Kobets T, Williams GM. Review of the evidence for thresholds for DNA-reactive and epigenetic experimental chemical carcinogens. Chemico-Biol Interact. 2019;301:88–111. https://doi.org/10.1016/j.cbi.2018.11.011.
82. Kobets T, Williams GM. Mechanisms of action of carcinogenic chemicals including occupational carcinogens. In: Paustenbach DJ, Farland W, Greim H, Klaunig J, Levy L, editors. Patty's toxicology; 2023. p. 1–22. https://doi.org/10.1002/0471125474.tox126.
83. Kobets T, Duan J-D, Brunnemann KD, Etter S, Smith B, Williams GM. Structure-activity relationships for DNA damage by alkenylbenzenes in turkey egg fetal liver. Toxicol Sci. 2015;150(2):301–11. https://doi.org/10.1093/toxsci/kfv322.
84. Kobets T, Duan J-D, Brunnemann KD, Iatropoulos MJ, Etter S, Hickey C, Smith B, Williams GM. In ovo testing of flavor and fragrance materials in Turkey Egg Genotoxicity Assay (TEGA), comparison of results to in vitro and in vivo data. Food Chem Toxicol. 2018a;115:228–43. https://doi.org/10.1016/j.fct.2018.03.015.
85. Kobets T, Iatropoulos MJ, Williams GM. Mechanisms of DNA-reactive and epigenetic chemical carcinogens: applications to carcinogenicity testing and risk assessment. Toxicol Res. 2018b;8(2):123–45. https://doi.org/10.1039/c8tx00250a.
86. Kobets T, Cartus AT, Fuhlbrueck JA, Brengel A, Stegmüller S, Duan J-D, Brunnemann KD, Williams GM. Assessment and characterization of DNA adducts produced by alkenylben-

zenes in fetal turkey and chicken livers. Food Chem Toxicol. 2019a;129:424–33. https://doi.org/10.1016/j.fct.2019.05.010.
87. Kobets T, Duan J-D, Brunnemann KD, Vock E, Deschl U, Williams GM. DNA-damaging activities of twenty-four structurally diverse unsubstituted and substituted cyclic compounds in embryo-fetal chicken livers. Mutat Res Genet Toxicol Environ Mutagen. 2019b;844:10–24. https://doi.org/10.1016/j.mrgentox.2019.06.004.
88. Kobets T, Duan JD, Vock E, Deschl U, Williams GM. Evaluation of pharmaceuticals for DNA damage in the Chicken Egg Genotoxicity Assay (CEGA). Int J Toxicol. 2022;41(4):297–311. https://doi.org/10.1177/10915818221093583.
89. Kontomanolis EN, Koutras A, Syllaios A, Schizas D, Mastoraki A, Garmpis N, Diakosavvas M, Angelou K, Tsatsaris G, Pagkalos A, Ntounis T, Fasoulakis Z. Role of oncogenes and tumor-suppressor genes in carcinogenesis: a review. Anticancer Res. 2020;40(11):6009–15. https://doi.org/10.21873/anticanres.14622.
90. Kortenkamp A, Faust M. Regulate to reduce chemical mixture risk. Science. 2018;361(6399):224–6. https://doi.org/10.1126/science.aat9219.
91. Kou F, Wu L, Ren X, Yang L. Chromosome abnormalities: new insights into their clinical significance in cancer. Mol Ther Oncolyt. 2020;17:562–70. https://doi.org/10.1016/j.omto.2020.05.010.
92. Kroes R, Galli C, Munro I, Schilter B, Tran LA, Walker R, Würtzen G. Threshold of toxicological concern for chemical substances present in the diet: a practical tool for assessing the need for toxicity testing. Food Chem Toxicol. 2000;38(2–3):255–312. https://doi.org/10.1016/s0278-6915(99)00120-9.
93. Ku WW, Bigger A, Brambilla G, Glatt H, Gocke E, Guzzie PJ, Hakura A, Honma M, Martus H-J, Obach RS, Roberts S. Strategy for genotoxicity testing – metabolic considerations. Mutat Res Genet Toxicol Environ Mutagen. 2007;627(1):59–77. https://doi.org/10.1016/j.mrgentox.2006.10.004.
94. Lee EY, Muller WJ. Oncogenes and tumor suppressor genes. Cold Spring Harbor Perspect Biol. 2010;2(10):a003236. https://doi.org/10.1101/cshperspect.a003236.
95. Llovet JM, Chen Y, Wurmbach E, Roayaie S, Fiel MI, Schwartz M, Thung SN, Khitrov G, Zhang W, Villanueva A, Battiston C, Mazzaferro V, Bruix J, Waxman S, Friedman SL. A molecular signature to discriminate dysplastic nodules from early hepatocellular carcinoma in HCV cirrhosis. Gastroenterology. 2006;131(6):1758–67. https://doi.org/10.1053/j.gastro.2006.09.014.
96. Loeb LA, Cheng KC. Errors in DNA synthesis: a source of spontaneous mutations. Mutat Res Rev Genet Toxicol. 1990;238(3):297–304. https://doi.org/10.1016/0165-1110(90)90021-3.
97. Loeb KR, Loeb LA. Significance of multiple mutations in cancer. Carcinogenesis. 2000;21(3):379–85. https://doi.org/10.1093/carcin/21.3.379.
98. Luijten M, van Benthem J, Morita T, Corvi R, Escobar PA, Fujita Y, Hemmerich J, Honarvar N, Kirkland D, Koyama N, Lovell DP, Mathea M, Williams A, Dertinger S, Pfuhler S, Pennings JLA. Evaluation of the standard battery of in vitro genotoxicity tests to predict in vivo genotoxicity through mathematical modeling: a report from the 8th International Workshop on Genotoxicity Testing. Environ Mol Mutagen. 2024; https://doi.org/10.1002/em.22640.
99. Mahadevan B, Snyder RD, Waters MD, Benz RD, Kemper RA, Tice RR, Richard AM. Genetic toxicology in the 21st century: reflections and future directions. Environ Mol Mutagen. 2011;52(5):339–54. https://doi.org/10.1002/em.20653.
100. Manevski N, Swart P, Balavenkatraman KK, Bertschi B, Camenisch G, Kretz O, Schiller H, Walles M, Ling B, Wettstein R, Schaefer DJ, Itin P, Ashton-Chess J, Pognan F, Wolf A, Litherland K. Phase II metabolism in human skin: Skin explants show full coverage for glucuronidation, sulfation, N-acetylation, catechol methylation, and glutathione conjugation. Drug Metab Disposition. 2015;43(1):126–39. https://doi.org/10.1124/dmd.114.060350.
101. Marchetti F, Cardoso R, Chen CL, Douglas GR, Elloway J, Escobar PA, Harper T Jr, Heflich RH, Kidd D, Lynch AM, Myers MB, Parsons BL, Salk JJ, Settivari RS, Smith-Roe SL,

Witt KL, Yauk C, Young RR, Zhang S, Minocherhomji S. Error-corrected next-generation sequencing to advance nonclinical genotoxicity and carcinogenicity testing. Nat Rev Drug Discov. 2023;22(3):165–6. https://doi.org/10.1038/d41573-023-00014-y.
102. Martin RJ, Denyer SP, Hadgraft J. Skin metabolism of topically applied compounds. Int J Pharmaceutics. 1987;39(1):23–32. https://doi.org/10.1016/0378-5173(87)90194-3.
103. Matsumura Y, Ananthaswamy HN. Toxic effects of ultraviolet radiation on the skin. Toxicol Appl Pharmacol. 2004;195(3):298–308. https://doi.org/10.1016/j.taap.2003.08.019.
104. McCally AW, Farmer AG, Loomis EC. Corneal ulceration following use of Lash-Lure. J Am Med Assoc. 1933;101(20):1560–1. https://doi.org/10.1001/jama.1933.27430450003009c.
105. McKelvey W, Jeffery N, Clark N, Kass D, Parsons PJ. Population-based inorganic mercury biomonitoring and the identification of skin care products as a source of exposure in New York City. Environ Health Perspect. 2011;119(2):203–9. https://doi.org/10.1289/ehp.1002396.
106. Menz J, Götz ME, Gündel U, Gürtler R, Herrmann K, Hessel-Pras S, Kneuer C, Kolrep F, Nitzsche D, Pabel U, Sachse B, Schmeisser S, Schumacher DM, Schwerdtle T, Tralau T, Zellmer S, Schäfer B. Genotoxicity assessment: opportunities, challenges and perspectives for quantitative evaluations of dose-response data. Arch Toxicol. 2023;97(9):2303–28. https://doi.org/10.1007/s00204-023-03553-w.
107. Morita T, Hamada S, Masumura K, Wakata A, Maniwa J, Takasawa H, Yasunaga K, Hashizume T, Honma M. Evaluation of the sensitivity and specificity of in vivo erythrocyte micronucleus and transgenic rodent gene mutation tests to detect rodent carcinogens. Mutat Res Genet Toxicol Environ Mutagen. 2016;802:1–29. https://doi.org/10.1016/j.mrgentox.2016.03.008.
108. Mukhtar H, Merk HF, Athar M. Skin chemical carcinogenesis. Clin Dermatol. 1989;7(3):1–10. https://doi.org/10.1016/0738-081x(89)90002-3.
109. Mukkanna KS, Stone NM, Ingram JR. Para-phenylenediamine allergy: current perspectives on diagnosis and management. J Asthma Allergy. 2017;10:9–15. https://doi.org/10.2147/jaa.S90265.
110. Neumann HG, Ambs S, Bitsch A. The role of nongenotoxic mechanisms in arylamine carcinogenesis. Environ Health Perspect. 1994;102:173. https://doi.org/10.2307/3432173.
111. New York State Department of Environmental Conservation, (NYSDEC). Amendments to Article 35 and Article 37 of the Environmental Conservation Law (ECL). Subpart 352-1. 1,4 Dioxane limits for household cleansing, personal care, and cosmetic products. 2023.
112. Niehues H, Bouwstra JA, El Ghalbzouri A, Brandner JM, Zeeuwen P, van den Bogaard EH. 3D skin models for 3R research: the potential of 3D reconstructed skin models to study skin barrier function. Exp Dermatol. 2018;27(5):501–11. https://doi.org/10.1111/exd.13531.
113. Nikki L, Khanh P, Yousuf M. Role of skin enzymes in metabolism of topical drugs. Metab Target Organ Damage. 2024;4(4):32. https://doi.org/10.20517/mtod.2024.17.
114. Nohmi T. Thresholds of genotoxic and non-genotoxic carcinogens. Toxicol Res. 2018;34(4):281–90. https://doi.org/10.5487/tr.2018.34.4.281.
115. Nohynek GJ, Antignac E, Re T, Toutain H. Safety assessment of personal care products/cosmetics and their ingredients. Toxicol Appl Pharmacol. 2010;243(2):239–59. https://doi.org/10.1016/j.taap.2009.12.001.
116. Oesch F, Herrero ME, Hengstler JG, Lohmann M, Arand M. Metabolic detoxification: implications for thresholds. Toxicol Pathol. 2000;28(3):382–7. https://doi.org/10.1177/019262330002800305.
117. Oesch F, Fabian E, Oesch-Bartlomowicz B, Werner C, Landsiedel R. Drug-metabolizing enzymes in the skin of man, rat, and pig. Drug Metab Rev. 2007;39(4):659–98. https://doi.org/10.1080/03602530701690366.
118. Ouedraogo G, Alexander-White C, Bury D, Clewell HJ, Cronin M, Cull T, Dent M, Desprez B, Detroyer A, Ellison C, Giammanco S, Hack E, Hewitt NJ, Kenna G, Klaric M, Kreiling R, Lester C, Mahony C, Mombelli E, Cosmetics E. Read-across and new approach methodologies applied in a 10-step framework for cosmetics safety assessment – a case study with parabens. Regul Toxicol Pharmacol. 2022;132:105161. https://doi.org/10.1016/j.yrtph.2022.105161.

119. Park BK, Kitteringham NR, Maggs JL, Pirmohamed M, Williams DP. The role of metabolic activation in drug-induced hepatotoxicity. Annu Rev Pharmacol Toxicol. 2005;45:177–202. https://doi.org/10.1146/annurev.pharmtox.45.120403.100058.
120. Pfuhler S, Kirst A, Aardema M, Banduhn N, Goebel C, Araki D, Costabel-Farkas M, Dufour E, Fautz R, Harvey J, Hewitt NJ, Hibatallah J, Carmichael P, Macfarlane M, Reisinger K, Rowland J, Schellauf F, Schepky A, Scheel J. A tiered approach to the use of alternatives to animal testing for the safety assessment of cosmetics: Genotoxicity. A COLIPA analysis. Regul Toxicol Pharmacol. 2010;57(2–3):315–24. https://doi.org/10.1016/j.yrtph.2010.03.012.
121. Pfuhler S, Fautz R, Ouedraogo G, Latil A, Kenny J, Moore C, Diembeck W, Hewitt NJ, Reisinger K, Barroso J. The Cosmetics Europe strategy for animal-free genotoxicity testing: project status up-date. Toxicol Vitro. 2014;28(1):18–23. https://doi.org/10.1016/j.tiv.2013.06.004.
122. Pfuhler S, van Benthem J, Curren R, Doak SH, Dusinska M, Hayashi M, Heflich RH, Kidd D, Kirkland D, Luan Y, Ouedraogo G, Reisinger K, Sofuni T, van Acker F, Yang Y, Corvi R. Use of in vitro 3D tissue models in genotoxicity testing: Strategic fit, validation status and way forward. Report of the working group from the 7th International Workshop on Genotoxicity Testing (IWGT). Mutat Res Genet Toxicol Environ Mutagen. 2020;850–851:503135. https://doi.org/10.1016/j.mrgentox.2020.503135.
123. Pfuhler S, Downs TR, Hewitt NJ, Hoffmann S, Mun GC, Ouedraogo G, Roy S, Curren RD, Aardema MJ. Validation of the 3D reconstructed human skin micronucleus (RSMN) assay: an animal-free alternative for following-up positive results from standard in vitro genotoxicity assays. Mutagenesis. 2021;36(1):1–17. https://doi.org/10.1093/mutage/geaa035.
124. Piccione M, Belloni Fortina A, Ferri G, Andolina G, Beretta L, Cividini A, De Marni E, Caroppo F, Citernesi U, Di Liddo R. Xeroderma Pigmentosum: general aspects and management. J Pers Med. 2021;11(11) https://doi.org/10.3390/jpm11111146.
125. Pitot HC. The molecular biology of carcinogenesis. Cancer. 1993;72(3 Suppl):962–70. https://doi.org/10.1002/1097-0142(19930801)72:3+<962::aid-cncr2820721303>3.0.co;2-h.
126. Pogribny IP, Rusyn I. Environmental toxicants, epigenetics, and cancer. Adv Exp Med Biol. 2013;754:215–32. https://doi.org/10.1007/978-1-4419-9967-2_11.
127. Poirier MC. DNA adducts as exposure biomarkers and indicators of cancer risk. Environ Health Perspect. 1997;105(Suppl 4):907–12. https://doi.org/10.1289/ehp.97105s4907.
128. Poirier MC, Beland FA. DNA adduct measurements and tumor incidence during chronic carcinogen exposure in rodents. Environ Health Perspect. 1994;102(Suppl 6):161–5. https://doi.org/10.1289/ehp.94102s6161.
129. Preston RJ, Williams GM. DNA-reactive carcinogens: mode of action and human cancer hazard. Crit Rev Toxicol. 2005;35(8–9):673–83. https://doi.org/10.1080/10408440591007278.
130. Ramaiahgari SC, Waidyanatha S, Dixon D, DeVito MJ, Paules RS, Ferguson SS. From the cover: three-dimensional (3D) HepaRG spheroid model with physiologically relevant xenobiotic metabolism competence and hepatocyte functionality for liver toxicity screening. Toxicol Sci. 2017;159(1):124–36. https://doi.org/10.1093/toxsci/kfx122.
131. Recio L, Kobets T. Genetic and epigenetic toxicology. In: Hayes AW, Kobets T, editors. Hayes' principles and methods of toxicology, vol. 2. 7th ed. CRC Press; 2023. p. 1409–54.
132. Reeder MJ. Allergic contact dermatitis to fragrances. Dermatol Clin. 2020;38(3):371–7. https://doi.org/10.1016/j.det.2020.02.009.
133. Reisinger K, Dony E, Wolf T, Maul K. Hen's Egg Test for Micronucleus Induction (HET-MN) [Research Support, Non-U S Gov't]. Methods Mol Biol. 2019:9646–9649_9610.
134. Rothfuss A, Honma M, Czich A, Aardema MJ, Burlinson B, Galloway S, Hamada S, Kirkland D, Heflich RH, Howe J, Nakajima M, O'Donovan M, Plappert-Helbig U, Priestley C, Recio L, Schuler M, Uno Y, Martus H-J. Improvement of in vivo genotoxicity assessment: Combination of acute tests and integration into standard toxicity testing. Mutat Res Genet Toxicol Environ Mutagen. 2011;723(2):108–20. https://doi.org/10.1016/j.mrgentox.2010.12.005.
135. Rubin CB, Brod B. Natural does not mean safe-The dirt on clean beauty products. JAMA Dermatol. 2019;155(12):1344–5. https://doi.org/10.1001/jamadermatol.2019.2724.

136. Seo K-Y, Jelinsky SA, Loechler EL. Factors that influence the mutagenic patterns of DNA adducts from chemical carcinogens. Mutat Res Rev Mutat Res. 2000;463(3):215–46. https://doi.org/10.1016/S1383-5742(00)00047-8.
137. Skowron K, Bauza-Kaszewska J, Kraszewska Z, Wiktorczyk-Kapischke N, Grudlewska-Buda K, Kwiecińska-Piróg J, Wałecka-Zacharska E, Radtke L, Gospodarek-Komkowska E. Human skin microbiome: impact of intrinsic and extrinsic factors on skin microbiota. Microorganisms. 2021;9(3):543. https://www.mdpi.com/2076-2607/9/3/543
138. Smith MT, Guyton KZ, Kleinstreuer N, Borrel A, Cardenas A, Chiu WA, Felsher DW, Gibbons CF, Goodson WH 3rd, Houck KA, Kane AB, La Merrill MA, Lebrec H, Lowe L, McHale CM, Minocherhomji S, Rieswijk L, Sandy MS, Sone H, Fielden M. The key characteristics of carcinogens: relationship to the hallmarks of cancer, relevant biomarkers, and assays to measure them. Cancer Epidemiol Biomark Prevent. 2020;29(10):1887–903. https://doi.org/10.1158/1055-9965.epi-19-1346.
139. Smythe P, Wilkinson HN. The skin microbiome: current landscape and future opportunities. Int J Mol Sci. 2023;24(4):3950. https://www.mdpi.com/1422-0067/24/4/3950
140. Solomon E, Borrow J, Goddard AD. Chromosome aberrations and cancer. Science. 1991;254(5035):1153–60. https://doi.org/10.1126/science.1957167.
141. Speit G. How to assess the mutagenic potential of cosmetic products without animal tests? Mutat Res. 2009;678(2):108–12. https://doi.org/10.1016/j.mrgentox.2009.04.006.
142. Srinivasan V, Antignac E. The safety assessment of plant-derived ingredients in cosmetics. In: Formulating, packaging, and marketing of natural cosmetic products; 2011. p. 123–47.
143. Staman JA. Enforcement of the Food, Drug, and Cosmetic Act: select legal issues. 2018. Retrieved March 25, 2025 from https://www.congress.gov/crs-product/R43609.
144. Storchova Z, Pellman D. From polyploidy to aneuploidy, genome instability and cancer. Nat Rev Mol Cell Biol. 2004;5(1):45–54.
145. Sutherland BM, Hacham H, Gange RW, Maytum D, Sutherland JC. DNA damage and repair in human skin: pathways and questions. Basic Life Sci. 1990;53:149–60. https://doi.org/10.1007/978-1-4613-0637-5_12.
146. Swenberg JA, Lu K, Moeller BC, Gao L, Upton PB, Nakamura J, Starr TB. Endogenous versus exogenous DNA adducts: their role in carcinogenesis, epidemiology, and risk assessment. Toxicol Sci. 2011;120(Suppl 1):S130–45. https://doi.org/10.1093/toxsci/kfq371.
147. Tcheremenskaia O, Battistelli CL, Giuliani A, Benigni R, Bossa C. In silico approaches for prediction of genotoxic and carcinogenic potential of cosmetic ingredients. Comput Toxicol. 2019;11:91–100. https://doi.org/10.1016/j.comtox.2019.03.005.
148. Teixeira M, De Wachter L, Ronsyn E, Goossens A. Contact allergy to para-phenylenediamine in a permanent eyelash dye. Contact Dermatitis. 2006;55(2):92–4. https://doi.org/10.1111/j.0105-1873.2006.00883.x.
149. Terradas M, Martín M, Tusell L, Genescà A. Genetic activities in micronuclei: is the DNA entrapped in micronuclei lost for the cell? Mutat Res Rev Mutat Res. 2010;705(1):60–7. https://doi.org/10.1016/j.mrrev.2010.03.004.
150. Thakkar Y, Kobets T, Api AM, Duan JD, Williams GM. Assessment of genotoxic potential of fragrance materials in the chicken egg assays. Environ Mol Mutagen. 2024;65(8):261–74. https://doi.org/10.1002/em.22627.
151. Towle KM, Hwang RY, Fung ES, Hollins DM, Monnot AD. Hair dye and risk of skin sensitization induction: a product survey and quantitative risk assessment for para-phenylenediamine (PPD). Cutan Ocul Toxicol. 2020;39(4):311–6. https://doi.org/10.1080/15569527.2020.1802740.
152. Tweats DJ, Scott AD, Westmoreland C, Carmichael PL. Determination of genetic toxicity and potential carcinogenicity in vitro – challenges post the Seventh Amendment to the European Cosmetics Directive. Mutagenesis. 2006;22(1):5–13. https://doi.org/10.1093/mutage/gel052.
153. Tweats DJ, Blakey D, Heflich RH, Jacobs A, Jacobsen SD, Morita T, Nohmi T, O'Donovan MR, Sasaki YF, Sofuni T, Tice R. Report of the IWGT working group on strategies and

interpretation of regulatory in vivo tests. Mutat Res Genet Toxicol Environ Mutagen. 2007;627(1):78–91. https://doi.org/10.1016/j.mrgentox.2006.10.005.
154. U.S. Environmental Protection Agency, (EPA). Integrated Risk Information System (IRIS) toxicological review of thallium and compounds (Final Report). 2009. https://iris.epa.gov/document/&deid=188550#:~:text=In%20the%20past%2C%20thallium%20was,risks%20associated%20with%20environmental%20contaminants
155. U.S. Food and Drug Administration, (FDA). FDA authority over cosmetics: how cosmetics are not FDA-approved, but are FDA-regulated. 2021. https://www.fda.gov/cosmetics/cosmetics-laws-regulations/fda-authority-over-cosmetics-how-cosmetics-are-not-fda-approved-are-fda-regulated
156. Vogel TA, Coenraads P-J, Bijkersma LM, Vermeulen KM, Schuttelaar M-LA, Group, o. b. o. t. E. F. S. p-Phenylenediamine exposure in real life – a case–control study on sensitization rate, mode and elicitation reactions in the northern Netherlands. Contact Dermatitis. 2015;72(6):355–61. https://doi.org/10.1111/cod.12354.
157. Waddell WJ, Fukushima S, Williams GM. Concordance of thresholds for carcinogenicity of N-nitrosodiethylamine. Arch Toxicol. 2005;80(6):305–9. https://doi.org/10.1007/s00204-005-0048-y.
158. Walmsley RM, Billinton N. How accurate is in vitro prediction of carcinogenicity? Br J Pharmacol. 2011;162(6):1250–8. https://doi.org/10.1111/j.1476-5381.2010.01131.x.
159. Washington State Legislature. House Bill (HB) 1694. Concerning logistical processes for the regulation of priority chemicals in consumer products. 2022. Retrieved from https://app.leg.wa.gov/billsummary?BillNumber=1694&Year=2021
160. Weisburger EK. Metabolic activation of chemical carcinogens. In: Jucker E, editor. Progress in Drug Research/Fortschritte der Arzneimittelforschung/Progrès des recherches pharmaceutiques. Basel: Birkhäuser; 1982. p. 143–66. https://doi.org/10.1007/978-3-0348-7111-2_4.
161. Wiegand C, Hewitt NJ, Merk HF, Reisinger K. Dermal xenobiotic metabolism: a comparison between native human skin, four in vitro skin test systems and a liver system. Skin Pharmacol Physiol. 2014;27(5):263–75. https://doi.org/10.1159/000358272.
162. Wielgus AR, Chignell CF, Miller DS, Van Houten B, Meyer J, Hu DN, Roberts JE. Phototoxicity in human retinal pigment epithelial cells promoted by hypericin, a component of St. John's Wort. Photochem Photobiol. 2007;83(3):706–13. https://doi.org/10.1562/2006-08-09-ra-1001.
163. Williams GM, Jeffrey AM. Oxidative DNA damage: endogenous and chemically induced. Regul Toxicol Pharmacol. 2000;32(3):283–92. https://doi.org/10.1006/rtph.2000.1433.
164. Williams GM, Iatropoulos MJ, Jeffrey AM. Thresholds for the effects of 2-acetylaminofluorene in rat liver. Toxicol Pathol. 2004;32(2_suppl):85–91. https://doi.org/10.1080/01926230490451716.
165. Williams GM, Iatropoulos MJ, Jeffrey AM. Thresholds for DNA-reactive (genotoxic) organic carcinogens. J Toxicol Pathol. 2005;18(2):69–77. https://doi.org/10.1293/tox.18.69.
166. Williams GM, Duan J-D, Brunnemann KD, Iatropoulos MJ, Vock E, Deschl U. Chicken fetal liver DNA damage and adduct formation by activation-dependent DNA-reactive carcinogens and related compounds of several structural classes. Toxicol Sci. 2014a;141(1):18–28. https://doi.org/10.1093/toxsci/kfu123.
167. Williams GM, Iatropoulos MJ, Enzmann HG, Deschl U. Carcinogenicity of chemicals: assessment and human extrapolation. In: Hayes A, Kruger CL, editors. Hayes Principles and methods of toxicology. 6th ed. Taylor and Francis; 2014b. p. 1251–303.
168. Williams GM, Kobets T, Iatropoulos MJ, Nolte T, Vock E. Carcinogenicity bioassays and related assays; human relevance. In: H. A. W. a. K. T, editor. Hayes' principles and methods of toxicology, vol. 2. 7th ed. CRC Press; 2023. p. 1455–96.
169. Witt KL, van Benthem J, Kobets T, Chen G, Kelber O, Krzykwa J, MacGregor JT, Mei N, Mitchell CA, Rietjens I, Sarigol-Kilic Z, Smith-Roe SL, Stopper H, Thakkar Y, Zeiger E, Pfuhler S. A proposed screening strategy for evaluating the genotoxicity potential of botanicals and botanical extracts. Food Chem Toxicol. 2025;197:115277. https://doi.org/10.1016/j.fct.2025.115277.

170. Wolf T, Luepke N-P. Formation of micronuclei in incubated hen's eggs as a measure of genotoxicity. Mutat Res Genet Toxicol Environ Mutagen. 1997;394(1–3):163–75. https://doi.org/10.1016/s1383-5718(97)00136-8.
171. Wolf T, Niehaus-Rolf C, Luepke N-P. Some new methodological aspects of the hen's egg test for micronucleus induction (HET-MN). Mutat Res Genet Toxicol Environ Mutagen. 2002;514(1–2):59–76. https://doi.org/10.1016/s1383-5718(01)00317-5.
172. Yang C, Barlow SM, Muldoon Jacobs KL, Vitcheva V, Boobis AR, Felter SP, Arvidson KB, Keller D, Cronin MTD, Enoch S, Worth A, Hollnagel HM. Thresholds of Toxicological Concern for cosmetics-related substances: new database, thresholds, and enrichment of chemical space. Food Chem Toxicol. 2017;109(Pt 1):170–93. https://doi.org/10.1016/j.fct.2017.08.043.
173. Zeller A, Pfuhler S, Albertini S, Bringezu F, Czich A, Dietz Y, Fautz R, Hewitt NJ, Kirst A, Kasper P. A critical appraisal of the sensitivity of in vivo genotoxicity assays in detecting human carcinogens. Mutagenesis. 2018;33(2):179–93. https://doi.org/10.1093/mutage/gey005.

Index

P. Elsner et al. (eds.), *Cosmetics*, https://doi.org/10.1007/978-3-032-14644-1

The manufacturer's authorised representative in the EU is Springer Nature Customer Service Centre GmbH, Europaplatz 3, 69115 Heidelberg, Germany. If you have any concerns regarding our products, please contact ProductSafety@springernature.com

Printed and bound by CPI Group (UK) Ltd, Croydon, CR0 4YY
16/09/2026
02217781-0003